THE THROMBOTIC PROCESS
IN ATHEROGENESIS

ADVANCES IN EXPERIMENTAL MEDICINE AND BIOLOGY

Recent Volumes in this Series

THE THROMBOTIC PROCESS IN ATHEROGENESIS

Edited by

A. Bleakley Chandler
Department of Pathology
Medical College of Georgia

Karl Eurenius
National Heart, Lung, and Blood Institute
National Institutes of Health

Gardner C. McMillan
National Heart, Lung, and Blood Institute
National Institutes of Health

Curtis B. Nelson
Division of Scientific Affairs
American Heart Association

Colin J. Schwartz
Department of Pathology
University of Texas, San Antonio

Stanford Wessler
Department of Medicine
New York University School of Medicine

PLENUM PRESS • NEW YORK AND LONDON

Library of Congress Cataloging in Publication Data

Workshop on Thrombotic Process in Atherogenesis, Reston, Va., 1977.
    The thrombotic process in atherogenesis.

    (Advances in experimental medicine and biology; v. 104)
    Sponsored by the Council on Thrombosis, American Heart Association and others.
    Includes indexes.
    1. Arteriosclerosis—Congresses. 2. Thrombosis—Congresses. I. Chandler, Arthur Bleakley,
1926-   II. American Heart Association. Council on Thrombosis. III. Title. IV. Series.
RC692.W67 1977   616.1'36'07   78-18939
ISBN 0-306-40022-7

Proceedings of the Workshop on The Thrombotic Process in Atherogenesis
held in Reston, Virginia, October 16–19, 1977

© 1978 Plenum Press, New York
A Division of Plenum Publishing Corporation
227 West 17th Street, New York, N.Y. 10011

Printed in the United States of America

PROGRAM COMMITTEE

Co-chairmen	A. B. Chandler and S. Wessler
Conceptual Aspects	C. J. Schwartz
Arterial Wall Workshops	H. Wolinsky, R. L. Nachman, W. A. Thomas
Lipid Workshops	D. J. Hanahan, J. B. Smith
Risk Factors	H. C. McGill, Jr.
Arterial Injury Workshops	C. G. Becker, D. L. Fry
Thrombotic Models Workshops	K. M. Brinkhous, E. J. W. Bowie
Clinical Assessment of Thrombotic Process	H. L. Nossel

American Heart Association	C. B. Nelson
National Heart, Lung, and Blood Institute	K. Eurenius J. C. Fratantoni G. C. McMillan

v

FOREWORD

Two informal meetings of consultants expert in hemostatic phenomena and in atherogenesis were held in Bethesda, Maryland, in December 1975 and February 1976 by the National Heart, Lung, and Blood Institute. Their purpose was to discuss the current status of knowledge concerning the thrombotic process in the pathogenesis of athcrosclcrosis.

It was readily agreed that thrombosis often played a major role in plaque building and in plaque complication. It was also commented, however, that the data were qualitative in nature and that quantitative information was remarkably sparse.

The term thromboatherogenesis was thought to be appropriate for those phenomena in which the full expression of the thrombotic process is manifest. At the same time, recent research was noted in which what appears to be an important pathway for the initiation of atherogenesis arises from the reaction of platelets with injured arterial endothelium and subendothelium without necessarily involving the complete classical thrombotic process. A name was not coined for this circumstance, but it was held that thromboatherogenesis was not a fully appropriate one.

A number of subjects were discussed, often in highly technical terms. Among them was the question of the need and feasibility of studying hemostatic variables as predictors or risk factors for thrombotic phenomena in relation to atherosclerotic disease, much as lipids or hypertension have been associated with coronary heart disease risk. Animal models were discussed at length, remarking *inter alia* that models which would suit the needs of research on many aspects of atherogenesis might offer little for research in hemostatic phenomena. Moreover, the former are often conducted as chronic experiments, the data being integrated over many months of time; while the latter are often brief, and involve rapid sequences of events. The special contribution that genetic variation might make to research involving these various processes was commented upon.

Many other topics were discussed. Their range and variety made it clear that not only was there much of pressing and mutual interest, but that communication was a problem. Experts in one field often had to pause and explain their thoughts more simply or in different terms to experts from other areas of interest, if misunderstandings were to be avoided and if concepts, limitations, and opportunities for research were to be appreciated in their full force and subtlety.

It was recognized that there were compelling opportunities for productive interaction and also significant needs in communication. The material discussed at these two meetings shaped much of the form and content of this workshop.

Gardner C. McMillan

PREFACE

The Workshop on the Thrombotic Process in Atherogenesis has explored many aspects of this emerging field. In view of current interest and significant new developments, it was considered timely to hold a broad-based, in-depth meeting of scientists representing the disciplines involved. In a series of conceptual review papers, the subject is placed in perspective, while other reviews provide background for the individual workshop sessions, which concentrate on recent work. Special note should be taken of an extensive survey on endothelium, the focal point of interaction between the constituents of the blood and vascular wall.

Over a number of years, much evidence has accrued from experimental studies and from observations in man that thrombi can contribute to the growth of atherosclerotic plaques, and at times, may initiate the lesions. The organization and incorporation of thrombi into atherosclerotic plaques is a direct, clear-cut mechanism for plaque growth. This concept has not previously been given substantial recognition as a factor in atherogenesis, in part because of the paradoxical nature of the process: recent thrombi that have formed on established atherosclerotic lesions are readily identified; but once formed, the thrombi may undergo organization and conversion by the arterial wall into plaque tissue no longer recognizable as thrombotic in origin.

The frequency, and consequently the morbidity and mortality, of arterial thrombosis alone has not been subject to accurate assessment for the very reason that thrombi intimately contribute to plaque formation and the progression of atherosclerosis. In contrast to deep vein thrombosis, which is often acute and frequently produces overt manifestations, arterial thrombosis may be chronic, extending over many years while plaques grow silently. Indeed, the question should be raised as to the desirability of considering thromboatherosclerosis as a distinct entity.

Collected data indicate a definite contribution to plaque growth by thrombi, but many fundamental gaps remain to be filled before proper attention can be given to environmental risk factors and to therapeutic and prophylactic approaches. Among the several outstanding questions to be addressed are the following:

What is the relative contribution of thrombosis to plaque growth?

When in the life of the individual and of the plaque does the process begin?

Are there subsets of the population in which thrombosis is, in fact, the dominant factor?

Another aspect of thromboatherogenesis that requires detailed consideration is the complex relationship between dietary and plasma lipids and thrombosis. Plasma lipids may affect thrombus formation and thrombolysis by several mechanisms that concern platelet reactivity and blood coagulation. Fat in thromboatherosclerotic plaques may be derived from entrapped plasma lipids as well as from lipids of thrombotic cellular elements. It is of particular relevance to this issue that fibromuscular and fatty plaques can form from experimental thrombi produced in normolipemic states.

Of special importance are recent observations relating arterial injury, the thrombotic process, and atherogenesis. For many years, investigators explored the idea that thrombosis initiates atherosclerosis, but found this possibility to be negligible in comparison to the effect of thrombi on plaque growth. However, it is now apparent that platelets and other components that share in the formation of thrombi might contribute to atherogenesis through initial injury to the arterial wall. Various factors involved in arterial damage including immunologic and hemodynamic injury must also take into account the associated effects of thrombotic components.

More recently, it has been demonstrated by sophisticated *in vitro* investigations that, in addition to being injurious to endothelium, platelets may release a mitogenic factor that stimulates proliferation of vascular smooth muscle, a feature of most plaques. These relationships involving platelet injury and the response of the arterial wall are further related through plasma lipids which may also initiate injury, and through a special class of lipids, the prostaglandins, that are concerned with platelet reactivity and interactions between platelets and the arterial intima.

The proceedings of this workshop brings together in a single document for the scientific community research relevant to the fields of thrombosis and atherogenesis. Recommendations have been developed for future research that will be helpful to individual investigators as well as to agencies that support research in these areas. It is hoped that this document will provide evidence to the Congress that basic research has yielded and continues to yield knowledge that will improve the health of the nation by attacking atherosclerosis early rather than in its terminal stages.

Finally, it is a goal of this publication to provide a basis for stimulating widened interest in these closely allied fields. Clearly, there is ample opportunity for fertile collaboration among lipidologists, thrombologists, atherologists, and flow engineers, to name only a few of the relevant disciplines.

A. Bleakley Chandler and Stanford Wessler

ACKNOWLEDGMENTS

The Workshop on the Thrombotic Process in Atherogenesis was sponsored by the Councils on Thrombosis and Arteriosclerosis of the American Heart Association and by the Divisions of Heart and Vascular Diseases and Blood Diseases and Resources of the National Heart, Lung, and Blood Institute. Financial support for several planning meetings and partial funding of the workshop were made possible by the American Heart Association. The National Heart, Lung, and Blood Institute provided substantial financial assistance for the organization and execution of the workshop as well as for the publication of the proceedings.

The endorsement of the Council Affairs Committee of the American Heart Association in this undertaking and the support and encouragement of Dr. Robert I. Levy, Director of the National Heart, Lung, and Blood Institute were key elements in the development of the workshop. The contributions of Dr. Mary Jane Jesse, the Director of the Division of Heart and Vascular Diseases and Dr. Wolf Zuelzer, the Director of the Division of Blood Diseases and Resources were also much appreciated.

The Planning Committee for this workshop consisted of Drs. Carl G. Becker, A. Bleakley Chandler, Joseph C. Fratantoni, Donald J. Hanahan, Henry C. McGill, Jr., Gardner C. McMillan, Curtis B. Nelson, Hymie L. Nossel, Colin J. Schwartz, Michael B. Stemerman, Harvey Weiss, Stanford Wessler, and Harvey Wolinsky. The Program Committee, which included many of those named above, also played a major role in the delineation of the final design and content of the workshop.

The generous contributions of all those participants who made this workshop so successful through their formal presentations and lively, productive discussions are gratefully acknowledged.

Lastly, it is a special pleasure to acknowledge the excellent and thoughtful administrative and logistical support for the workshop provided by Mrs. Sally Simpson and her associates of Kappa Systems, Inc., and to thank Mrs. Claire Doyle, also of Kappa Systems, Inc., for her careful guidance of the manuscripts through the many steps required for publication of this proceedings.

CONTENTS

FIRST PLENARY SESSION
CONCEPTUAL ASPECTS

Colin J. Schwartz, *Session Chariman*

Research Division
Cleveland Clinic Foundation
Cleveland, Ohio

ATHEROGENESIS: THE PROCESS FROM NORMAL TO LESION

G.C. McMillan

Division of Heart and Vascular Diseases
National Heart, Lung, and BLood Institute
National Institutes of Health
Bethesda, Maryland

Arteriosclerosis is an ancient lesion found in mummies, illustrated by da Vinci and only clearly designated as a disease distinct from aging processes early in this century. (1, 2) The modern period of research, that is, since about 1930, has seen a progressive emphasis on two major theories of atherogenesis.

One of these theories is the lipid hypothesis. It bases its credibility on the frequent occurrence of excessive amounts of cholesterol and lipids in lesions; on the positive association between elevated serum lipids and atherogenesis in man and in animals; on the association between dietary saturated fats and cholesterol and atherogenesis in man and in experimental animals; and on associations between specific diseases and genetic disorders that affect lipid metabolism and atherogenesis.

The lipid hypothesis has several variants which propose specific mechanisms through which it may operate, but it regards atherogenesis as a process intimately concerned with and due to abnormal lipid metabolism. The information which relates to this theory is enormous; most of it is supportive and caveats have been few. The theory has had worldwide acceptability but it has been particularly popular in the United States where it has dominated research on atherogenesis.

The second major theory regards atherogenesis as a process involving the conversion through tissue organization of arterial mural thrombi into atherosclerotic plaques. This theory, the Duguid-Rokitanski concept, has rested its credibility largely on pathological observations in man that show morphological evidence compatible with this view of atherogenesis. Such evidence is easily found, but it has been most convincing in relation to the mid- or late development of plaques rather than to their early stages. Consequently, many commentators have regarded this as a theory, albeit a most important one, or plaque progression or complication rather than as a theory of plaque initiation. The demonstration that platelets are capable of interacting with intimal smooth muscle cells to stimulate them to proliferate has now extended this theory beyond its original boundaries to encompass the initiation of atherogenesis without necessarily invoking the complete classical sequence of thrombosis. The theory has lacked the support of correlative geographic, metabolic or other pathophysiologic associations in atherogenesis and until the past decade, has lacked any but the most artificial experimental animal systems in which it could be studied. This theory, too, has had worldwide acceptance but it has been most popular in Western Europe, particularly the United Kingdom.

There has been some tendency for the proponents of one or other of these theories to emphasize the rather exclusive importance of their particular hypothesis not only in special cases but for atherogenesis in general. Moreover, when other factors have been found to be of great importance for atherogenesis, for example, cigarette smoking, arterial hypertension, or diabetes, they have often been subsumed under one or the other theory as independent factors that promote lipid or thrombotic atherogenesis.

Yet the view has persisted that atherogenesis is best accounted for by the known facts if it is regarded as polyetiologic and polypathogenetic. Indeed, the last decade has seen a rapprochement of the two major theories within one of the major divisions of classical pathology, namely that of injury and of the tissue reactions to injury. These reactions include exaggerated or defective cellular function, pathological differentiation, degeneration, proliferation, excess production of cellular products, necrosis, and the basic attributes of inflammation and repair in connective tissue.

Injury and the tissue reactions to it are venerable concepts of atherogenesis, but until recently they were concepts so broad as to have little value for an understanding of the process. Now, however, the experimental techniques are available to pose and answer meaningful questions within the concepts and to test ideas with precision. The result has been a growing sense of compatibility of the major theories of atherogenesis under this rubric and of a remarkable and rapidly developing body of qualitative information about the most fundamental aspects of atherogenesis. As yet, equivalent quantitative information is scant.

The conference speakers and workshops will present a wealth of pathogenetic data that will be highly informative. Obviously,

I cannot provide here as adequate a view of atherogenesis as you will hear in the next days. (3-6) But Dr. Colin Schwartz asked if I would comment on certain specific current findings. I do so with the proviso that my perspectives may be as insubstantial as a reflection and as transient as the moment.

Recently the Benditts found that samples from individual fibrous plaques were uniform for one or other of the sex-linked isoenzymes of 6-GPD. Others have confirmed the finding. This enzymatic monotypism or monoclonality could mean that each mature plaque derives from a single cell. This in turn raises specula-tions about cell transformation and a possible role for chemical or viral mutagens in the initiation of plaques. (7-9) The finding is the basis for a genuinely new theory of atherogenesis; it de-serves our most thoughtful consideration. Moreover, the theory provides a prior condition to other theories such as the lipid or thrombopathic hypotheses, since it designates the cells that will react to stimulation and form plaques.

It has also been observed that fatty streaks are not monotypic (10) and that thin plaques tend to be heterotypic while thicker ones from the same aorta tend to isoenzymic monotypism. (11) A different explanation for plaque monotypism is that it arises from the selective survival and proliferation of a line of cells as a particular plaque develops over time and that phenomena of cell adaptation and selection rather than of transformation are the basis for plaque monotypism.

It is apparent that more sophisticated studies of cell dif-ferentiation, probably using techniques available in the areas of embryology and neoplasis, will be needed to settle these questions to everyone's satisfaction. Nevertheless, the known facts bring several issues into sharper focus. Given the cellular homogeneity implied under either explanation for the monotypism of mature plaques, what significance should be attached to the pleomorphism (12, 13) seen within and between plaques of advanced lesions?

Since fatty streaks are heterotypic and mature plaques are monotypic does this mean, as has been suggested, that mature plaques do not derive from the fatty streaks of childhood? (10) Or, does it mean that the fatty streak possesses options for cel-lular adaptation that it loses as it becomes a monotypic advanced plaque? The possible evolution of childhood lesions to those of adult life to become plaques of clinical consequence is one of the most important utilitarian questions in atherogenesis today and it is unresolved. The studies needed to help resolve the Benditts' hypothesis may help to resolve this issue too. Moreover, their hypothesis legitimizes both an interest in viruses or chemical agents from the environment that may have transformational impact on arterial smooth muscle cells as well as an interest in the

host's defenses against such agents. There has been little or no
basis for such interests prior to the presentation of their theory.

     Both the lipid and thrombopathic theories share an interest
in the arterial endothelium and its integrity of function. Most
lipid theories have required that lipid traverse the arterial endothelium in some fashion prior to its accumulation in the plaque.
Thrombopathic theories have regarded endothelial participation as
primary or secondary, but as essential phenomena in either case.
In studies that may have been stimulated by a renewed interest in
examining the arterial endothelium en face (14, 15) and by investigations on arterial platelet microthrombi, new data have been
gathered to show that the endothelium is the guardian or gate
keeper of the intima and of access to the arterial smooth muscle
cell. Transmission and scanning electronmicroscopy data indicate
that endothelial damage or cell loss manifest either as increased
permeability to macromolecules, or as injury, loss and platelet
adhesion, aggregation and release at the site, are probably atherogenic stimuli.

     These areas of research are of considerable technical diffi-
culty, contain artifacts and have interpretive obscurity. Nevertheless, there has emerged a synthesis that places the failure of
endothelial integrity from whatever ictus or circumstance as the
initiating tissue step in atherogenesis. The changes may be mild,
and reparable and without additional consequence, or they may be
followed by events congruent with atherogenesis.

     The sequence appears to be that the intima becomes exposed
to plasma rather than to an ultrafiltrate and that platelets may
adhere and release their contents to diffuse into the intima.
The plasma exposure may exceed the tissue capacity for homeostatic
metabolism of, for example, lipoproteins or fibrinogen. It is
suggested, moreover, that the exposure may also be mitogenic for
smooth muscle cells and it can be speculated that it may also
shape the lesion by modulating the cellular production of collagen
and glycosaminglycans. Exposure to platelets clearly is mitogenic
and an appropriate factor has been isolated from them. It has
been 50 years since Okuneff (16) used Trypan blue as an intravital
stain for the aorta and drew an analogy between the staining patterns that he saw and the location and genesis of atherosclerotic
lesions. About 30 years ago Duff and I described mitotic activity
in the plaques of experimental arteriosclerosis and suggested
that cell proliferation in situ could account for plaque building.
(17) Another paper showed that plaque cells could be phagocytic
of a thorium dioxide tracer. (18) These three early descriptive
papers had theoretical interest. Now, however, recent investigations of great elegance have begun to provide detailed analyses
and mechanisms for such findings and indeed, recent research brings

us very close to understanding the basic principles of atherogenesis *ab initio*.

The appreciation that damage to endothelial integrity may comprise the earliest changes that in some circumstances can initiate atherogenesis requires us to consider the next pathogenetic steps and the further circumstances of atherogenesis. It becomes necessary to account for such characteristics as localization, cellularity, lipid accumulation, and the desmoplastic nature of plaques.

The recognition of growth factors and means by which they may contact and stimulate foci of cells to proliferate in the intima can be expected to create a parallel interest in the role of growth regulators. One anticipates that studies in atherogenesis will increasingly draw upon the information and techniques to study growth and growth regulation that have been developed in the fields of cellular biology, embryology, and neoplasia.

Cellular products such as glycosaminoglycans, collagens and elastins make up an important part of plaques. We know very little about these phenomena except in terms of descriptive biochemistry or histochemistry. There is a fairly detailed taxonomy of the products, but the pathogenetic events leading to their cellular production and accumulation in plaques are obscure. It is reasonable to speculate that there may be close analogies with similar accumulations in the reactions of wound healing and of chronic or granulomatous inflammation and repair in connective tissue, but, in fact, not much information is available regarding their pathogenesis and control.

A number of pathogenetic mechanisms have been offered for the accumulation of lipid in plaques including the *in situ* synthesis of phospholipids and the accumulation of structural lipids from necrotic or effete smooth muscle cells, platelets or red blood cells in appropriate circumstances. There is no reason to question that these mechanisms may operate, but the most popular hypothesis has involved the percolation of lipids from the plasma into the vessel wall. According to this view, an injured endothelial barrier admits excessive amounts of lipoproteins, particularly low density lipoproteins, to the intima. These are internalized by smooth muscle and other connective tissue cells, are digested too slowly and fail to efflux rapidly from the cells. Liberated sterol may fail to find adequate high density lipoprotein to accept it and transport it from the intima. Cellular necrosis can spill accumulated lipid into the extracellular plaque area where it is relatively isolated from cellular processes. Thus lipid accumulates intra- and extra-cellularly and acts as a local agent of injury.

This sequential concept is one of inadequate barrier function, overload with failure of homeostasis, and pathological adaptation.

A considerable amount of experimental data has been gathered in
support of the chain of events. Although the data are often provided by artificial models and are demonstrably of limited applicability, nevertheless, this pathogenetic theme with suitable
variations is the most credible explanation for the presence of
lipids in the generality of atherosclerotic lesions.

There is, however, a possible paradox that may provide a potentially serious challenge to this view of pathogenesis. The concept should apply to early or minor lesions as well as to later or
more advanced ones. Yet the fatty flecks and streaks of infancy
and childhood can occur under conditions in which low density lipoprotein concentrations are below those that are atherogenic in
adults and in circumstances where levels of high density lipoproteins are relatively increased. Moreover, endothelial integrity
in early childhood is not challenged by hypertension or by smoking
and its capacity for repair should be high. Consequently, the
concepts of injury, overload and failed homeostasis seem less
persuasive. Unless suitable age-related phenomena such as the
presence in childhood of a less effective endothelial barrier, or
a less effective lysosomal digestive system in intimal cells, or
some other appropriate difference in childhood or adult life is
elicited, it will be difficult to maintain the credibility of the
foregoing pathogenetic explanation for lipid accumulation. Of
course, if the childhood and adult lesions are unrelated, there
will be no paradox, but it would appear to be essential to gather
data and to test hypotheses in settings related to age or development.

Another brief comment should be made for the purposes of
this conference. Whatever the pathogenetic interplay of platelet
pathophysiology and of blood coagulation may finally prove to encompass for the nascent atherosclerotic lesion, the potent role
of mural thrombotic encrustation in the mid- and late-stage pathogenesis of many plaques should be emphasized. There is no reasonable doubt that such encrustation is a frequent and at times dominant element in the progression of plaques. It deserves better
documentation than it has had, and more emphasis on research. We
know too little about it.

While important principles may be within our grasp, it is
already clear that their quantitation, their alternative pathways
and their integration to explain particular examples of atherogenesis are going to be complex and difficult to understand. For example, it is known that endothelium and arterial smooth muscle
cells can respond differently to different growth factors. Dr.
Minick and his colleagues have evidence from in vivo experiments
with cholesterol-fed rabbits following aortic endothelial denudation that lipid accumulates where aortic endothelium is regenerating rather than where it has already regenerated or where it is

still denuded. (19) Dr. Theodore Spaet and his colleagues have shown in vivo that the proliferative activity is suppressed by hypophysectomy, but that it can be restored by non-specific stimuli such as a sterile subcutaneous abscess or indeed, even by the passage of time (personal communication). There are, therefore, multiple themes and variations that can be invoked for the processes of cellular proliferation and lipid accumulation in atherogenesis and it will be a complex matter to ascertain which ones may have meaning for the initiation and progression of plaques under the ordinary circumstances of life. The post-initiation phenomenon of atherogenesis will not prove to be simple.

In my view, what is happening today in research on atherogenesis is that two major theories are being found not merely to be debatable alternatives, but that rather they are being found to be compatible and to share common phenomena at the most basic initiating stages of atherogenesis. In the qualitative sense an appreciation of some of the most primitive principles of atherogenesis appears to be almost within our grasp.

At the same time, difficult and complex tasks remain to quantify, integrate and relate these phenomena to the realities of atherogenesis, and most important, to understand the host's defensive mechanisms against the initial steps of plaque development. The challenge for research on the pathogenesis of plaques will be changing its emphasis from seeking to understand initiating events to understanding the progression that follows initiation.

REFERENCES

1. Long, E.R. (1967) A Survey of the Problem, Cowdry's Athero-sclerosis, 2nd Ed. (Blumenthal, H.T., Ed.), Thomas, Springfield, Ill., pp. 5-20.

2. Lebowitz, J.O. (1970) The History of Coronary Heart Disease The Univ. of California Press, Berkeley and Los Angeles.

3. Ross, R., and Glomset, J.A. (1976) N. Engl. J. Med. 295, 369-377, 420-425.

4. Wissler, R.W., Jesselinovitch, D., and Getz, G.S. (1976) Progr. Cardiovasc. Dis. 18, 341-369.

5. Wolinsky, H. (1976) Cardiovasc. Med., September, 41-54.

6. McGill, H.C., Jr. (Paoletti, R. and Gotto, A.M., Jr., Eds.) (1977) in Atherosclerosis Reviews, Vol. 2.

7. Benditt, E.P., and Benditt, J.M. (1973) <u>Proc. Nat. Acad. Sci.
    USA</u> 70, 1753-1756.

8. Benditt, E.P. (1974) <u>Circulation</u> 50, 650-652.

9. Benditt, E.P. (1977) <u>Sci. Am.</u>, February, 74-85.

10. Pearson, T.A., Wang, A., Solez, K., and Heptinstall, R.H.
    (1975) <u>Am. J. Pathol</u>. 81, 379-388.

11. Thomas, W.A., Janakidevi, K., Reiner, J.M., and Lee, K.T.
    (1976) <u>Circulation</u> 54, No. 4, October II-137, abstract no.
    0540.

12. McMillan, G.C. (1955) <u>Minnesota Med.</u> 38, 746-748.

13. Osborn, G.R. (1973) <u>The Incubation Period of Coronary Throm-
    bosis</u>, Butterworths, London.

14. Duff, G.L., McMillan, G.C., and Ritchie, A.C. (1957) <u>Am. J.
    Pathol</u>. 33, 845-873.

15. Poole, J.C.F., and Florey, H.W. (1958) <u>J. Path. Bact.</u> 75, 245-
    251.

16. Okuneff, N. (1926) Virchow's <u>Arch. Path. Anat.</u> 259, 685-697.

17. McMillan, G.C., and Duff, G.L. (1948) <u>Arch. Pathol</u>. 46, 179-
    182.

18. Duff, G.L., McMillan, G.C., and Lautsch, E.V. (1954) <u>Am. J.
    Pathol</u>. 30, 941-955.

19. Minick, C.R., Stemerman, M.B., and Insull, W., Jr. (1977)
    <u>Proc. Nat. Acad. Sci. USA</u> 74, 1724-1728.

THE GEOGRAPHIC PATHOLOGY AND TOPOGRAPHY OF ATHEROSCLEROSIS AND RISK FACTORS FOR ATHEROSCLEROTIC LESIONS

Jack P. Strong, Douglas A. Eggen, and Richard E. Tracy

Department of Pathology
Louisiana State University Medical Center
New Orleans, Louisiana

Any theory of the pathogenesis of atherosclerosis must fit with observed distributions of lesions within and among arterial systems and among populations of diverse economic, ethnic or social circumstance. It must also be consistent with the known effects of various factors (risk factors) on the extent of atherosclerotic lesions. Thus, a review of the topography and geographic pathology of atherosclerosis and of risk factors for atherosclerotic lesions would seem appropriate as a preliminary to discussions on the role or thrombosis in the pathogenesis of atherosclerosis.

In this report we will not attempt a detailed review of all of the earlier reports on the distribution of atherosclerosis but will refer the reader to previous reviews of this material. The basic material to be presented on the topography of atherosclerotic lesions will be taken from investigations in our laboratory, from the volume reporting the principal results of the International Atherosclerosis Project (IAP) (1), and from subsequent reports based on the IAP material. This material is limited to the aorta, coronary arteries, and arteries supplying the brain. In addition, we refer to the preliminary results of recent long-term epidemiological studies of cardiovascular disease with autopsy follow-up to summarize the latest information on the geographic pathology of atherosclerotic lesions as related to antecedent risk factors.

CLASSIFICATION OF LESIONS

Most of the material to be reviewed involves studies of arterial specimens that were stained grossly with Sudan IV. The following working definitions are offered for different types of atherosclerotic lesions detectable grossly in such specimens. Although this classification implies a pathogenetic sequence, it can be used as a descriptive classification regardless of the ideas of pathogenetic interrelationships among the lesions.

Fatty streak. A fatty intimal lesion that is stained distinctly by Sudan IV and shows no other underlying change. Fatty streaks are flat or only slightly elevated and do not significantly narrow the lumina of blood vessels.

Fibrous plaque. A firm, elevated intimal lesion which in the fresh state is gray white, glistening, and translucent. The surface of the lesion may be sudanophilic, but usually is not. Human fibrous plaques characteristically contain fat. Often a thick fibrous connective tissue cap containing varying amounts of lipid covers a more concentrated 'core' of lipid. If a lesion also contains hemorrhage, thrombosis, ulceration, or calcification, that lesion is classified according to one of the next two categories.

This classification of lesions based on gross examination does not permit distinction between those plaques with and without a core of degenerated or necrotic lipid-rich debris. Those plaques with necrotic lesions and ulceration of the surface would of course be classified as complicated lesions. The plaques with necrotic centers and intact intimal surfaces ("atheroma" according to some classifications) would be classified as fibrous plaques. Microscopic examination is usually necessary to distinguish various subtypes of fibrous plaques.

Complicated lesion. An intimal plaque in which there is hemorrhage, ulceration, or thrombosis with or without calcium.

Calcified lesion. An intimal plaque in which insoluble mineral salts of calcium are visible or palpable without overlying hemorrhage, ulceration, or thrombosis.

The term raised atherosclerotic lesion is sometimes used to indicate the sum of fibrous plaques, complicated lesions, and calcified lesions. Raised lesions are contrasted with fatty streaks which typically show little or no elevation above the surrounding intimal surface.

Use of the word atheroma is not consistent among investigators and authors. Some use it for the lesion described above - a plaque with a pool of degenerated or necrotic lipid-rich debris. Others use atheroma to refer to the process of atherosclerosis or arteriosclerosis. Still others have used the term to refer to various lesions - from a fatty streak to a complicated lesion. To avoid ambiguity when one uses the term, it should be qualified or modified so that its meaning is perfectly clear. We will not use it here.

Other lesions which are sometimes considered as atherosclerosis or as lesions predisposing to atherosclerosis include fibromuscular intimal thickening, gelatinous or edematous intimal lesions, and organizing mural thrombi on an otherwise normal intima. The pathogenetic relationship of these lesions to atherosclerosis and its clinical manifestations is less well established and quantitative information related to topography and geographic pathology are not available. Dr. Haust will discuss these lesions in her report on the light and ultrastructural morphology of atherosclerosis.

GEOGRAPHIC PATHOLOGY OF ATHEROSCLEROSIS

Early Studies

In the middle 1950's, in addition to observing persons from a single autopsy population, pathologists began to compare atherosclerosis in two or more populations. The principal objective was to determine the environmental conditions associated with preclinical lesions. Earlier epidemiologic impressions of clinical disease related to atherosclerosis were generally confirmed. This method of investigation also confirmed the relevance of atherosclerosis to coronary heart disease (CHD). The higher the CHD mortality and morbidity rates were in a population, the more extensive and severe were the lesions of atherosclerosis in autopsied persons from that population. This finding was particularly true of the advanced stages (fibrous plaques, calcification, stenosis and thrombosis). However, some puzzling inconsistencies remained, particularly with regard to the earlier lesions of atherosclerosis, such as fatty streaks.

In 1958 several pathologists and biometricians who had been involved in earlier attempts to compare atherosclerotic lesions among different populations proposed a project to answer questions raised by previous studies and to correct faults in earlier comparisons. Previous comparisons had involved only two or three populations at a time; numbers of cases had been relatively small; and grading methods were not uniform and would have permitted grader bias to influence the results. The problems of enlisting cooperation of interested pathologists and developing workable methods were solved and collection of specimens for this project, to be known as the International Atherosclerosis Project (IAP), began in May, 1960 and continued until September, 1965.

Major Findings of the International
Atherosclerosis Project

In the IAP a group of cooperating pathologists examined 23,000 aortas and coronary arteries collected from autopsied persons in fourteen countries. The principal findings of this extensive investigation have been published in detail (1) and summarized recently (2).

Only a brief description of the methods will be given here (3). Arterial specimens were collected at autopsy following a standard procedure, fixed in a flattened position, packed in plastic bags, and shipped to a central laboratory, where they were stained grossly with Sudan IV under standardized conditions.

The coded specimens were evaluated by a team of pathologists who visually estimated the percentage of the surface covered by different types of lesions. Periodic checks of reproducibility and reliability of the grading procedure were conducted to control inter- and intra-observer variability.

Racial and geographic comparisons among these populations have been reported (4). Figure 1 shows the mean extent of intimal surface involvement with fatty streaks and raised atherosclerotic lesions in the coronary arteries from nineteen location race groups of autopsied men classified by geographic location and race and dying at fifteen to sixty-four years of age. The extent of involvement varied among these groups at all ages. Variation was greater for raised lesions than for fatty streaks. Involvement by raised lesions was most extensive in the New Orleans and Oslo groups.

In Table 1 these nineteen "location-race" groups are ranked according to a composite measure of extent involvement with raised atherosclerotic lesions (4). This composite is an average of the mean percent surface in each of five arterial segments (3 coronary arteries, 2 segments of aorta) for cases grouped by sex and age (a crude sort of age-sex adjustment). Geographic and ethnic differences in average extent of coronary atherosclerosis were large. On the average, cases from populations such as New Orleans and Oslo had about three times as much intimal surface involvement with raised lesions as did those from Guatemala and the Durban (South Africa) Bantu. Mortality rates from coronary heart disease (CHD) are not available for all of these populations, but where such data are available, the measures of atherosclerotic lesions rank the populations in much the same order as do the mortality rates.

When the nineteen location-race groups were ranked by extent of lesions in coronary arteries alone, in the aorta alone, in each sex alone, and in each decade alone, a substantially similar rank

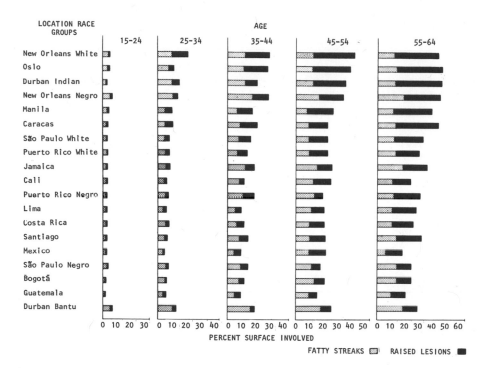

Figure 1. Mean percentage of intimal surface involved with fatty streaks and raised atherosclerotic lesions in coronary arteries of men. (From reference 4, with permission).

was obtained. We concluded that populations with more extensive lesions in the aorta tend to have more lesions in the coronaries and that those with more extensive lesions in men also tend to have more extensive lesions in women at the same age.

TOPOGRAPHIC DISTRIBUTION

Atherosclerosis in Different Arterial Systems

The topographic distribution of atherosclerotic lesions has been described qualitatively in the earliest literature on arterio-sclerosis. It was reviewed by Duff and McMillan in their classical seminar on the pathology of atherosclerosis in 1951 (5) and by Glagov and Ozoa (6). Schwartz and Mitchell (7) described selective involvement of some arteries and areas of localization of arterial plaques in their necropsy survey. Early studies were generally

Table 1. Nineteen location-race groups ranked by mean extent of raised lesions. Data from International Atherosclerosis Project (4).

location-race group	rank	mean intimal surface with raised lesions*	arbitrary classification
		%	
New Orleans, white	1	18.3	high
Oslo	2	17.3	high
Durban Indian	3	14.6	medium-high
New Orleans, black	4	14.5	medium-high
Manila	5	12.8	medium
Caracas	6	12.1	medium
São Paulo, white	7	10.8	medium-low
Puerto Rico, white	8	9.6	medium-low
Jamaica, black	9	9.5	medium-low
Cali	10	9.1	medium-low
Puerto Rico, black	11	8.8	medium-low
Lima	12	8.5	medium-low
Costa Rica	13	8.4	medium-low
Santiago	14	8.2	medium-low
Mexico	15	7.9	medium-low
São Paulo, black	16	7.4	low
Bogotá	17	6.7	low
Guatemala	18	6.5	low
Durban Bantu	19	6.2	low

*The value given is an unweighted mean of the 40 mean values for raised lesion obtained in each location-race group, i.e., the means for percent with raised lesion in each of 5 arteries (3 coronary, 2 aorta) for cases classified into 2 sexes and 4 ten-year age groups (25 to 64 years) were averaged.

consistent in the finding that lesions occurred earliest and most extensively in the aorta. Lesions developed later and less extensively in the coronary and cerebral arteries, and the renal, mesenteric and pulmonary arteries were the least susceptible to atherosclerotic lesions. A diagrammatic representation of localization of arterial involvement by atherosclerosis is depicted in Figure 2 taken from the NHLI task force report of Arteriosclerosis (8).

The studies in the IAP led to the following conclusions concerning atherosclerosis in the aorta and the coronary, carotid, vertebral and intracranial arteries (9).

The severity of atherosclerosis in one artery does not predict the severity in another artery for an individual case. On a cross cultural basis, however, the average predilection to raised lesions in one artery is correlated with the predilection in another artery. The location-race groups in the IAP are ranked in approximately the same order, regardless of whether the ranking is based on raised lesions in one of the three major coronary arteries, the thoracic aorta, the abdominal aorta, or the cerebral arteries. This finding is consistent with the idea that environmental conditions predominantly determine the severity of atherosclerosis in a population, despite large differences in susceptibility to lesions among individuals or among different anatomic loci within the arteries of each person.

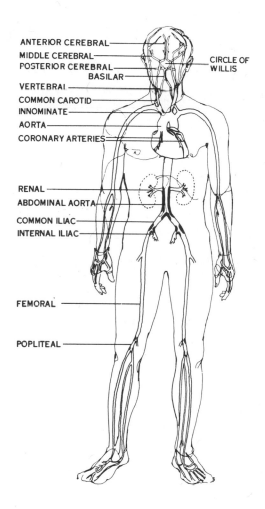

Figure 2.   Common sites of atherosclerotic lesions.   (From reference 8).

The arteries are involved by atherosclerosis in a definite
sequence. The aorta is first involved beginning in infancy with
fatty streaks which increase rapidly during puberty. Fatty streaks
begin in the coronary arteries during puberty, but begin to increase significantly and become converted into fibrous plaques in
the third decade of life in high risk populations. The carotid
arteries begin to be involved with fatty streaks at approximately
the same age as the aorta, and the other cerebral arteries begin
at approximately the same age as the coronary arteries. Raised
lesions develop in the carotid arteries at roughly the same age as
in the aorta, but do not develop in the vertebral and intracranial
arteries until much later.

Distribution of Lesions Within Arterial Systems

In addition to the descriptive reports on the topographic distribution of lesions among arterial systems, detailed quantitative
or morphometric studies have been reported on the distribution of
lesions within the aorta, coronary arteries and arteries supplying
the brain.

Aorta. Holman, McGill, Strong, and Geer in 1958 (10) described the topographic distribution of early aortic atherosclerotic
lesions (evaluated in autopsied persons 1 to 40 years of age) in
qualitative and quantitative terms. Figures 3 and 4 taken from
their report show the quantitative development of fatty streaks
and fibrous plaques in the different segments of the aorta. They
gave the following description of the topographic development of
lesions: "...the aortic ring was the first to be involved by
fatty streaks. The sudanophilic deposits encountered in this area
were scattered along a line at the upper edge of the valvular com-
missures. The aortic valve leaflets themselves were not affected,
and fatty streaks deep within the sinuses of Valsalva were rarely
found. Although not sought systematically in this study, fatty
deposits were frequently noted on the ventricular surface of the
anterior leaflet of the mitral valve.

"The involvement of the aortic arch was similar to that of
the ring. Here the fatty deposits usually occurred in small discrete foci conforming to no particular pattern, except that they
seemed to be more frequent about the orifices of the large branches
arising from the arch.

"The descending thoracic and abdominal portions of the aorta
set the distinctive pattern of increasing lesions ... that has
been previously demonstrated in terms of total percentage of surface involved. Of the two, the abdominal aorta was consistently
the more severely affected. The same relationship of the various

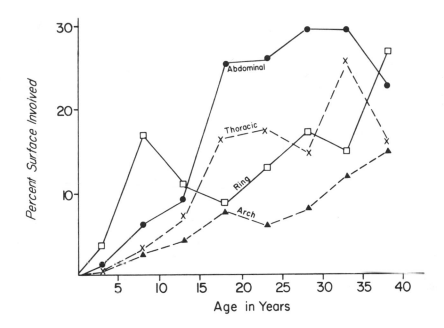

Figure 3. Aortic atherosclerosis, New Orleans. Average per cent surface covered by fatty streaks by anatomic region in 184 white cases (from reference 10, with permission).

segments of aorta to one another was also present with regard to fibrous plaques. The abdominal segment was most severely involved, the descending thoracic was next and the ring and arch were least.

"In the descending thoracic aorta, fatty streaks - especially the extensive ones appearing in the second decade - occurred as parallel, linear, longitudinal streaks localized along the posterior portion of the aorta, between and to each side of the orifices of the intercostal vessels. About each orifice there was a small area which was characteristically spared. In contrast, in the abdominal portion the fatty streaks occurred as larger irregular areas, often confluent so as to cover fairly uniformly rather extensive portions of the intimal surface."

In the thoracic portion of the descending aorta fibrous plaques tend to concentrate in the posterior surface and often appear to be centered on the orifices of the intercostal arteries. There appears

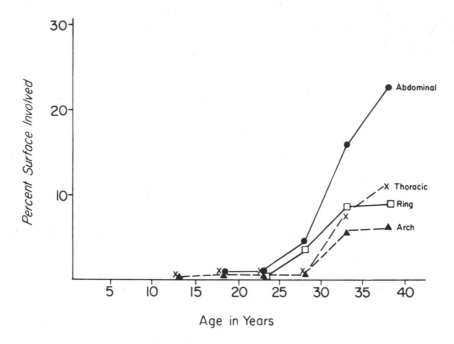

Figure 4. Aortic atherosclerosis, New Orleans. Average per cent surface covered by fibrous plaques by anatomic region in 184 white cases. (From reference 10, with permission).

to be a greater propensity for formation of fibrous plaque in the abdominal aorta than in the thoracic aorta and the plaques are more uniformly distributed over the circumference, involving posterior, anterior and both lateral walls.

Recent observations in our laboratory have indicated other additional sites of predilection for formation of fibrous plaques in the aorta. One site is the left anterolateral wall of the thoracic aorta in the region from about the third to the seventh intercostal orifice; a second is the left posterolateral wall of the abdominal aorta just proximal to the bifurcation of the iliacs. A further detailed quantitative study of the topography of lesions in a large number of unselected specimens will be required, however, before the validity and significance of these tentative observations are established, and whether or not these same areas are sites of predilection for fatty streak.

Topographic analyses have yielded differences of opinion concerning the interrelationships of fatty streaks and fibrous plaques
in the aorta. Holman and colleagues (10) indicated that there was
sufficient fatty change to serve as a basis for all the fibrous
plaques encountered at later ages and concluded that the conversion
of fatty streaks to fibrous plaques in the aorta required at least
15 years. Mitchell and Schwartz (7, 11) after their study of topographic distribution of lesions, concluded that aortic fatty streaks
should not be considered precursors of fibrous plaques.

These discrepancies and the growing controversy concerning the
relationships of fatty streaks to fibrous plaques (12) led to additional systematic approaches to topography of lesions in other arterial segments.

Coronary Arteries. Montenegro and Eggen (13) analyzed the axial
distribution of atherosclerosis in the coronary arteries in detail
for fatty streaks, fibrous plaques, and complicated lesions in 2964
human coronary artery specimens from Durban, Guatemala, New Orleans,
Santiago, and Sao Paulo. The presence or absence of each type of
lesion was recorded for each one centimeter segment for each of the
three main coronary artery branches from autopsied persons aged 10
to 69 years. Prevalence of each type of lesion by axial segment was
examined for consistency of pattern among geographic location, race,
sex, and age groups.

In the left coronary artery, prevalence of lesions of all types
was greatest near the bifurcation. A marked decrease in prevalence
of lesions occurred as one moved distally from the bifurcation along
both the circumflex and the anterior descending branches (Fig. 5).

The maximum prevalence of lesions in the right coronary artery
also occurred in the region just distal to the orifice (Fig. 5) but
this maximum was lower than that at the bifurcation of the left
coronary. The decrease in prevalence distally from the maximum was
much less pronounced in the right coronary artery than in either
branch of the left coronary artery. There was an indication of a
second, but lower, peak in prevalence of lesions at about 8 to 10
cm from the orifice of the right coronary artery.

This pattern of distribution along the axis of each artery was
similar for both sexes, all five location groups, all three race
groups, and all ages. The patterns were also similar for fatty
streaks and fibrous or complicated lesions. This finding lends support to the hypothesis that there is a close pathogenetic association between fatty streak and the more advanced lesions.

Carotid and Vertebral Arteries. Solberg and Eggen (14) examined the axial distribution of fatty streak, fibrous plaque, calci-

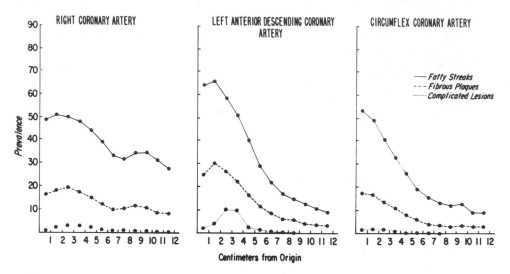

Figure 5.   Percentage of positive cases with fatty streaks, fibrous plaques, and complicated lesions in the first 12 cm of the three coronary arteries in 2964 sets of arteries from five locations, three race groups, and both sexes. (From reference 13, with permission).

fied lesions and complicated lesions in the carotid and vertebral arteries of 961 autopsied patients, aged 25-69 years, from Guatemala and Oslo, Norway. The common carotid and internal carotid arteries were each divided into five equal segments and the vertebral arteries into seven equal segments. The presence or absence of each type of lesion was assessed for each segment by visual examination of the sudan stained artery or, of a soft x-ray radiograph of the artery (for calcified lesions). Prevalence of each type of lesion in each segment was computed for 10-year age groups by geographic location and sex for both right and left paired arteries.

The pattern of axial distribution was characteristic for each of the three major arteries. Lesions were most prevalent near the bifurcation of the common carotid and in the distal segment of the internal carotid artery (Fig. 6). At any age the prevalence of lesions in a given segment of the carotid artery decreased successively in the proximal direction from these maxima. The trend with age and the distribution from segment to segment indicated that the atherosclerotic process begins at the bifurcation and in the siphon region of the internal carotid artery and progresses proximally from there along the common or the internal carotid artery.

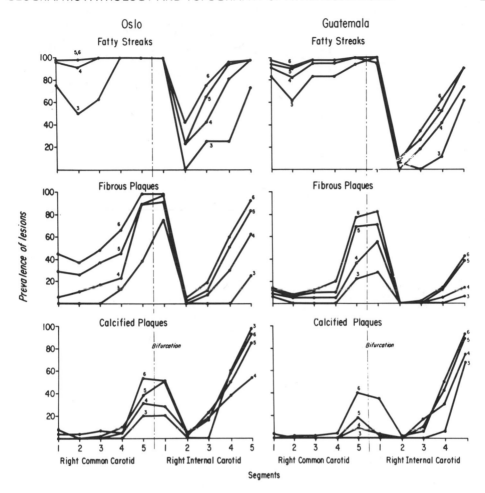

Figure 6. Percentage of positive cases with fatty streaks, fibrous plaques and calcified lesions in segments of right common carotid and right internal carotid arteries from autopsied men in Oslo, Norway and Guatemala, C.A. Numbers along side curves represent 10 year age groups as follows: 3 = 5-24 years, 4 = 35-44 years, 5 = 45-54 years and 6 = 55-64 years (From reference 14, by permission of the American Heart Association, Inc.).

Lesions in the vertebral arteries were much more uniformly distributed along the axis; however, the prevalence was somewhat higher in the distal and proximal segments than in the five central segments.

These patterns of axial distribution in the carotid and vertebral arteries were consistent for both left and right arteries, in all age groups, in both sexes and in both geographic locations. Since the patterns were also similar for all types of lesions, these authors suggest that their data support the hypothesis that fatty streaks are precursors of fibrous plaques and more advanced lesions.

RISK FACTORS AND ATHEROSCLEROSIS

Epidemiologic investigation of living populations has disclosed characteristics of persons which are associated with increased risk of developing coronary heart disease (CHD). A plenary session of this workshop on the thrombotic process in atherogenesis is devoted to the relationship of risk factors for atherosclerosis and CHD to thrombosis. We shall review here the relationship of some of these risk factors for CHD to the atherosclerotic lesions (15). Lesions in the coronary arteries will be the principal focus.

Of all risk factors age has the strongest and most consistent association with lesions. The average extent of atherosclerosis increased with age in each sub-group of all the populations of the IAP (nineteen location-race groups in fourteen countries) (16).

In a supplemental study in the IAP ethnically similar groups in geographically distinct locations with vastly different ways of life were compared (17). On grouping the nineteen location-race groups into five arbitrary categories of average extent, athero- sclerotic involvement in the white populations was high in New Orleans (USA) and Oslo (Norway), medium in Sao Paulo (Brazil), and medium-low in Puerto Rico, Costa Rica, and Santiago (Chile). Atherosclerosis in the black population was medium-high in New Or- leans, medium-low in Jamaica and Puerto Rico, and low in Sao Paulo, and Durban. A strong gradient in coronary atherosclerosis existed both among black populations from New Orleans, Puerto Rico, Jamai- ca, Sao Paulo, and Durban and among the white populations from New Orleans, Oslo, Puerto Rico, Sao Paulo, Santiago, and Costa Rica. Thus environmental background seemed more important than racial background in determining the extent of coronary atherosclerosis.

Coronary atherosclerosis is generally considered to be more extensive in men than in women (17). The average extent of coro- nary lesions in men and women from the IAP and the ratio of lesions in men and women supported this view for the white populations; however, this sex difference was less striking or absent in the black populations. Also, there was little or no sex difference in aortic atherosclerosis (17). Thus, the differences in athero- sclerosis between sexes are not consistent.

An indication of possible racial differences was obtained by examining lesions in three locations in the IAP that have both black and white populations, i.e., New Orleans, Puerto Rico, and São Paulo (17). The black groups in these geographic locations have somewhat less extensive lesions than the white groups, particularly in the men. Any genetic or racial effect, however, is undoubtedly confounded with socio-economic differences between the races in any one geographic location.

Table 2 summarizes the relationship of atherosclerosis as measured in the IAP to serum cholesterol and diet as determined by Scrimshaw and Guzman from available literature (18). The correlation of rank of lesions with rank of serum cholesterol is 0.75 which is significantly greater than zero (P < 0.01). The correlation of rank based on raised lesions and rank by per cent of calories from fat in these populations is also statistically significant. The correlations between rank based on raised lesions and rank by per cent of animal fat in total fat or by sugar consumption are not statistically significant.

Although studies indicated a relationship of atherosclerotic lesions to diet and serum lipids when comparing geographically or racially distinct populations, there were, at the time of the IAP, no conclusive data for positive association between atherosclerotic lesions and serum lipids or diet among individual subjects within such a population. In the more recent past, prospective studies have been initiated with careful documentation of serum lipid levels and, in some instances, of dietary patterns, and with standardized evaluation of atherosclerotic lesions at autopsy. Tentative results concerning antecedent risk factors and extent of atherosclerotic lesions at autopsy have been reported (19-23) and are summarized in Table 3. These studies for the first time show, on a case related basis, significant positive relationships between the extent of atherosclerosis as measured at autopsy and serum lipid values carefully measured during life (24).

Data from the IAP confirm many studies which have reported aggravation or acceleration of atherosclerotic lesions in persons with hypertension and diabetes (25). Raised lesions in the coronary arteries were greater in the known hypertensive persons than in those without hypertension in all of these populations. Similar results were obtained when comparing lesions in persons with and without diabetes. Thus, hypertension and diabetes accelerate the natural progression of atherosclerosis in all populations. The recent epidemiological studies with autopsy follow-up (Table 3) show highly significant correlations of antecedent blood pressure measurements and extent of atherosclerosis as measured carefully after autopsy.

Table 2:   Twelve location-race groups ranked by mean extent of raised lesions, serum cholesterol, and per cent of calories from fat.   Data from International Atherosclerosis Project (from reference 17).

location-race group	rank				
	raised lesions	serum cholesterol	percent calories from fat	percent animal fat in total fat	sugar consumption
New Orleans white	1	1	2	8	6
Oslo	2	2	1	5	3
New Orleans black	3	3	4	9	4
Manila	4	6	6	7	10
Puerto Rico	5	4	3	1	7
Cali	6	8	11	11	8
Lima	7	10	5	10	2
San Jose	8	11	12	2	1
Santiago	9	5	10	4	12
Bogotá	10	9	8	12	5
Guatemala	11	12	9	6	9
Durban Bantu	12	7	7	3	11

Table 3:   Association between major CHD risk factors and extent of atherosclerosis as assessed at autopsy (from reference 24).

principal investigator (year)	location	number of cases	major CHD risk factors		
			serum cholesterol	blood pressure	cigarette smoking
Garcia-Palmieri (1977)	Puerto Rico	92	+	+	+
Hatano (1977)	Tokyo	186	+	+	+
Solberg (1977)	Oslo	49	+	+	±
Stemmermann (1977)	Honolulu	124	+	+	+
Sternby (1977)	Malmo	33	+	+	-

+ positive and significant relationship
± positive relationship but not statistically significant
- negative relationship

Although there is considerable evidence that physical activity, obesity, and mineral content of drinking water are related to CHD mortality, most studies have failed to find a consistent association between these risk factors and atherosclerotic lesions per se. Reports from the IAP (26) and our local studies in New Orleans have also failed to detect consistent relationships between these risk factors and atherosclerotic lesions. The relationship between obesity and lesions will be investigated further in the on-going epidemiological studies. In one of them (22) obesity and lesions are significantly correlated in the data collected to date.

We examined the mean extent of coronary raised lesions in relation to cigarette smoking in autopsied New Orleans white and black men (27, 28). The average extent of raised atherosclerotic lesions was greater in the heavy smokers than in the non-smokers within each ten-year age group. Studies by Auerbach (29, 30) have also indicated that advanced coronary atherosclerosis is much more prevalent in heavy smokers than in non-smokers and that there is regular progression in severity of atherosclerotic lesions with increasing rate of smoking. Thus, the propensity for heavy smokers of cigarettes to develop CHD can, at least in part, be attributed to atherosclerotic lesions in the arterial wall. The effect of cigarette smoking on CHD is not limited to the terminal occlusive episode.

An intriguing finding is the wide variation in the extent of lesions among individuals in the most homogeneous sub-groups (31). Even after selecting cases according to race, sex, age, disease, and level of cigarette consumption, there is much variability in the extent of atherosclerosis. This variability should be investigated intensively by epidemiologic, pathologic, genetic, and other methods, for this unexplained variability indicates the existence of undiscovered etiologic agents or risk factors.

CONCLUDING REMARKS

Investigators concerned with the role of the thrombotic process in atherogenesis and readers of the proceedings of this workshop symposium should take into account these findings, because it is essential that any factor involved in the pathogenesis of atherosclerosis be compatible with the known distribution of lesions among human populations and among and within the various arteries of individuals. If thrombosis has a role in the early pathogenesis of atherosclerosis (in addition to its well recognized role as an occlusive process superimposed on pre-existing atherosclerotic lesions) this early role should be compatible and explainable in relationship to the findings reviewed here. Some key questions

follow. Can thrombosis explain the propensity of lesions to form
more readily in the abdominal aorta than in the thoracic aorta or
at the bifurcation of the left coronary artery rather than in the
more distal regions of the interior branch of this artery? Can
thrombosis be responsible for some population groups having more
raised lesions than others? Can thrombosis explain why, in some
populations, a sex difference occurs in some arteries but not in
others? Many other similar questions come to mind.

In considering thrombosis as a factor in the pathogenesis of
atherosclerotic lesions we should be considering its potential in-
terrelationship to risk factors such as age, sex, race, serum lipoprotein levels, levels of blood pressure, smoking habits, physical
activity, obesity, etc. The findings summarized in this report
concerning the relationship of smoking habits to the development
of mural atherosclerotic lesions, while indicating that the effect
of smoking is not limited to the terminal occlusive episode, are
not evidence that there is no such relationship. Searching out
relationships of any of the known or suspected risk factors for
atherosclerosis and coronary heart disease to the process of thrombosis is a worthwhile and potentially rewarding goal. A segment
of this workshop is devoted to possible relationships of risk factors and thrombosis, and this material is covered elsewhere in this
volume.

REFERENCES

1. McGill, H.C., Jr., Editor (1968) The Geographic Pathology of
    Atherosclerosis: The Williams and Wilkins Co., Baltimore.
    or Lab. Invest. 18, 463-653.

2. Strong, J.P. (1977) Atherosclerosis, A Preventable Disease?
    Autopsy Evidence. Proceedings of the International Symposium
    on the State of Prevention and Therapy in Human Atherosclerosis
    and in Animal Models. Munster, Aug., 1977.

3. Guzman, M.A., McMahan, C.A., McGill, H.C., Jr., Strong, J.P.,
    Tejada, C., Restrepo, C., Eggen, D.A., Robertson, W.B., and
    Solberg, L.A. (1968) Selected methodologic aspects of the
    International Atherosclerosis Project. Lab. Invest. 18, 479-497.

4. Tejada, C., Strong, J.P., Montenegro, M.R., Restrepo, C., and
    Solberg, L.A. (1968) Distribution of coronary and aortic
    atherosclerosis by geographic location, race, and sex. Lab.
    Invest. 18, 509-526.

5. Duff, G.L., and McMillan, G.C. (1951) Pathology of atheroscle-
    rosis. Am. J. Med. 11, 92-108.

6. Glagov, S., and Ozoa, A.K. (1968) Significance of the rela-
    tively low incidence of atherosclerosis in the pulmonary, renal
    and mesenteric arteries. Ann. N.Y. Adad. Sci. 149(2), 940-955.

7. Schwartz, C.J., and Mitchell, J.R.A. (1962) Observations on
    the localization of arterial plaques. Circ. Res. 11, 63-73.

8. Arteriosclerosis: Report by NHLI task force on Arteriosclero-
    sis. Volume 1. (1971) DHEW Publication Number (NIH) 72-137.
    U.S. Dept. of Health, Education, and Welfare, Public Health
    Service.

9. McGill, H.C., Jr., Arias-Stella, J., Carbonell, L.M., Correa,
    P., de Veyra, E.A., Jr., Donoso, S., Eggen, D.A., Galindo, L.,
    Guzman, M.A., Lichtenberger, E., Loken, A.C., McGarry, P.A.,
    McMahan, C.A., Montenegro, M.R., Moossy, J., Perez-Tamayo, R.,
    Restrepo, C., Robertson, W.B., Salas, J., Solberg, L.A.,
    Strong, J.P., Tejada, C., and Wainwright, J. (1968) The Geo-
    graphic Pathology of Atherosclerosis: The Williams and Wilkins
    Co., Baltimore. pp. 38-42, or Lab Invest. 18, 498-502.

10. Holman, R., McGill, H.C., Jr., Strong, J.P., and Geer, J.C.
    (1958) The natural history of atherosclerosis: The early
    aortic lesions as seen in New Orleans in the middle of the
    20th century. Am. J. Pathol. 34, 209-235.

11. Mitchell, J.R.A., and Schwartz, C.J. (1965) Arterial Disease,
    F.A. Davis Co., Philadelphia.

12. Robertson, W.B., Geer, J.C., Strong, J.P., and McGill, H.C.,
    Jr. (1963) The fate of the fatty streak. Exp. Molec. Path.
    2 (Suppl. 1), 28-39.

13. Montenegro, M.R., and Eggen, D.A. (1968) Topography of athero-
    sclerosis in the coronary arteries. Lab. Invest. 18, 586-593.

14. Solberg, L.A., and Eggen, D.A. (1971) Localization and se-
    quence of development of atherosclerotic lesions in the caro-
    tid and vertebral arteries. Circulation 43, 711-724.

15. Strong, J.P., and Eggen, D.A. (1970) Risk factors and athero-
    sclerotic lesions. In Atherosclerosis (R.J. Jones, Ed.)
    Springer-Verlag, New York, pp. 355-364.

16, Eggen, D.A., and Solberg, L.A. (1968) Variations of athero-
    sclerosis with age. Lab. Invest. 18, 571-579.

17. Strong, J.P. (1972) Atherosclerosis in human population.
    Atherosclerosis 16, 193-201.

18. Scrimshaw, N.S., and Guzman, M.A. (1968) Diet and atheroscle-
     rosis. Lab. Invest. 18, 623-628.

19. Garcia-Palmieri, M.R., Castillo, M.I., Oalmann, M.C., Sorlie,
     P.D., and Costas, R., Jr. (1977) The relation of antemortum
     factors to atherosclerosis. Proceedings of the Fourth Inter-
     national Symposium on Atherosclerosis, Tokyo. In press.

20. Hatano, S., and Matsuzaki, T. (1977) Atherosclerosis in re-
     lation to personal attributes of a Japanese population in homes
     for the aged. Proceedings of the Fourth International Symposium
     on Atherosclerosis, Tokyo. In press.

21. Solberg, L.A., Hjermann, I., Helgeland, A., Holme, I., Leren,
     P.A., and Strong, J.P. (1977) Association between risk factors
     and atherosclerotic lesions based on autopsy findings in the
     Oslo study: A preliminary report. Proceedings of the Fourth
     International Symposium on Atherosclerosis, Tokyo. In press.

22. Stemmermann, G.N., Rhoads, G.G., and Blackwelder, W.C. (1977)
     Atherosclerosis and its risk factors in the Hawaiian Japanese.
     Proceedings of the Fourth International Symposium on Athero-
     sclerosis, Tokyo. In press.

23. Sternby, N.H. (1977) Atherosclerosis and risk factors.
     Proceedings of the Fourth International Symposium on Athero-
     sclerosis, Tokyo. In press.

24. Strong, J.P. (1977) An introduction to the epidemiology of
     atherosclerosis. Proceedings of the Fourth International
     Symposium on Atherosclerosis, Tokyo.

25. Robertson, W., and Strong, J.P. (1968) Atherosclerosis in
     persons with hypertension and diabetes mellitus. Lab. Invest.
     18, 538-551.

26. Strong, J.P., Correa, P., and Solberg, L.A. (1968) Water hard-
     ness and atherosclerosis. Lab. Invest. 18, 620-622.

27. Strong, J.P., Richards, M.L., McGill, H.C., Jr., Eggen, D.A.,
     and McMurry, M.T. (1969) On the association of cigarette
     smoking with coronary and aortic atherosclerosis. J. Athero-
     sclerosis Res. 10, 303-317.

28. Strong, J.P., and Richards, M.L. (1976) Cigarette smoking and
     atherosclerosis in autopsied men. Atherosclerosis 23, 451-476.

29. Auerbach, O., Carter, H.W., Garfinkel, L., and Hammond, E.C.
     (1976) Cigarette smoking and coronary artery disease. Chest
     70, 697-705.

30. Auerbach, O., Hammond, E.C., and Garfinkel, L. (1965) Smoking
     in relation to atherosclerosis of the coronary arteries. N.
     Engl. J. Med. 273, 775-779.

31. Strong, J.P. (1977) Unexplained variability in extent of athe-
     rosclerosis in homogenous subgroups of human populations.
     Proceedings of the Fourth International Symposium on Athero-
     sclerosis, Tokyo. In press.

Supported in part by grants from NHLBI (HL-08974 and HL-14496)

LIGHT AND ELECTRON MICROSCOPY OF HUMAN
ATHEROSCLEROTIC LESIONS

M. Daria Haust

Departments of Pathology and Pediatrics
University of Western Ontario and the
Children's Psychiatric Research Institute
London, Ontario, Canada

Ever since the clinically important arterial fibrous plaques were described in the past century on the basis of their gross and light microscopic appearance, there has been general agreement that these plaques represent the hallmark of atherosclerosis. Subsequent use of modern methods and tools in the examination of these lesions has yielded much new biochemical and structural data on their nature and has stimulated a broadening of concepts concerning the fibrous plaque and the disease as a whole.

Despite the enormous advances made in the field of atherosclerosis (1, 2), many aspects of the lesions remain controversial or unknown. Among these are the following problems:

a. How does the fibrous atherosclerotic plaque begin and progress?

b. Do all plaques arise from a single, identical precursor lesion, or alternatively, does a plaque represent the outcome of several different precursor lesions which at one point or another enter an ultimate common pathway?

c. In either a. or b., what constitutes the early or earliest lesion of atherosclerosis?

d. Are the earliest lesions as characteristic of the disease as is the atherosclerotic plaque?

e. Is it paramount, or alternatively irrelevant, to the evolution of the plaque that several different processes

and tissue reactions be "operational" synergistically at
the level of inception and progression?

f.   What extramural factors directly or indirectly influence
     the composition of the precursor lesions and the rate
     of their progression to the plaque?

g.   Are all plaques identical in their composition at one
     phase of at all stages of their development and diversify
     their appearance only upon reaching a uniform "endpoint"
     in their progression?

These questions represent but a small number of the open
issues that pertain to atherosclerotic lesions. They are of more
than academic interest because attempts at preventing the inception of lesions or retarding their growth may be expected to suc-
ceed only when based on knowledge of the processes involved.

Following is a review of the available morphological data on
the three different precursor lesions believed to represent the
earliest phase in the inception of atherosclerosis, and the clinically important atherosclerotic plaques, with the exception of complicated forms. Whenever possible, the morphological findings
will be discussed based on present knowledge of the pathogenesis
of the lesions and of the factors implicated in the disease.

I.   EARLY LESIONS

In this and earlier presentations (3, 4) early lesions of
atherosclerosis are defined according to their combined gross,
light and electron microscopic appearance, although one of these
lesions may not always be recognizable on gross examination.
Lesions are considered early based on knowledge of general pathology
and of tissue reactions. They may occur in one of three forms, each
believed to reflect a stage of inception: the fatty dots and
streaks (the basic tissue change is fatty metamorphosis of intimal
smooth muscle cells); gelatinous elevations (the basic tissue
change is focal intimal edema = insudation); and microthrombi
(focal microthrombosis; may not be apparent on gross inspection).
Not all investigators agree that either one or both of the latter
lesions are precursors of the atherosclerotic plaque, but support
for the above delineation has been growing in recent years. As
a result, the following account may be more acceptable now than
it would have been a decade ago.

All forms and stages of atherosclerotic lesions have been
delineated and the relevant terminology defined elsewhere (5).

A. Fatty Dots and Streaks

The lesions are visible on gross examination of the intimal surface as well circumscribed, round or elongated, flat or slightly elevated yellow areas measuring up to 0.5 cm in diameter. Larger areas involved may represent the confluence of enlarging adjacent small lesions. In the aorta, the fatty streaks appear within a few months after birth above the aortic valve ring and in the region of the ductus scar, and appear later just distal to the ostia of the intercostal arteries (6). Subsequently, areas of the arch and the posterior wall of the thoracic aorta become involved with lesions that in time spread anteriorily. In the abdominal aorta, the lesions begin to appear in the first decade of life and the intimal involvement increases steadily in the second decade (7, 8).

In the coronary arteries, fatty streaking appears in the proximal segments of the major branches approximately at the time of puberty. Thus, there exists a definite time sequence in which fatty dots and streaks appear not only in different arteries but also in various segments of the same vessel (for reviews, see 7 and 9).

The microscopic appearance of the fatty streaks is quite variable and depends upon their size. A small lesion may consist in essence of only a few fat-containing (= foam) cells grouped together immediately beneath the endothelium, or separated from each other in the superficial intimal layers (Fig. 1). The former may be present as a slightly elevated lesion, the latter as a flat one. The intracellular fat droplets are large and confined to the cytoplasm of elongated cells whose nature cannot be determined by light microscopy. Cells containing numerous tiny fat droplets may be occasionally observed. The connective tissues are not detectably altered, and a finely dispersed extracellular lipid may be present similar in appearance and distribution to that in a normal, diffusely thickened intima. In the large fatty streaks (Fig. 2) there are many cells containing fat in the form of both large and small droplets. The small droplet-containing cells are found in the deeper layers and often are globular and of considerable size. Occasionally, fat-free ovoid cells resembling macrophages may be observed in the subendothelial region (Fig. 2). There is a considerable amount of finely distributed extracellular fat; it increases proportionately to the size of the lesion. The fibers of the connective tissues may be distorted or frayed.

By fluorescent antibody techniques, albumin (3, 10-12), fibrin (3, 10, 11, 13, 14), and various classes of lipoproteins (3, 10, 11, 15) may be identified in the lesions in amounts that are variable, increase with the size of lesions, and are negligible in the normal arterial intima. The more prominent the lesion,

the more marked is the increase in fibrin and beta-lipoproteins.
The accumulation of plasma proteins is often accompanied by dis-
tortion and fraying of the intimal connective tissue fibers.

Electron microscopy of small lesions (Fig. 3) shows that fat
is present in cells having all or some of the characteristics of
smooth muscle cells (SMC's) (4, 16-18). The cells are elongated;
the nucleus is cigar-shaped with typical fence-like indentations
and marginal chromatin distribution; a partial or complete basal
lamina envelops the cell; and the cytoplasm shows numerous caveolae
cellulares, myofilaments, and triangular and fusiform densities.
The lipid inclusions are large but not uniform in size, and vary
also in number and texture. They may consist of a moderately
electron-dense homogeneous substance with smooth or scalloped bor-
ders, and be associated with electron-opaque, irregularly shaped
materials that are interpreted as lipopigments (9). Other lipid
inclusions may appear reticulated, and/or have a central electron-
lucent core (4). The individual lipid droplets may fuse with
each other. Not all intimal SMC's contain lipid includions in
the small lesions (Fig. 3).

Electron microscopy of the large streaks (Fig. 4) shows that
the number of fat-containing cells is increased and usually paral-
lels the size of the lesion. In addition to the cells with large
lipid droplets recognizable as SMC's, other cells with numerous
tiny lipid inclusions are present, being particularly numerous in
the deeper layers; these often have no recognizable features of
SMC's (4, 17). They are oval or globular, and the chromatin distribution of the nucleus may not be characteristic of that found
in SMC's. The cells occasionally have microvillar processes extending into the surrounding tissues and no basal lamina is apparent
(4, 9). The small lipid inclusions in these cells appear partly
or entirely empty and occasionally are enclosed by a rim of a
slightly electron-lucent substance. In addition, various round or
irregular electron-opaque bodies, probably representing lipopigments, may be present in the cytoplasm. It is not possible to
identify the nature of these cells when they are filled with numerous, largely empty lipid inclusions. Occasionally, cells with
identical nuclear and cytoplasmic features, but with either a few
or no lipid inclusions are also present in the lesions (Fig. 5);
they are also observed at times in the immediate subendothelial
area and may be detectable on light microscopic examination (Fig.
2). It is probable that most of the ovoid cells containing the
numerous tiny lipid vacuoles and other inclusions are derived
from these inclusion-free cells. Whether they exclusively represent macrophages derived from blood monocytes, or alternatively
another cell type, has been discussed in detail elsewhere (4).
In addition to the SMC's containing lipid droplets, i.e., the so-
called myogenic foam cells (17), and the ovoid or globular cells,

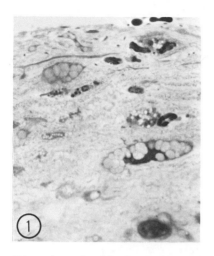
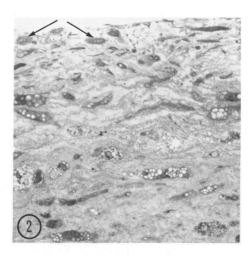

Fig. 1. Small fatty streak. Large fat droplets in a few elongated intimal cells. Toluidine blue stain; X 540.
Fig. 2. Large fatty streak. Many large and tiny droplets containing intimal cells. Subendothelial mononuclear cells (arrows)
are fat-free. Toluidine blue stain; X 210.

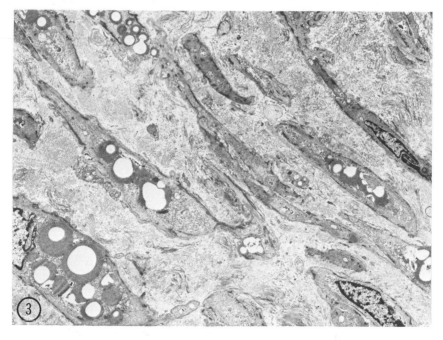

Fig. 3. Small fatty streak. Fat droplets confined to some, not
all smooth muscle cells. Electron micrograph; X 3,700.

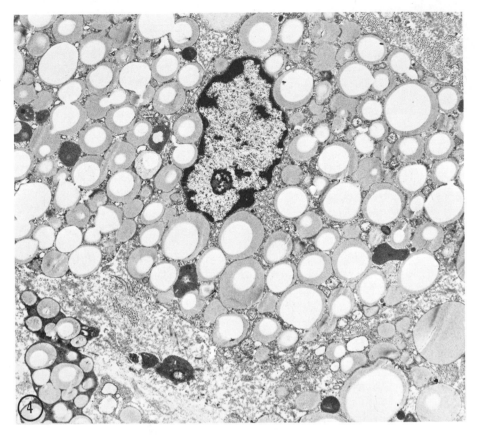

Fig. 4. Large fatty streak. Many tiny fat droplets in myogenic foam cells and interstitium. Electron micrograph; X 9,200.

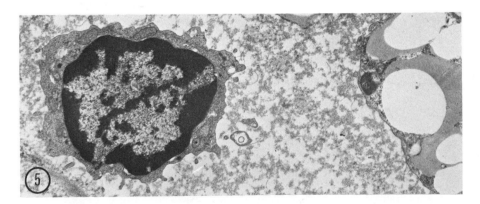

Fig. 5. Large fatty streak. A fat-free mononuclear cell has villous extensions (left). Electron micrograph; X 9,200.

with and without lipid droplets, probably representing macrophages, mast cells also have been observed in fatty streaks (4).
The endothelium overlying fatty streaks is often remarkably free
of detectable morphological alterations; on occasion it may contain a few small cytoplasmic lipid and lipopigment inclusions (4).
The possible origin of all cells in the fatty streaks and the
pathogenesis of the intracellular lipid accumulation is discussed
in detail in another publication (4).

The electron microscopic counterparts of the finely dispersed
extracellular lipids are considered to be the small electron-dense
bodies or particles of various appearance, size and shape (4, 19,
20). There is general agreement that these bodies contain lipids,
at least in part. Some investigators believe that in the small,
pure fatty streak, these extracellular fat aggregates do not
exceed those observed in the normal, diffusely thickened intima,
and are only increased in larger lesions. The large lipid droplets
in the extracellular space are indistinguishable from inclusions in
the SMC's (Fig. 4) and, no doubt, are derived from necrosis of
these cells.

In some of the larger fatty streaks, fibrin is present in
clumps and strands in the extracellular space. These clumps are
often extremely electron-dense and structureless, but in other preparations the typical axial periodicity of fibrin (200-200Å) is
easily visualized (3, 21). In such areas the connective tissues,
particularly the elastic tissue elements, are distorted and permeated by edema fluid; the small electron-dense bodies often penetrate into the substance of the distorted elastic tissue elements
(9). By electron microscopy, fibrin also may be identified in fatty streaks by the ferritin-conjugated antibody technique (21).

It is not known with certainty what all the mechanisms are
that culminate in the formation of fatty dots and streaks. Accumulation of lipids in the intimal SMC's may represent a fatty metamorphosis analogous to degenerative changes in other cells, but
the etiological factors remain largely unknown. It was believed
that the intracellular fat accumulation is peculiar to arterial
SMC's, but recently similar changes were observed under pathological
conditions in the SMC's elsewhere in the body (22).

The pure forms of fatty dots and streaks are of no clinical
consequence. They may become significant only when they progress
to fibrous atherosclerotic plaques. The accumulation of fat in
any of the cells in the fatty streaks may ultimately lead to cellular necrosis and release of lipids into the extracellular space,
thus contributing to the extracellular lipid pool. The phenomenon
of cell necrosis is often observed in advanced fatty streaks. It
is reasonable to assume that this induces the macrophages in the

area to migrate into the lesion and phagocytize the lipids, the
debris of connective tissues that may be damaged in the process,
and the fibrin that may have gained access with other blood constituents into the lesion, as a result of a secondarily induced
altered permeability of the area. Phagocytosis alone may not suffice to clear the accumulating debris. Furthermore, when the
native connective tissues are damaged, the arterial wall may
attempt to replace them. In the course of these events, the endothelium overlying the fatty streak may be altered and either thrombosis or a recurrent insudation (see below) of blood constituents
may ensue. Therefore, a simple fatty streak may be converted into
a rather complex lesion which ultimately results in the formation
of an atherosclerotic plaque. However, not all fatty streaks
necessarily progress to a clinically important lesion as is evident
from the distribution of fatty streaks on the one hand and of advanced lesions on the other. Observations on the racial and sex
differences of the occurrence of fatty streaks are just the opposite of what would be expected were the childhood fatty streak
invariably the precursor of the adult fibrous atherosclerotic
plaque (7). Thus, some fatty streaks in man may regress (3).

B. Gelatinous (Insudative) Lesions

These lesions (Figs. 6-9) have a grayish-translucent gelatinous appearance on gross inspection and resemble a blister. They
may be slightly or prominently elevated, vary in size from 2 to 10
mm in diameter, and may be round or, more often, elongated in the
direction of the blood flow. They are either isolated or present
at the apex of a fully developed, atherosclerotic plaque. Occasionally, there is a slight yellow tinge in some parts of the
lesions. The gelatinous elevations may be observed on an intima
also showing the presence of fatty dots and streaks. A study on
the distribution of these lesions in childhood aortas has been
initiated recently by the author and her colleagues.

On cross section the lesions appear as a focal intimal swelling. Light microscopic examination shows the presence of intimal
edema which represents an insudate (3, 11, 23). It separates the
extracellular connective tissue components with accompanying dis-
tortion and fraying of collagen and elastic fibers (Fig. 7). In a
small lesion, only the superficial layers of the intima are affected; in prominent lesions the changes usually involve most of the
intimal width (Fig. 8). Electron microscopic examination of these
lesions (Fig. 6) confirms the presence of frayed elastic tissue
elements; other areas, particularly those that consist of only
partially fused units (24) are permeated by edema fluid (Fig. 6)
(23). The intimal cells in the lesions usually do not contain fat,
but finely dispersed lipid present in association with elastic
fibers in diffuse intimal thickening (4) may be observed in the

deeper layers in the form of tiny, electron-dense, unstructured round or oval bodies (9, 23). A change, interpreted as a swelling of the glycosaminoglycans-rich ground substance, accompanies the separation of the connective tissue fibers (Fig. 6) (23). The widened interfibrillar spaces often contain a fine proteinaceous precipitate (Figs. 6 and 7). In the prominent lesions a variable amount of fibrin is present in the intimal edema fluid (Figs. 8 and 9). At times, the fibrin is found only in the superficial layers and in small aggregates, but in other lesions it may be a prominent feature of the insudate (Fig. 8). The endothelial cells overlying the prominent lesions may be swollen, partly damaged and separated from each other (9). They may also contain lipopigments (9). The morphological identification of fibrin is not possible when it appears in the form of extremely electron-dense clumps, but in other preparations the characteristic axial periodicity of fibrin (21) is evident (Fig. 9). Occasionally, processes of SMC's in the area of insudation are swollen (23).

In addition to the above changes, gelatinous elevations with a yellow tinge show microscopically the presence of a moderate number of fat-containing SMC's. It is impossible to establish in such instances whether these represent primary fatty streaks that subsequently became edematous, or whether the latter change preceded the former.

Pathogenetically, the gray gelatinous elevations are important since they represent a serous or serofibrinous insudate following local intimal injury. Many factors may be injurious to the endothelium or the intima and thus initiate this process. These factors may act from the lumen (hormones; altered levels of vitamins; toxins; certain lipids, biological agents; heavy metals), may result from altered dynamics of the circulation (hypertension; increased viscosity), or may originate in the abnormal homeostasis of the artery itself (various genetic diseases; changed neurovascular mechanisms) (5, 25). They may act either singly or in combination to alter the selective permeability of the endothelial lining with consequent indiscriminate entry of blood constitutents into the intima. The lesion may contain only a serous insudate when the endothelial damage is not extensive (5, 25). Alternatively, when the damage to the endothelium is severe, large-size molecules may enter the intima (fibrinogen and beta-lipoproteins). Presumably, a serous edema may be reabsorbed, but it would be difficult in the absence of capillaries and lack of the immediate availability of macrophages for the intima to clear itself of the large molecular substances. In addition, the thromboplastic properties of the intima effect the conversion of soluble fibrinogen to fibrin. Macrophages are necessary for the removal of the fibrin, but they are not a prominent feature of these lesions. Massive insudation also may affect the intimal SMC's and result in

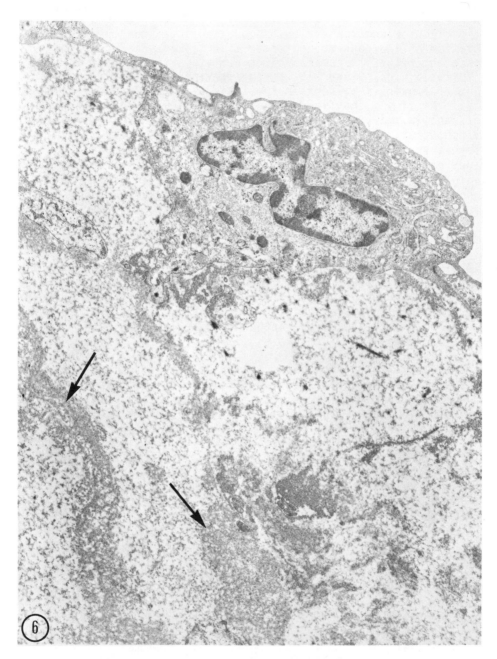

Fig. 6. Gray gelatinous elevation. Endothelium (top) well preserved. Elastic elements (arrows) and interstitium permeated by
fine floccular substance. Electron micrograph; x 11,200.

fatty metamorphosis, a change occasionally observed in these cells in serofibrinous insudates (3).

The serofibrinous insudate not absorbed or removed may be organized to connective tissue. The intimal SMC's play a key role in this process (26, 27). The organizing forces in the intima might not be sufficiently fast, particularly when there is a considerable amount of serofibrinous insudate. Thus, unorganized fibrin-containing substances remain and may induce fat accumulation in the area (Figs. 8 and 9) (28), a phenomenon observed also in mural thrombosis (see below).

Even the completely organized insudative lesion represents a focus of altered structure and a site likely to be subjected to further pathological changes, i.e., fatty metamorphosis of its SMC's or thrombus deposition. Thus, a chain of events may be initiated that ultimately may culminate in the formation of the fibrous atherosclerotic plaque. Frequently, one may observe lesions representing the outcome of two or more episodes of insudation with subsequent organization. Therefore, insudation may play a role not only in the inception, but also in the progression of atherosclerotic lesions (5).

Many investigators are reluctant to recognize the existence of the gelatinous lesion, while others, accepting that such a lesion exists, are not convinced that it is relevant to the process of atherosclerosis. The recent biochemical data of Smith and her colleagues (29) strongly support the morphological observations on the occurrence and composition of these gelatinous lesions, and their relation to the established atherosclerotic plaque.

C. Microthrombi

It has been known for a long time that occlusive arterial thrombi are associated with the clinical manifestations of atherosclerosis and its sequelae. However, it took approximately a century to accept von Rokitansky's theory (30) that arterial thrombi also contribute to the growth and progression of atherosclerotic lesions (31-35). Moreover, evidence is slowly accumulating that tiny mural thrombi occurring in the arteries of animals and man (3, 9, 36-38) found early in human life (3, 9) may also represent a form of inception of atherosclerotic lesions.

The microthrombi may be present on a normal intima (Fig. 10) with minimal or moderate diffuse intimal thickening (3) in the coronary arteries and aorta. They may consist largely of platelets, or fibrin, or more often, mixed (platelet-fibrin) in composition (3, 9). They may be partially or totally organized or

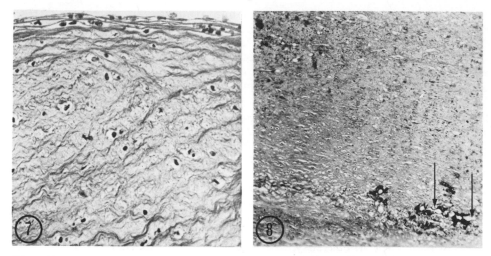

Fig. 7.   Gelatinous lesion.   Serous insudate separates and dis-
torts intimal collagen and elastic fibers.   Pentachrome II; X 360.
Fig. 8.   Gelatinous lesion.   Serofibrinous insudate permeates the
entire intimal width.   Lipid vacuoles (arrows) around conglomer-
ates of fibrin above media.   Heidenhain's azan stain; X 92.

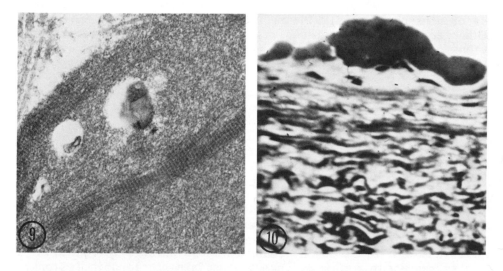

Fig. 9.   Electron micrograph of area corresponding to left lower
corner of Fig. 8.   200-200 Å axial periodicity of fibrin still
demonstrable.   X 62,000.
Fig. 10.   A microthrombus (top) on thin aortic intima with slight
edema in the diffuse thickening.   Masson's Trichrome stain; X 580.

hyalinized, and are usually overgrown by endothelium (3, 35). The
small size of the thrombi and their presence upon a largely unal-
tered intima supports the interpretation that they represent an
early stage of atherosclerotic lesions. The size and the shape
of the microthrombi vary. They may be narrow and small, flattened
and molded into the substance of the artery (3, 9), or they may
protrude into the lumen. The flat microthrombi may extend over
a considerable intimal surface (3). On microscopic examination,
it is not known whether the microthrombi that are not endothelialized will be ultimately dislodged. It is of interest that the
pattern of distribution of microthrombi around the orifices of
the intercostal vessels and the bifurcation on the aortic intima
of normal pigs are similar to those of atherosclerotic lesions in
these animals and to those of the precipitates that form in extracorporeal shunts (39). It is believed that, in the intact circulation of man and animals, fibrin forms and is removed constantly
by fibrinolysins (40). The delicate balance between the formation and lysis of these deposits may be disturbed by many factors
that either promote coagulation or inhibit fibrinolytic activity.
The endothelium also possesses fibrinolytic activity (41).

The formation of microthrombi is intimately associated with
the dynamics and status of platelets in the circulation. In addition to playing a role in thrombosis, platelets may relate to
atherosclerosis by releasing various substances capable of increasing vascular permeability, i.e., the intermediates of arachidonate
metabolism, nucleotides, prostaglandins, serotonin, and a cationic
protein (42). The platelets may form or release an elastase (43)
acting upon the arterial elastic tissue; and when activated,
release a collagenase that may digest collagen (44). Finally,
the platelets may release a factor believed to stimulate the proliferation of SMC's (45) and fibroblasts (46). The absence of
platelets from a microthrombus does not necessarily indicate that
upon degranulation the platelets may have disintegrated within
the thrombus, nor that they were not present in the thrombus a
priori; it has been shown that platelets engaged in the process
of thrombosis may be returned to the circulation (47).

Platelets may also represent a link between blood coagulability and such risk factors as cigarette smoking, dietary hyperlipoproteinemia and hypertension. Thus, factors that promote
coagulability, e.g., food rich in dairy fats and eggs, and smoking, also shorten the survival, and increase the turnover and
adhesiveness of platelets. Stress and catecholamines influence
the properties of platelets, and also have been implicated in
atherogenesis. Hypertension is thought to relate to the role of
platelets in atherosclerosis in several ways. Platelets collide
with each other, with red blood cells, and with endothelium more
often in hypertension than under normotensive conditions, thus

increasing the release of adenosine diphosphate that promotes
aggregation of platelets and the likelihood of their deposition upon
the endothelial surface. The platelets deposited on endothelium
may initiate thrombosis or induce permeability changes, as well
as cellular proliferation (45) in the underlying intima. Indeed,
on occasion slight edema may be observed in the intima immediately
beneath the microthrombus (9).

Several factors implicated in atherogenesis are also known
to promote thrombosis, e.g., a high content of dairy fat in the
diet and hyperlipidemia, phospholipids rich in phosphatidyl
enthanolamine, saturated long-chain fatty acids, stress, epinephrine, and tobacco smoking. Fibrinolytic activity may be inhibited by alimentary hyperlipemia and the intake of butter. It
was believed in the past that platelets also contribute significantly to the lipid component of the developing lesion; however,
this is less certain at present. (For reviews on the above subjects see: 3, 5, 11, 42, 47, 48.)

Once the microthrombus is established and persists it represents a nidus upon which repeated precipitation of thrombi may
occur; this build-up of thrombotic substances may result in the
formation of the clinically important atherosclerotic lesion.
The persisting microthrombus may become secondarily altered or
induce changes in the underlying intima. Thus, the microthrombus,
whether organized or not, may permit a considerable influx of
plasma proteins into its substance. When the microthrombus is
rich in platelets, substances released from thrombocytes may increase local arterial permeability and result in focal intimal
edema. Alternatively, intimal edema (insudation) may precede
the precipitation of a microthrombus. An organized microthrombus
that is incorporated into the intima may influence the nutritional
state and the metabolism of the SMC's in the subjacent area with
consequent fatty metamorphosis of these cells. Indeed, fat-containing SMC's, similar to those observed in fatty streaks, are
at times present in the intima with a superimposed, not very
recent, microthrombus. In such instances, it is not possible to
determine whether the microthrombus was deposited upon a pre-
existing small fatty streak, or alternatively, if the appearance
of lipid in the intimal SMC's followed the deposition of the
microthrombus. Thus, several tissue changes may be induced by
the deposition of even a small thrombus and these changes may
result in complex interactions conceivably culminating in the
formation of a typical atherosclerotic plaque.

The difficulty in establishing the incidence of microthrombi
in man may reflect the fact that they are invisible on gross
inspection and are found only incidentally on microscopic examination. There are very few studies on the occurrence of microthrombi in man (3, 9, 33, 36, 49-52). Systematic search for

microthrombi in arteries of normal young subjects in the first
decades of life has been undertaken only rarely. In one study
aimed at establishing incidence, no thrombi were found in grossly
normal aortas in the vicinity of the origin of the renal artery
of infants and children (52). In another study, microthrombi
were found in seven serially sectioned segments of left coronary
arteries obtained at autopsy from nine patients ranging in age
from 12 to 30 years (49). In six instances the microthrombi were
superimposed upon an underlying intimal lesion and only in three
were they present on a seemingly normal intima. It is apparent
that further prospective studies are required for the assessment
of the place of microthrombi in atherosclerosis.

II.   ADVANCED LESIONS

The delineation and terminology of advanced lesions that
represent and denote the progression of the disease has been provided in detail elsewhere (5). For this presentation, these
lesions are considered under the generic term "atherosclerotic
plaques" and for simplicity will be used interchangeably with
the term "fibrous plaques."

Atherosclerotic (Fibrous) Plaques

Whereas these lesions have been the hallmark of atherosclerosis and are the least controversial of all forms, the term
refers only to the gross appearance without reference to specific,
or even consistent, microscopic features which are, indeed, quite
variable (Figs. 11-15). On gross examination (32), the color
varies slightly from pearly-white to white-opaque, and the size
from a few millimeters to over a centimeter in length. The
lesions are prominent, protrude above the intimal surface and in
the smaller arteries, e.g., the coronary arteries, may encroach
considerably upon the lumen. The plaques usually are elongated
in the direction of the longitudinal axis of the artery. On
cross-section a typical lesion shows yellow, gruel-like material
at the basal center immediately above the media representing the
atheroma, and a superficial, firm, pearly-white or gray fibrous
layer cap (Fig. 11). Many of the plaques are composed of several
such basic pair-units, i.e., an atheroma and a fibrous layer,
each interpreted as representing a distinct episode in the formation of the lesion. This feature is prominent in the coronary
artery and is less often observed in the aorta. Not all grossly
typical fibrous plaques contain a centro-basal atheroma, and are
thus exclusively fibrous in nature (Fig. 12) (26, 32). The
distribution, incidence, time of appearance, and the extent of
surface involvement varies in different arteries and at various
levels of the same vessel. This variation has been well documented
(53).

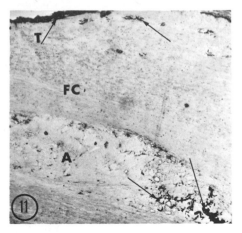 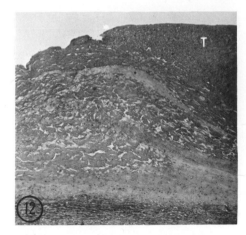

Fig. 11. Aortic atherosclerotic plaque. Superimposed narrow
thrombus (arrowed T) merges with fibrous cap (FC) overlying the
atheroma (A). Fibrinous remnants in both (arrows). PTAH stain;
X 36.
Fig. 12. Aortic atherosclerotic plaque without atheroma consists
of several layers of partly organized thrombus. Recent thrombus
(T) is superimposed. Replacing connective tissues are light gray
in photograph. Pentachrome II stain; X 36.

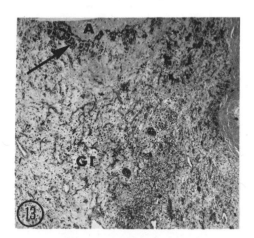 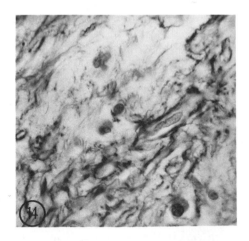

Fig. 13. Organization of thrombus deposited on fibrous plaque in
coronary artery by an avascular process from lumen (A) and granulation tissue at base (GT). Thrombotic remnants between (black
in photograph) (arrow). PTAH stain; X 36.
Fig. 14. Smooth muscle cell from avascular tissues (A in Fig. 13)
and fibrous cap (FC in Fig. 11) in close association with elastic
fibers. Pentachrome II stain; X 510.

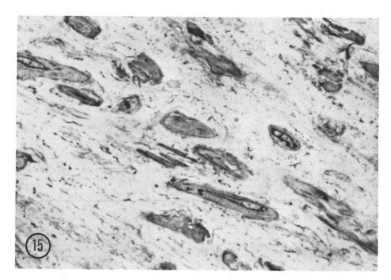

Fig. 15. Details of a young fibrous cap. Fat-free SMC's are embedded in avascular connective tissues. Toluidine blue stain; X 780.

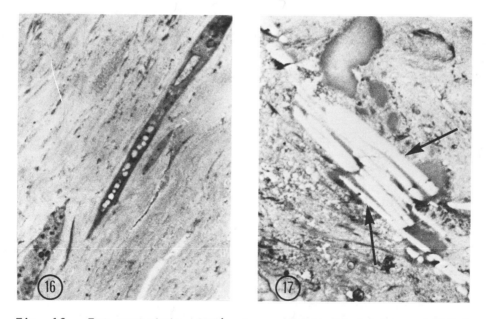

Fig. 16. Fat-containing SMC's in an old hyalinized cap. Toluidine blue stain; X 820.
Fig. 17. An atheroma contains cholesterol crystals (arrows) and nondescript tissue debris. Toluidine blue; X 820.

Light microscopic examination of fibrous plaques (4, 11, 26, 28, 32, 33, 54) discloses many variable features (Figs. 11-17). The typical, mature, uncomplicated atherosclerotic plaque, occurring usually in the third and fourth decade of life, is composed of a core-atheroma and overlying fibrous connective tissue (Fig. 11). The atheroma consists of a pool of acellular, amorphous and ill-defined material which contains lipids, cholesterol crystals (Fig. 17), some stainable proteoglycans, fibrin, and unidentifiable proteins. The fibrous cap is covered by endothelium and consists of avascular extracellular connective tissues in which are embedded elongated smooth muscle cells (Figs. 14-16) (11, 18, 26, 27). The connective tissue contains glycosaminoglycans, rich ground substance, elastic and collagenous fibers, and reticulin fibrils. Each component varies considerably from lesion to lesion depending upon the maturation and aging of the connective tissue cap and the simplicity or complexity of the lesion. In a young fibrous cap, the SMC's, except those immediately adjacent to the central atheroma, usually are free of demonstrable intracellular lipid (Figs. 14 and 15), but myogenic foam cells (Fig. 16) (17) may be present in older fibrous caps. In the latter, the collagen is dense and hyalinized and the SMC's atrophied (18, 26). The connective tissue components, however, are seldom in the same stage of maturation throughout the width of the cap; special stains reveal that a cap almost invariably consists of layers, each representing tissues of a different age. Superficial areas of the plaque often exhibit morphologic features and consequences of insudation that are identical with those observed in gray gelatinous elevations (see above). Albumin (55), fibrin (56) and alpha- and beta-lipoproteins (15) all have been demonstrated in the fibrous cap by fluorescent antibody techniques; the amount of the former two varies inversely with the maturity of the connective tissues of the cap.

Frequently, mural thrombi not identified on gross inspection of the lesion show an intimate association with the fibrous plaque on microscopic examination, particularly with its cap component (Figs. 11 and 12). On occasion, remnants of a mural thrombus may be present either in the deep or superficial layers of the fibrous cap (Figs. 11 and 12). At other times a mural thrombus, fresh or in various stages of organization, may be observed on a pre-existing plaque, often blending with its substance (Fig. 11). In other instances, several layers of thrombi superimposed upon each other and in various stages of organization (Fig. 12) comprise the plaque itself; on gross examination such a plaque appears as a white opaque lesion (26, 32, 54).

A relatively thin thrombus may be replaced (i.e., organized) entirely by avascular tissue, whereas in large, prominent mural thrombi, replacement takes place by two different but simultaneously ongoing processes (26, 32, 54). At the base of the thrombus,

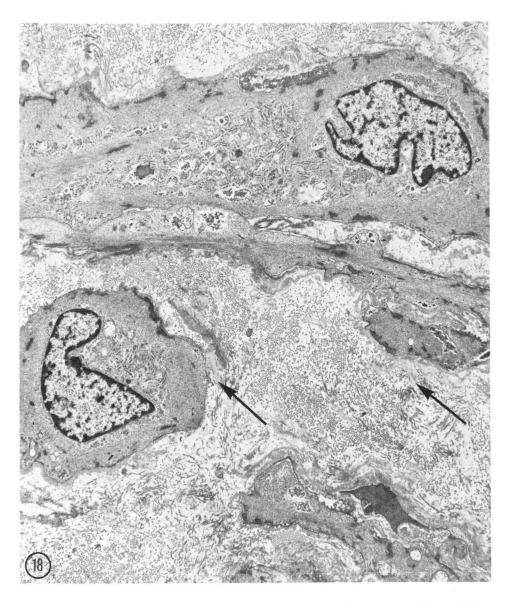

Fig. 18. Details of a young fibrous cap. SMC's have a fence-like nucleus, bundles of myofilaments, and oblong and triangular densities. A basal lamina envelops SMC's and extends into extracellular space which also contains numerous collagen fibrils and elastic tissue elements (arrows). Electron micrograph; X 8,000.

i.e., the part closest to the media, organization progresses by
the orthodox formation of granulation tissue that contains capillaries and fibroblasts. The superficial layers of the thrombus
in contact with the arterial lumen are organized by an avascular
process (Fig. 13). Thus, the connective tissue replacing the
thrombus becomes devoid of capillaries. The cellular elements in
this tissue are SMC's rather than fibroblasts (11, 18, 26, 27).
They are associated with all extracellular connective tissue components in the same fashion as observed in the typical fibrous
cap (Fig. 14). Since the SMC's are the only cells present in such
areas it is reasonable to conclude that they are capable of organizing the mural thrombus (at least its most superficial layers) and
elaborating all connective tissue components usually present in
an artery (27). When the organizing forces of the above two processes are successful, the entire thrombus may be converted into
a fibrous plaque. However, it appears that at times the two processes (one progressing from the lumen, the other from the base
of the thrombus) do not meet, leaving a remnant of unorganized
thrombotic substance between them (Fig. 13) (28, 54). This seems
to be a particularly common feature in the coronary artery. Foam
cells are almost invariably associated with the unorganized remnants of thrombotic substances amidst the fibrous tissue. It
has been postulated (28) that these foam cells represent an unsuc-
cessful attempt by tissue macrophages at removing the remnants of
the thrombus. Presumably, these cells phagocytize the remnants
and undergo fatty metamorphosis. Just what the pathway of conversion of the presumably phagocytosed thrombus to fat may be, or
whether this could ever be possible, is entirely unknown; such an
assumption may even be considered unreasonable on purely biochemical grounds. Nevertheless, the observation that fat-containing
cells gather around unorganized thrombotic substances in the depths
of a fibrous lesion is an attractive basis for the belief that
this phenomenon may represent one of the ways by which an atheroma
develops. In further support of this theory is the finding that
remnants of fibrinous substances may be present in a well-established atheroma (Fig. 11) (28).

Electron microscopy of atherosclerotic plaques (Fig. 18)
(11, 25, 57-59) in various stages of development and maturation
largely confirms the light microscopic observations and histochemical studies with respect to the nature of the cells, i.e., they
are SMC's that elaborate connective tissues. The reticulin-posi-
tive fibrils that are produced by the SMC's (along with other
connective tissue components) may be identified by electron microscopy as the microfibrils of the extracellular space (60). Microfibrils are the smallest structured elements which may either
exist free or as one of the two components of the structured,
organized elastic tissues (24, 61). Moreover, abundant basal
lamina-like substances are observed which are not necessarily asso-

ciated with the SMC's. Well-formed elastic tissue components are
fewer in number than may be assumed on the basis of light microscopic examination. There is seldom intracellular lipid in the
SMC's in the superficial layers of the fibrous cap, but in the
vicinity of the centro-basal atheroma, the cells do contain lipid
droplets. The cytoplasmic fat accumulation varies considerably
from cell to cell, but it appears to be inversely related to the
distance from the atheroma. Cells filled with fat droplets appear
to disintegrate in the immediate vicinity of the atheroma.
Occasionally, structurally typical fibrin and extracellular electron-dense lipid material similar to that observed in advanced
fatty streaks (19, 21) may be found in the interstitium of the
fibrous cap.

The atheromatous core itself consists largely of electron-
dense, granular lipid substances identical to those present in
the extracellular space of advanced fatty streaks and in the interstitium of the fibrous cap (4). Intermingled with these substances
may be electron-lucent clefts, i.e., empty spaces corresponding
to the cholesterol crystals lost in the course of tissue processing.
A variable number of electron-dense crystals may be observed in
the atheromata; these are interpreted as representing a form of
calcium (4).

The morphological accounts above refer to atherosclerotic
plaques that are considered by the majority of investigators to be
lesions of an uncomplicated nature in contra-distinction to those
that are complicated by other processes, i.e., calcification,
ulceration, hemorrhage and occlusive thrombosis. For details on
the morphology of these complicated lesions the reader is referred
to the monograph of Morgan (62). In its uncomplicated form, the
prominent fibrous atherosclerotic plaque may be of little consequence in large elastic arteries unless it is situated close to
the origin of an artery supplying a vital organ or tissue. However, in medium sized arteries, e.g., the coronary and cerebral,
the same lesion may seriously impair the circulation no matter
where it occurs. In addition, once established, all plaques are
potential sites of change that may lead to events precipitating
the clinical manifestations of the disease (5).

III. COMMENTS

Our present understanding of how the various factors implicated in atherosclerosis relate to lesions and to the clinical
manifestations of the disease has been discussed in detail elsewhere (5). Atherosclerosis develops and progresses through stages
involving a certain sequence of events (3, 63). The lesions may
begin in infancy as one of the three earliest forms, i.e., the

fatty dot and streak, microthrombus or gelatinous elevation. In
the first two decades of life only the early lesions are encountered.
The second stage of the lesions, i.e., the fibrous atherosclerotic
plaque, may develop at the end of the second but is usually established at the beginning of the third decade of life. The so-called
complicated third-stage lesions (5, 62) develop in the fourth and
subsequent decades. Since the clinical manifestations of the
disease are preceded by stages in the evolution of the lesion over
at least two to three decades, it is understandable that attention
has been directed recently towards early life in the hope of
retarding the conversion of the earliest lesions to the advanced,
fibrous atherosclerotic plaques. Identification of the factors
instrumental in this conversion thus becomes important in the
study of atherosclerosis, particularly in view of the fact that
at present we are not capable of preventing the inception of the
early lesion, or of treating the advanced lesions and their sequelae.

In man, the difficulty in unravelling the above problems is
compounded by many factors, which may be eliminated in experimental animals. One cannot study serially the evolution of the
emerging, complex human lesion at various time intervals. A given
population, no matter how similar the constituent subjects, can
never be as homogeneous in a biological sense as inbred animals
of the same litter. The reactions of the highly individualistic
homo sapiens to his environment and to the factors considered to
be important in atherosclerosis; e.g., food, occupation, cultural
background, physical activities, other habits, and geography, are
expected to vary from one person to another, as do the lesions,
even of the same type. It is therefore doubtful whether it will
ever be possible to provide answers to questions and problems
rasied in the Introduction, at least with respect to the human
lesion. Notwithstanding these limitations, and on the basis of
our knowledge of general tissue reactions, it is reasonable to
postulate the following course of events in the natural history
of the atherosclerotic lesion.

Various factors relating to the make-up of the arterial wall,
the prevailing hemodynamic conditions, and the status of the circulating blood may be injurious either to the endothelium or to
the elements in the underlying intima (5, 25). Injury to the
endothelium may be followed by an influx (insudation) of plasma
constituents into the intima to form a gelatinous elevation, or by
deposition of a microthrombus, or both (25). Both processes may
induce fatty metamorphosis of the SMC's in the underlying intima
and in addition the insudation may cause mechanical damage to the
intimal connective tissues. The failure to remove or organize
the insudate and/or the thrombus may furnish substances that induce
further lipid accumulation and provide stimuli for SMC's to proliferate in the area. The latter phenomenon may be enhanced in part

by platelet factors (45) and by the nature of the lipoproteins in the insudate (64).

The native SMC's accumulating lipid droplets may continue on that course beyond their ability to survive. Necrosis follows and the intracellular lipids, released into the extracellular space, contribute to the lipid component of the lesion. Once established, lesions of any one of the three basic types appear to promote the development of some or all features of the two other forms. The tendency to repeated episodes of mural thrombosis and insudation, and the simultaneously ongoing proliferative and reparative phenomena in the area contribute further to the complexity of the process.

Present knowledge of the morphogenesis of the lesions, while not sufficiently advanced to permit the prevention of their inception, may be considered to be at a stage that provides some basis for rational intervention of their growth, or retardation of their progression to fibrous atherosclerotic plaques and their complicated forms.

Acknowledgments. This work was supported by grants-in-aid of research T.3-11 from the Ontario Heart Foundation, Toronto, Ontario, and MT-1037 from the Medical Research Council of Canada. The author wishes to thank Ms. Irena Wojewodzka for her skillful technical assistance and Miss Delight Downham for typing the manuscript.

REFERENCES

1. Schettler, G., Goto, Y., Hata, Y., and Klose, G. (Eds.), (1977) Atherosclerosis IV, Springer-Verlag, Berlin-Heidelberg.

2. Manning, G.W., and Haust, M.D. (Eds.) (1977) Atherosclerosis: metabolic, morphologic and clinical aspects, Adv. Exper. Med. Biol. 82, Plenum Press, New York.

3. Haust, M.D. (1971) Human Pathol. 2, 1-29.

4. Geer, J.C., and Haust, M.D. (1972) Smooth Muscle Cells in Atherosclerosis, S. Karger, Basel.

5. Haust, M.D., and More, R.H. (1972) in The Pathogenesis of Atherosclerosis (Wissler, R.W. and Geer, J.C., Eds.) The Williams and Wilkins Co., Baltimore, pp. 1-19.

6. Schwartz, C.J., Ardlie, N.G., Carter, R.F., and Paterson, J.C. (1967) Arch. Pathol. 83, 325-332.

7. McGill, H.C., Jr. (1968) Lab. Invest. 18, 560-564.

8. Strong, J.P., and McGill, H.C., Jr. (1969) J. Atheroscl. Res. 9, 251-265.

9. Haust, M.D. (1978) in Perspectives in Pediatric Pathology (Bolande, R.P. and Rosenberg, H.S., Eds.), Year Book Publ., Chicago, Ill. In press.

10. Haust, M.D. (1968) in Progr. Biochem. Parmacol. Vol. 4 (Miras, C.J., Howard, A.N. and Paoletti, R., Eds.), S. Karger, Basel, pp. 429-437.

11. Haust, M.D. (1971) in Concepts of Disease: A Textbook of Pathology (Brunson, J.G. and Gall, E.A., Eds.), Macmillan Co., New York, pp. 451-487.

12. Haust, M.D., Choi, J., Wyllie, J.C., and More, R.H. (1965) Circulation 32 (II), 17.

13. Wyllie, J.C., More, R.H., and Haust, M.D. (1964) J. Pathol. Bact. 88, 335-338.

14. Woolf, N., and Crawford, T. (1960) J. Pathol. Bact. 80, 405-408.

15. Kao, C.K., and Wissler, R.W. (1965) Exp. Molec. Pathol. 4, 465-479.

16. Geer, J.C., McGill, H.C., and Strong, J.P. (1961) Am. J. Pathol. 38, 263-287.

17. Balis, J.U., Haust, M.D., and More, R.H. (1964) Exp. Molec. Pathol. 3, 511-525.

18. Haust, M.D., and More, R.H. (1963) in Evolution of the Atherosclerotic Plaque (Jones, R.J., Ed.), The University of Chicago Press, Chicago, pp. 51-63.

19. Haust, M.D., More, R.H., Bencosme, S., and Balis, J.U. (1967) Exp. Molec. Pathol. 6, 300-313.

20. Geer, J.C. (1965) Lab. Invest. 14, 1764-1783.

21. Haust, M.D., Wyllie, J.C., and More, R.H. (1965) Exp. Molec. Pathol. 4, 205-216.

22. Haust, M.D., Las Heras, J., and Harding, P.G. (1977) Science, 195, 1353-1354.

23. Haust, M.D. (1977) in Progr. Biochem. Pharmacol. Vol. 13
     (Sinzinger, H., Auerswald, W., Jellinek, H. and Feigel, W.,
     Eds.), S. Karger, Basel, pp. 203-207.

24. Haust, M.D., More, R.H., Bencosme, S.A., and Balis, J.U.
     (1965) Exp. Molec. Pathol. 4, 508-524.

25. Haust, M.D. (1970) in Atherosclerosis (Jones, R.J., Ed.),
     Springer-Verlag, New York, pp. 12-20.

26. Haust, M.D., More, R.H., and Movat, H.Z. (1959) Am. J. Pathol.
     35, 265-273.

27. Haust, M.D., More, R.H., and Movat, H.Z. (1960) Am. J. Pathol.
     37, 377-389.

28. More, R.H., and Haust, M.D. (1961) Am. J. Pathol. 38, 527-537.

29. Smith, E.B., and Smith, R.H. (1976) in Atherosclerosis Reviews,
     Vol. 1 (Paoletti, R. and Gotto, A.M., Eds.), Raven Press, New
     York, pp. 119-136.

30. Rokitansky, C., von (1852) in A Manual of Pathological Anatomy,
     Vol. 4 (Day, G.E., Transl.), The Sydenham Society, London,
     p. 272.

31. Duguid, J.B. (1946) J. Pathol. Bact. 58, 207-212.

32. More, R.H., Movat, H.Z., and Haust, M.D. (1957) Arch. Pathol.
     63, 612-620.

33. Haust, M.D., and More, R.H. (1960) Heart Bull. 9, 90-92.

34. Chandler, A.B. (1969) in Thrombosis (Sherry, S., Brinkhaus,
     K.M., Genton, E. and Stengle, J.M., Eds.), Nat. Acad. Sci.
     Washington, pp. 279-299.

35. Haust, M.D. (1977) in Der Herzinfarkt (Schettler, G., Horsch,
     A., Mörl, H., Orth, H. and Weizel, A., Eds.), F.K. Schattauer
     Verlag, Stuttgart, pp. 120-135.

36. Movat, H.Z., Haust, M.D., and More, R.H. (1959) Am. J. Pathol.
     35, 93-101.

37. French, J.E., Jennings, M.A., and Florey, H.W. (1965) Ann.
     N.Y. Acad. Sci. 127, 780-797.

38. Geissinger, H.D., Mustard, J.F., and Rowsell, H.C. (1962)
     Can. Med. Ass. J. 87, 405-408.

39. Murphy, E.A., Rowsell, H.C., Downie, H.G., Robinson, G.A., and Mustard, J.F. (1962) Can. Med. Ass. J. 87, 259-274.

40. Astrup, T. (1959) in Connective Tissue, Thrombosis, and Atherosclerosis (Page, I.H., Ed.), Academic Press, New York, pp. 223-237.

41. Todd, A.S. (1964) Brit. Med. Bull. 20, 210-212.

42. Mustard, J.F. (1976) Trans. Am. Clin. Climatol. Assoc. 87, 104-127.

43. Robert, B., Robert, L., Legrand, Y., Pignaud, G., and Caen, J. (1971) Series Haemat. 4, 175-185.

44. Chesney, C. McI., Harper, E., and Coleman, R.W. (1974) J. Clin. Invest. 53, 1647-1654.

45. Rutherford, R.B., and Ross, R. (1976) J. Cell Biol. 69, 196-203.

46. Kohler, N., and Lipton, A. (1974) Exp. Cell Res. 87, 297-301.

47. Mustard, J.F. (1967) Exp. Molec. Pathol. 7, 366-377.

48. Haust, M.D. (1975) in Platelets, Drugs and Thrombosis (Hirsh, J., Ed.), S. Karger, Basel, pp. 94-110.

49. Chandler, A.B. (1974) in Atherosclerosis and Coronary Heart Disease (Likoff, W., Segal, B.L., Insull, W., Jr. and Moyer, J.H., Eds.), Grune and Stratton, Inc., New York, p. 28.

50. Chandler, A.B. (1974) Throm. Res. Suppl. 1, 4, 3-23.

51. Chandler, A.B., and Pope, J.T. (1975) in Blood and Arterial Wall in Atherogenesis and Arterial Thrombosis (Hautvast, J.G. A.J., Hermus, R.J.J. and Van Der Haar, F., Eds.), E.J. Brill, Leiden, Netherlands, pp. 111-118.

52. Hudson, J., and McCaughey, W.T.E. (1974) Atherosclerosis 19, 543-553.

53. McGill, H.C., Jr. (Ed.) (1968) Geographic Pathology of Atherosclerosis, Williams and Wilkins, Baltimore, p. 653.

54. More, R.H., and Haust, M.D. (1961) in Anticoagulants and Fibrinolysins (MacMillan, R.L. and Mustard, J.F., Eds.), Macmillan Co., Toronto, pp. 143-153.

55. Choi, J.H., Haust, M.D., Wyllie, J.C., and More, R.H. (1966) Lab. Invest. 15, 1125-1126.

56. Haust, M.D., Wyllie, J.C., and More, R.H. (1964) Am. J. Pathol. 44, 255-267.

57. Haust, M.D., and More, R.H. (1966) Circulation 34, 14.

58. Ghidoni, J.J., and O'Neal, R.M. (1967) Exp. Molec. Pathol. 7, 378-400.

59. Marshall, J.R., Adams, J.G., O'Neal, R.M., and DeBakey, M.E. (1966) J. Atheroscler. Res. 6, 120-131.

60. Haust, M.D. (1965) Am. J. Pathol. 47, 1113-1137.

61. Haust, M.D., and More, R.H. (1966) Laval Med. 37, 551-557.

62. Morgan, A.D. (1956) The Pathogenesis of Coronary Occlusion, Blackwell, Oxford.

63. Strong, J.P., Eggen, D.A., and Oalmann, M.C. (1974) in The Pathogenesis of Atherosclerosis (Wissler, R.W. and Geer, J.C., Eds.), the Williams and Wilkins Co., Baltimore, pp. 20-40.

64. Fischer-Dzoga, K., Jones, R.M., Vesselinovitch, D., and Wissler, R.W. (1974) in Atherosclerosis III (Schettler, G. and Weizel, A., Eds.), Springer-Verlag, Berlin, pp. 193-195.

THE PLASMA LIPOPROTEINS: CURRENT CONCEPTS OF METABOLISM AND STRUCTURE WITH CLINICAL IMPLICATIONS

Antonio M. Gotto, Jr.

Baylor College of Medicine and The Methodist Hospital
Houston, Texas

The work I will summarize on the plasma lipoproteins comes
from many laboratories and has been recently reviewed in considerable detail (1-5). I will emphasize information which is pertinent
to structure and metabolism with clinical medicine, beginning with
definitions and classifications. All of the plasma lipoproteins appear spherical in negatively stained electron micrographs (Fig. 1).
The chylomicrons, which carry dietary triglyceride, are the largest
of the particles and are elevated in Type I and V hyperlipoproteinemia by the Fredrickson, Levy and Lees typing system. The very low
density lipoproteins (VLDL) are the second largest in size. They
carry the triglyceride made endogenously in the body and are increased in concentration in types IIb, III, IV and V hyperlipoproteinemia. The low density lipoproteins (LDL) carry one-half to two-
thirds of the cholesterol and are high in types IIa and IIb. The
high density or alpha-lipoproteins do not enter the typing classification but may be very important in atherosclerosis. There is also
a family called intermediate density lipoproteins (IDL), which have
a density between VLDL and IDL. Clinical interest in lipoproteins
in recent years is due largely to the known risk of hyperlipoproteinemia in the development of premature atherosclerosis.

Each family of lipoproteins is heterogeneous in its lipid and
protein or apoprotein composition (Table 1). ApoA-I and apoA-II are
present in HDL and in chylomicrons. ApoA-I is a predominant component of HDL in all species studies thus far. ApoB is a major protein
constituent in LDL and VLDL. The apoC's are found in chylomicrons,
in VLDL and HDL. ApoD, or the thin-line protein, is found in HDL.
ApoE, or the "arginine-rich" protein, is in VLDL and in trace quantities in HDL. Each of the apoproteins has special functions in addi-

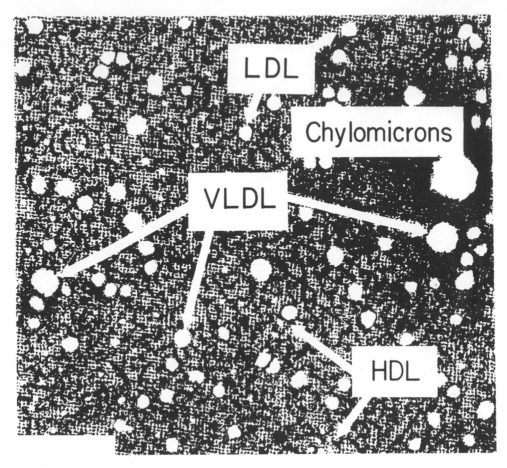

Figure 1: Drawing of the family of lipoproteins as seen in an
electron microscopic photograph. (Published by permission: Baylor College of Medicine.)

tion to contributing to lipid transport. ApoB has a special role in
cholesterol and triglyceride transport from the gut and liver to the
plasma. In abetalipoproteinemia, apoB is absent and the normal
transport of cholesterol and triglyceride is virtually absent.
ApoA-I and apoC-I are activators of lecithin cholesterol acyltransferase, a liver enzyme released in the plasma which is responsible
for the formation of most of the cholesteryl ester in the blood.
ApoC-II activates adipose tissue lipoprotein lipase, a key enzyme
involved in the catabolism of the triglyceride-rich lipoproteins.
ApoE is present in high concentrations in type III hyperlipoproteinemia and in hypothyroidism, is induced in animals by cholesterol
feeding and may play a special role in cholesterol transport. As
far as atherosclerosis is concerned, LDL-cholesterol is atherogenic,

Table 1: Composition of human plasma lipoproteins

Properties	Chylo-microns	VLDL	IDL	LDL	HDL
Major Apoproteins	ApoA-I ApoB ApoC	ApoB ApoC-I ApoC-II ApoC-III ApoE	ApoB	ApoB	ApoA-I ApoA-II
Minor Apoproteins	ApoA-II ApoE[1]	ApoA-I ApoA-II ApoD[2]	ApoC-I ApoC-II ApoC-III ApoE		ApoC-I ApoC-II ApoC-III ApoD ApoE

[1]Also termed "arginine-rich" protein.
[2]Also termed "thin-line" protein and apoA-III.

VLDL and triglyceride may be, while HDL is related inversely to the risk of coronary heart disease (6-10).

I would like to present a brief summary of lipoprotein metabolism. As far as is known, the assembly and secretion of the plasma lipoproteins occurs only in the liver and intestine. Once secreted, the plasma lipoproteins undergo rapid modification and catabolism occurs by at least three distinct processes. One is the physical transfer and exchange of lipid and apoprotein components, second is the change in composition induced by the enzyme lecithin cholesterol acyl transferase (LCAT) and lipoprotein lipase (LPL) and third is cellular uptake through receptor mediated and non-specific mechanisms (Fig. 2).

Chylomicrons are synthesized in the gut and they are transported to the blood through the lymph. Chylomicrons and VLDL are catabolized in two phases. Phase I occurs in peripheral or non-hepatic tissues where the lipoproteins are hydrolyzed through the influence of LPL, an enzyme released into the blood from the endothelium after intravenous injection of heparin. ApoC-II is required in this phase of chylomicron catabolism and is transferred from HDL. A triglyceride-depleted and cholesteryl ester-enriched particle is formed which in phase II of chylomicron catabolism is taken up and further degraded by the liver. There is also an hepatic lipase, but its role is unknown and it is not activated by apoC-II. Chylomicron remnants are important for several reasons. One is that they appear to be a major regulator of cholesterol synthesis in the liver (11, 12), which is the body's main source of blood cholesterol. Second, there

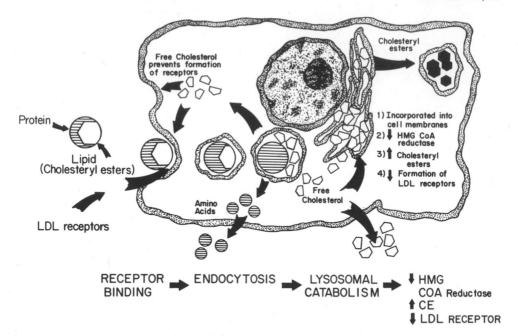

Figure 2: LDL metabolism by non-hepatic tissues. This pathway for
metabolism of LDL by peripheral tissues is based on studies with
fibroblasts grown in tissue culture. Please refer to the text for
a description of the individual steps shown in the figure. Theoretically, HDL could interfere with LDL uptake by the receptor or could
promote the loss of cholesterol from the cell. No in vivo evidence
exists to support these postulated mechanisms; however, in experiments with isolated cells, HDL can exert both of these actions.
(Published by permission: Gotto, A.M., and Jackson, R.L. (1978)
Plasma lipoproteins and atherosclerosis. In Atherosclerosis Reviews,
Volume III (Gotto, A.M. and Paoletti, R., Eds.), Raven Press, New
York, in press.)

is evidence from tissue culture studies, that the chylomicron remnants may be the most atherogenic of all the lipoprotein particles
(13). Zilversmit has postulated that the rate of hydrolysis of
the triglyceride-rich particles at the endothelial surface may be
an important determinant in the development of atherosclerosis (13).

    The liver synthesizes and secretes most of the plasma VLDL (14,
15) (Fig. 3). As VLDL are catabolized through the influence of LPL
at an endothelial cell site, a remnant is formed which may be converted to LDL or which may be taken up and catabolized by the liver.
VLDL catabolism represents the major pathway for the formation of
LDL in man.

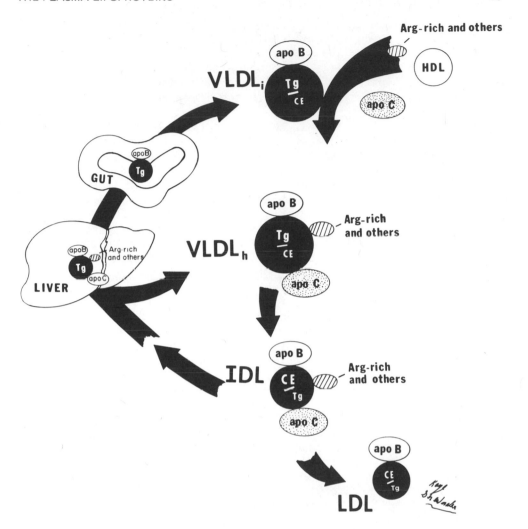

Figure 3: VLDL transport endogenously synthesized triglyceride.
Its primary source is the liver, although some plasma VLDL originate from the gut. Animal studies suggest that the hepatic VLDL
contain a group of proteins called apoC, while those from the gut
do not; gut VLDL acquire apoC by transfer from HDL after reaching
the plasma. VLDL metabolism is thought to be regulated by lipoprotein lipase in peripheral tissues which catalyzes the hydrolysis of
triglyceride. An intermediate density lipoprotein (IDL) is formed
which can be further catabolized to LDL, or which can be taken up
and catabolized by the liver. (Published by permission: Gotto,
A.M., and Jackson, R.L. (1978) Plasma lipoproteins and atherosclerosis. In Atherosclerosis Reviews, Volume III (Gotto, A.M. and
Paoletti, R., Eds.), Raven Press, New York, in press.)

A nascent form of HDL is secreted by the liver, which is a substrate for LCAT which converts cholesterol to cholesterol ester.
Arginine-rich proteins and apoC from HDL are transferred to the triglyceride-rich lipoproteins. HDL may also serve the function of
transporting cholesterol from peripheral tissues, including the
reticulo-endothelial system, back to the liver (16).

The next question is what happens to LDL? Most evidence suggests that in men the major sites of LDL removal and catabolism are
in peripheral or non-hepatic tissues. The effective concentration
of LDL to which peripheral tissues are exposed is more accurately
reflected by the concentration of this lipoprotein in lymph, where
it is present at about 1/10-1/15 the plasma level (17).

I have touched on two of the three mechanisms which modulate
lipoprotein catabolism, namely the transfer of lipid and apoprotein
components, and the action of LCAT and lipoprotein lipase. Now we
come to the third category, that of cellular uptake and catabolism.
Brown and Goldstein have intensively studied receptor mediated uptake of LDL in tissue culture, initially in fibroblasts, also now
in a variety of other cells, including smooth muscle cells (5).
The LDL particle is bound to a specific receptor on the cell surface.
Through the process of endocytosis LDL reach the lysosomes, they are
degraded to amino acids, cholesterol and fatty acids. The major
effects of the increase in cellular content of cholesterol are as
follows: 1) a decrease in the formation of new LDL receptors, 2)
a suppression of cholesterol synthesis effected by decreasing HMG
CoA reductase, the rate-limiting step in cholesterol biosynthesis,
and 3) a stimulation of cholesterol esterification, the acyl cholesterol acyl transferase reaction. The cell has only a limited
number of ways in which it can dispose of an increased amount of
cholesterol. One is to incorporate it into membranes; another is
to deposit it as cholesteryl ester, but both of these processes
have finite capacities. A third alternative is to remove cholesterol
from the cell. HDL could exert its effect in protecting against
atherosclerosis, by acting as a shuttle mechanism for the cholesterol
excreted from the cell, which must be transported back to the liver
(16). Alternatively, HDL could compete with or interfere with LDL
binding to the cell (18).

A well-established relationship exists between familial hypercholesterolemia and premature coronary heart disease. In at least
some of these patients, there is a deficiency, defectiveness or complete absence of the LDL receptor, as measured by binding experiments (19-23). An alternative hypothesis based on leukocyte studies
is that the cell is unable to retain its intracellular cholesterol
(24). Under ordinary circumstances, when a cell is placed in tissue
culture and exposed to LDL cholesterol in the medium, there is an
inverse relationship between the concentration of extracellular

cholesterol and the rate of cholesterol synthesis within the cell.
This phenomenon does not hold in patients with familial hypercholesterolemia. If these patients have a defect in the LDL receptor,
since they are susceptible to atherosclerosis, and since other patients with hypercholesterolemia are also susceptible to atherosclerosis, the question arises as to whether such receptors on
smooth muscle cells within the arterial wall could contribute to
the pathogenesis of atherosclerosis (25). Patients with low levels
of LDL-cholesterol have a diminished risk of developing atherosclerosis. Low levels of circulating LDL-cholesterol should promote a
very rapid intracellular synthesis of cholesterol. When smooth muscle cells are exposed over a long period of time to high concentrations of LDL, they do not accumulate cholesterol (26). The cells
may be induced to accumulate cholesterol by structurally damaging
the LDL, so that it bypasses the receptor mechanism. The major contribution of the LDL receptor to the pathophysiology of atherosclerosis in my opinion is to regulate the rate of the catabolism of this
lipoprotein class which, together with rate of the synthesis, controls the concentration of LDL. Goldstein and Brown have suggested
that as much as one-third of LDL is catabolized by a non-specific
mechanism, that is, other than by the LDL-receptor mechanism (27).
We are left with several incompletely resolved questions: 1) What
is the physiological role of the receptor? 2) Can the receptor defect account for the hypercholesterolemia of familial hypercholesterolemia? 3) Do receptors on smooth muscle cells in the arterial
wall play a role in atherogenesis?

The clinical relevance of information about lipoprotein structure is often less apparent than that concerning lipoprotein metabolism. It is difficult for us to relate much of the knowledge that
has been gained in recent years about lipoprotein structure at this
time to clinical atherosclerosis. The amino acid sequences of five
of the apoproteins, apoA-I, apoA-II, apoC-I, apoC-II and ApoC-III,
have been determined. All are water soluble in the lipid-free state.
They combine readily with phospholipids to form stable complexes
which can be isolated by centrifugation or column chromatography.
Very little cholesteryl ester and triglyceride is bound by apoproteins unless phospholipid is present; this finding has lead to the
conclusion that the primary lipid-protein interaction in lipoproteins is between the apoprotein and the phospholipid constituents.
For the interaction to occur, the fatty acyl chain of the phospholipid is in the melted or liquid crystalline state and associates
with certain hydrophobic or non-polar regions of the apoproteins.

All of the five proteins sequenced to date contain regions
called the amphipathic helix as shown for apoC-I (Fig. 4). This apoprotein has three such regions, which can be shown in a space-filling
three-dimensional model. We believe that these are the sites where
binding of phospholipid and protein most likely occurs. The amphi-

pathic helix has two faces, a polar one which is exposed to the
exterior of the lipoprotein maintaining water solubility and a non-
polar one which binds to the fatty acyl of the phospholipids.

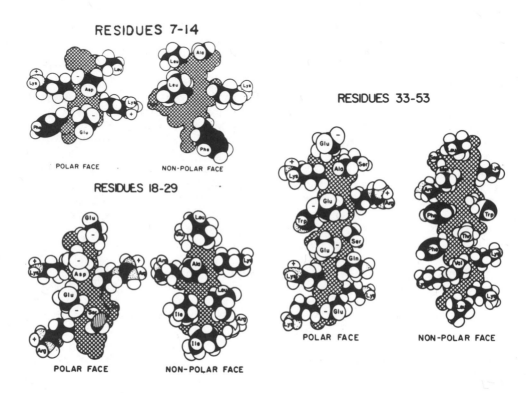

Figure 4:   The α-helical surface topography of amphipathic regions
of apoC-I.   Each helix was built with Ealing CPK space-filling models.
A right-handed α-helical backbone with 3.6 residues per turn was
constructed.   For each amphipathic region amino acid residues were
added onto the α-carbons in their proper order.   Each helix is shown
with its axis oriented parallel to the plane of the page and its
NH$_2$-terminal end toward the top of the page.   The polar and apolar
face of each helix, rotated around the helix axis by 180° relative
to one another, are shown.   (Published by permission of the American
Society of Biological Chemists.   Jackson, R.L., Morrisett, J.D.,
Sparrow, J.T., Segrest, J.P., Pownall, H.J., Smith, L.C., Hoff, H.F.,
and Gotto, A.M. (1974) The interaction of apolipoprotein-serine
with phosphatidylcholine.   J. Biol. Chem. 249, 5314-5320.)

Acidic amino acids are located in a narrow strip in the center of the polar face, while the basic ones are oriented at the periphery between the non-polar and polar faces. The role of the charged groups has not yet been determined. It is possible that they could orient the phospholipid to the apoprotein or simply maintain the solubility of the lipoprotein. Computer analysis with the apoproteins has predicted an evolutionary similarity between them, and, in particular, has identified a repeating unit of 11 amino acids in the amphipathic region of apoA-I (28).

How can the amphipathic structures account for phospholipid binding? In a model for HDL, the amphipathic helical region associates with hydrated phospholipid by partially submerging at the interface between the hydrocarbon chains and the polar head groups of the phospholipid (29). In this model the α-helix is oriented perpendicular to the direction of the phospholipid fatty acyl chains. The main driving force for the association in this model is the hydrophobic interaction between the non-polar face of the amphipathic helix and the methylene groups of the fatty acyl chains of the phospholipid.

Sparrow et al. have provided a different type of evidence to support the importance of hydrophobic binding. They have prepared synthetic peptides predicted to contain the amphipathic helix (30). Peptide II (Fig. 5) is a 16 residue peptide with a hydrophobicity index of 791. It contains alanines at residues 7 and 8. By substituting tyrosine and tryptophan at residues 7 and 8 the hydrophobicity index is increased from 791 to 1031 (Fig. 6). Peptide III readily binds phospholipids, whereas peptide II does not. This experiment shows the contribution of hydrophobicity to phospholipid binding. In order to further test the amphipathic helical theory, a number of other analogs are being synthesized, some of which are being specifically substituted in the charged amino acids on the polar face to determine the significance of these residues in the binding of phospholipids.

One of the postulated mechanisms for the protection by HDL against atherosclerosis, based on studies of Stein et al. (31, 32), is that HDL apoproteins in association with phospholipid can effect a net removal of cholesterol from cells. Synthetic peptides can exert a similar effect. One problem with this approach is that while cholesterol is removed from the cell, there is a marked stimulation of HMG CoA reductase. Nonetheless, there is a net removal of cellular cholesterol.

I would like to give one example of the relationship between apoprotein structure and metabolism. ApoC-II obviously presents interesting opportunities since it both binds lipids and activates LPL. The amino acid sequence of apoC-II has been recently completed

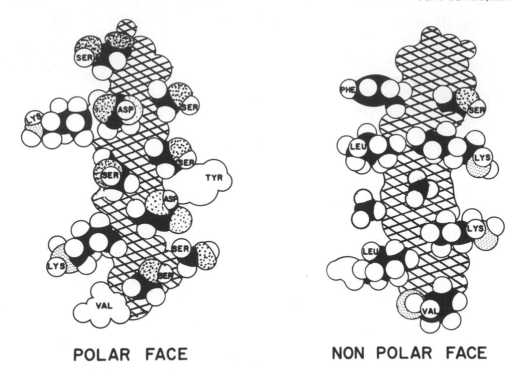

POLAR FACE   NON POLAR FACE

Figure 5:   Drawing of the CPK model of synthetic peptide II showing
the polar and nonpolar faces of the amphipathic helix (hydrophobicity index = 791). (Published by permission: Baylor College of
Medicine.)

by Jackson et al. (33) (Fig. 7).   It contains 78 amino acids and
shows an increase in α-helix upon binding to phospholipids. ApoC-II
has two methionines at residues 9 and 59. Kinnunen et al. (34) have
addressed the question of the minimum sequence necessary for activation of lipoprotein lipase, using fragments produced by cyanogen
bromide cleavage and trypsin hydrolysis and by using synthetic fragments prepared by solid phase peptide synthesis. A synthetic peptide fragment representing the residues 55-78 exhibits almost the
same activity as the intact apoC-II. Figure 8 represents the region
of apoC-II involved in activation. The charged amino acids at the
carboxyl terminus probably have an important role as potential sites
for ionic interaction. Interestingly, the amino terminal half of
the molecule contains the amphipathic helix, while the carboxyl terminal half does not. The amino terminal end most likely is involved
in phospholipid binding and the carboxyl terminal end with enzymic
activation. Thus, in this apoprotein, it is possible to separate
and distinguish between these two different functions of the protein.

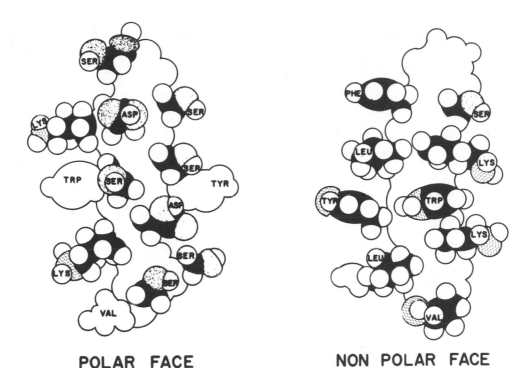

POLAR FACE   NON POLAR FACE

Figure 6:   Drawing of the CPK model of synthetic peptide III showing
the polar and non-polar faces of the amphipathic helix (hydrophobicity index = 1031). (Published by permission: Sparrow, J.T., Morrisett, J.D., Pownall, H.J., Jackson, R.L., and Gotto, A.M. (1975)
The mechanism of lipid binding by the plasma lipoproteins: Synthesis of model peptides. In Peptides: Chemistry, Structure and
Biology (Walter, R. and Meienhofer, J., Eds.), Ann Arbor Science,
Ann Arbor, pp. 597-602.)

These speculations are summarized in Figure 9, which shows lipoprotein lipase bound to a sulfated glycosaminoglycan receptor on
endothelial cells. Because of the charged interaction with the carboxyl terminus, LPL interacts with the apoC-II, which also is able
to bind the lipids. The configuration of the LPL is changed, thereby permitting it to attack VLDL and chylomicrons to bring about the
catabolism. Zilversmit has postulated that the rate at which this
phenomenon occurs at the endothelial site may be the most important
determinant for atherosclerosis (13). It is at this point that the
potentially atherogenic remnant particles are formed. It is conceivable that appropriate structural modifications of the apoC proteins could influence the rate and direction of this process and
thus put one in a position to test in a more direct way its influence on the pathogenesis of atherosclerosis.

THR-GLU-GLN-PRO-GLN-GLN-ASP-GLU-MET-PRO
5   10

SER-PRO-THR-PHE-LEU-THR-GLU-VAL-LYS-GLU
15   20

TRP-LEU-SER-SER-TYR-GLN-SER-ALA-LYS-THR
25   30

ALA-ALA-GLN-ASN-LEU-TYR-GLU-LYS-THR-TYR
35   40

LEU-PRO-ALA-VAL-ASP-GLU-LYS-LEU-ARG-ASP
45   50

LEU-TYR-SER-LYS-SER-THR-ALA-ALA-MET-SER
55   60

THR-TYR-THR-GLY-ILE-PHE-THR-ASP-GLN-VAL
65   70

LEU-SER-VAL-LEU-LYS-GLY-GLU-GLU
75

Figure 7: The amino acid sequence of humna apoC-II as described by
Jackson et al. (33). (Published by permission: Baylor College of
Medicine.)

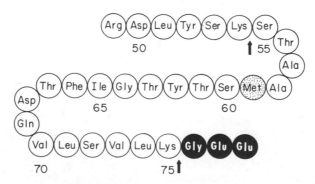

Figure 8: Residues 55-78 of apoC-II appear to contain the active
site for stimulation of lipoprotein lipase, according to Kinnunen
et al. (34). (Published by permission: Baylor College of Medicine.)

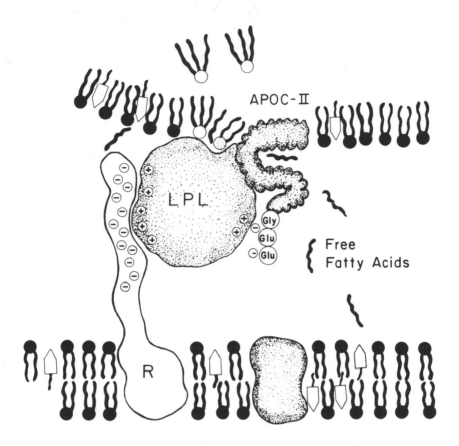

ENDOTHELIAL CELL

Figure 9: ⟨ = phospholipid: ⟨⟩ = cholesterol; ⟨⟩ = triglyceride; ⟨⟩ = hydrolyzed triglyceride; R = glycosaminoglycan receptor.
Postulated interaction of lipoprotein lipase (LPL) and apoC-II, resulting in activation of the triglyceride hydrolyzing potential of
the enzyme. LPL is shown as bound to glycosaminoglycan receptors
on the surface of the endothelial cell. The substrate is a triglyceride-rich lipoprotein, either chylomicrons or VLDL. Please see
text for further details. (Published by permission: Baylor College of Medicine.)

ACKNOWLEDGMENTS

The author gratefully acknowledges the work of his colleagues
Joel D. Morrisett, Richard L. Jackson, Louis C. Smith, Henry J.
Pownall, James T. Sparrow, William A. Bradley, and Josef R. Patsch
described in this manuscript and expresses his thanks to Ms. Kaye
Shewmaker for assistance in drawing the figures and Ms. Barbara
Allen for editorial assistance in the preparation of the manuscript.

Work from the author's laboratory described in this paper was
supported in part by grants from the National Institutes of Health
for a National Heart and Blood Vessel Research and Demonstration
Center (HL-17269) and for a Lipid Research Clinic (NIH 71-2156).

REFERENCES

1. Smith, L.C., Pownall, H.J., and Gotto, A.M., Jr. (1977) Ann.
    Rev. Biochem. In press.

2. Morrisett, J.D., Jackson, R.L., and Gotto, A.M., Jr. (1975)
    Ann. Rev. Biochem. 44, 183-207.

3. Jackson, R.L., Morrisett, J.D., and Gotto, A.M., Jr. (1976)
    Physiol. Rev. 56, 259-316.

4. Scanu, A.M., Edelstein, C., and Keim, P. (1975) in The Plasma
    Proteins: Structure, Function and Genetic Control (Putnam, F.
    W., Ed.), Academic Press, New York, pp. 317-391.

5. Goldstein, J.L., and Brown, M.S. (1977) Ann. Rev. Biochem. 56,
    259-316.

6. Miller, G.J., and Miller, N.E. (1975) Lancet 1, 16-19.

7. Berg, K., Børresen, A.-L., and Dahlen, G. (1976) Lancet 1,
    499-505.

8. Bang, H.O., Dyerberg, J., and Nielsen, A.B. (1971) Lancet 1,
    1143-1145.

9. Rhoads, G.G., Gulbrandsen, C.L., and Kagan, A. (1976) N. Engl.
    J. Med. 294, 293-300.

10. Castelli, W.P., Doyle, J.T., Gordon, T., Hames, C.G., Hjortland,
    M.C., Halley, S.B., Kagan, A., and Zukel, W.J. (1977) Circula-
    tion 55, 767-772.

11. Andersen, J.M., and Dietschy, J.M. (1977) J. Biol. Chem. 252, 3652-3659.

12. Glomset, J.A., Norum, K.R., Nichols, A.V., King, W.C., Mitchell, C.D., Applegate, K.R., Gong, E.L., and Gjone, E. (1975) Scand. J. Clin. Lab. Invest. 35 (Suppl. 142), 3-30.

13. Zilversmit, D.B. (1973) Circ. Res. 33, 633-638.

14. Havel, R.J., Felts, J.M., and Van Duyne, M. (1962) J. Lipid Res. 3, 297-308.

15. Windmueller, H.G., Herbert, P.N., and Levy, R.I. (1973) J. Lipid Res. 14, 215-223.

16. Glomset, J.A. (1972) in Blood Lipids and Lipoproteins: Quantitation, Composition and Metabolism (Nelson, G.J., Ed.), Wiley, New York, pp. 745-787.

17. Reichl, D., Myant, N., Brown, M.S., and Goldstein, J.L. (1978) J. Clin. Invest. In press.

18. Stein, O., and Stein, Y. (1976) Biochim. Biophys. Acta 431, 363-368.

19. Goldstein, J.L., and Brown, M.S. (1975) Am. J. Med. 58, 147-150.

20. Goldstein, J.L., Dana, S.E., and Brown, M.S. (1974) Proc. Natl. Acad. Sci. USA 71, 4288-4292.

21. Goldstein, J.L., Dana, S.E., Brunschede, G.Y., and Brown, M.D. (1975) Proc. Natl. Acad. Sci. USA 72, 1092-1096.

22. Avigan, J., Bathena, S.J., and Schreiner, M.E. (1975) J. Lipid Res. 16, 151-154.

23. Breslow, J.L., Spaulding, D.R., Lux, S.E., Levy, R.I., and Lees, R.S. (1975) N. Engl. J. Med. 293, 900-902.

24. Fogelman, A.M., Edmond, J., Seager, J., and Popjak, G. (1975) J. Biol. Chem. 250, 2045-2055.

25. Goldstein, J.L., and Brown, M.S. (1975) Arch. Pathol. 99, 181-184.

26. Goldstein, J.L., Anderson, R.G., Buja, L.M., Basu, S.K., and Brown, M.S. (1977) J. Clin. Invest. 59, 1196-1202.

27. Goldstein, J.L., and Brown, M.S. (1977) Metabolism 26, 1257.

28. Fitch, W.M. (1977) Genetics 86, 623-644.

29. Segrest, J.P., Jackson, R.L., Morrisett, J.D., and Gotto, A.M.,
     Jr. (1974) FEBS Lett. 38, 247-253.

30. Sparrow, J.T., Morrisett, J.D., Pownall, H.J., Jackson, R.L.,
     and Gotto, A.M., Jr. (1975) in Peptides: Chemistry, Structure
     and Biology, (Walter, R. and Meinhofer, J., Eds.), Ann Arbor
     Science, Ann Arbor, pp. 597-602.

31. Stein, Y., Glangeaud, M.C., Fainaru, M., and Stein, O. (1975)
     Biochim. Biophys. Acta 380, 106-118.

32. Jackson, R.L., Stein, O., Gotto, A.M., Jr., and Stein, Y. (1975)
     J. Biol. Chem. 250, 7204-7209.

33. Jackson, R.L., Baker, H.N., Gilliam, E.B., and Gotto, A.M., Jr.
     (1977) Proc. Natl. Acad. Sci. USA 74, 1942-1945.

34. Kinnunen, P.K.M., Jackson, R.L., Smith, L.C., Gotto, A.M., Jr.,
     and Sparrow, J.T. (1977) Proc. Natl. Acad. Sci. USA. In press.

PROGRESSION AND REGRESSION OF ATHEROSCLEROTIC LESIONS

Robert W. Wissler

Department of Pathology and Specialized Center of
Research in Atherosclerosis
The University of Chicago
Chicago, Illinois

The most important concepts in understanding the progression and regression of clinically significant coronary atherosclerosis and the ways in which this disease process produces its most common clinical effects have been changing rapidly.

Developing knowledge regarding the pathogenesis of the advanced atherosclerotic plaque has been reviewed in some detail recently (1-4). Evidence for regression of the advanced atherosclerotic plaque (5-7) has also been recently summarized.

In this report we will outline the major advances in our understanding of the factors influencing the progression and regression of the advanced coronary atherosclerotic plaque.

The space-occupying features of this plaque are well documented (Figure 1) (8). They are composed of two major components. The first is the deposited cholesterol and lipid, often largely extracellular, in an acellular, soft grumous core of the atheroma, and the second is proliferated smooth muscle cells in the intima. The cells are usually mixed with variable quantities of collagen and elastin, as well as glycoproteins and/or glycosaminoglycans (GAGs). This "fibrous and cellular cap" can vary greatly in relative and absolute mass and thickness and in the extent of fibrosis (density). It can also contain a variable amount of intracellular and extracellular lipid, a considerable portion of which may still include identifiable apolipoprotein B (9).

Much of the recent work from this laboratory reported in this paper was supported in part by a grant from the National Heart, Lung, and Blood Institute, No. A/S HL 15062.

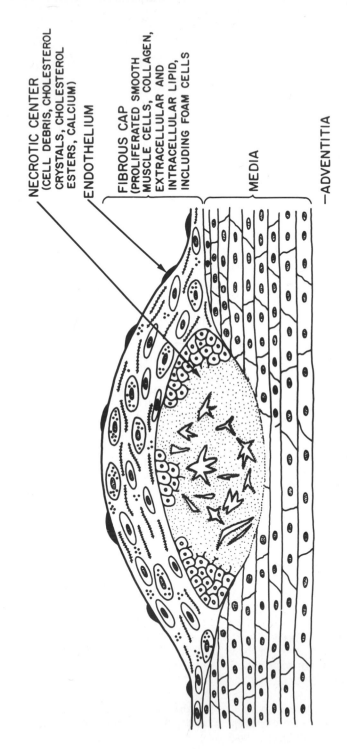

NECROTIC CENTER
(CELL DEBRIS, CHOLESTEROL
CRYSTALS, CHOLESTEROL
ESTERS, CALCIUM)

ENDOTHELIUM

FIBROUS CAP
(PROLIFERATED SMOOTH
MUSCLE CELLS, COLLAGEN,
EXTRACELLULAR AND
INTRACELLULAR LIPID,
INCLUDING FOAM CELLS

MEDIA

—ADVENTITIA

Figure 1. Diagram of an Atherosclerotic Plaque (after P. Constantinides)

Other components contributing to the space occupying mass of the coronary atherosclerotic plaque are "foam cells," fibrin and/or fibrinogen, and calcium.

Of these components, the acellular lipid-rich center with its high concentrations of cholesterol ester and the accumulating smooth muscle cells are probably the most important in determining the common life-threatening clinical effects of the advanced coronary plaque, namely stenosis and coronary thrombosis (Figure 2).

The most impressive recent advances have been in understanding the factors involved in stimulating the arterial smooth muscle cells to proliferate in the arterial intima and the factors responsible for the entrance of serum lipids into the artery wall and accumulation of lipid in the plaque.

Relatively little understanding has been gained as yet about the mechanisms responsible for cell death in relation to the acellular core of the atheroma. The factors which influence the relative amounts of collagen, elastin and GAGs that are produced by the smooth muscle cells in the fibrous cap are also largely still to be elucidated. Our knowledge will be enhanced substantially when these additional responses of the arterial smooth muscle cells to injury, namely necrosis and synthesis of their major extracellular products, are better understood.

CURRENT CONCEPTS OF ATHEROGENESIS

The major advances that have occurred in the past 10-15 years involve the interaction of the artery wall with blood serum or plasma factors. Thus far they have been focused primarily on five important premises as follows:

1. The arterial medial smooth muscle cell is the principal cell involved in the development of the progressive atherosclerotic plaque by means of its multifunctional mesenchymal reactions of:

   a. cell proliferation
   b. taking up lipid
   c. synthesis of collagen, elastin or glycosaminoglycans
   d. necrosis

2. Most of the cholesterol accumulation in the plaque is derived from low density lipoproteins (LDL) from the blood.

3. Arterial endothelial damage or destruction, particularly when sustained or repeated, are important determinants of plaque localization and progression.

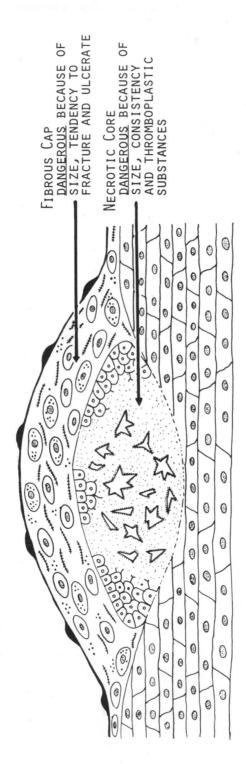

FIBROUS CAP
DANGEROUS BECAUSE OF
SIZE, TENDENCY TO
FRACTURE AND ULCERATE

NECROTIC CORE
DANGEROUS BECAUSE OF
SIZE, CONSISTENCY
AND THROMBOPLASTIC
SUBSTANCES

Figure 2. Relation of Plaque Components to Clinical Effects

4.   Low density lipoproteins from hyperlipidemic serum have been found to stimulate stationary cultures of rabbit, monkey and human arterial smooth muscle cells:

   a.   to proliferate excessively
   b.   to accumulate unusual quantities of cholesterol ester.

5.   The platelet, or factors transported by the platelet, stimulates arterial smooth muscle cell proliferation under some conditions.

Arterial Smooth Muscle Cell as the Principal Cell of the Atherosclerotic Lesion

Much of the evidence for the importance of arterial smooth muscle cells in the development of the atherosclerotic plaque comes from studies of the lesions of human subjects using electron microscopy (10-13). This developing evidence, along with studies in our own laboratory (14, 15), led us in 1968 to implicate this cell type as the principal cell type in the lesion, not only in relation to excessive proliferation (hyperplasia), but also in several other ways. This prompted us to refer to it as a multifunctional medial mesenchymal cell and to summarize the evidence that it is also the principal cell responsible for collagen, elastin and GAGs synthesis in the lesion, as well as for lipoprotein uptake and metabolism, and for necrosis (16). Subsequent studies by Ross and coworkers (17, 18) and in our laboratory (19) have helped to document the synthetic capacity of this arterial cell.

Recent studies by Dr. Chen (20-22) and Dr. Bates (23) in our laboratory have added to our appreciation of the importance of this cell type in lipoprotein metabolism and cholesterol ester accumulation. Furthermore, Dr. Chen has presented further evidence (21, 24-27) that hyperlipidemic serum and LDL fractions derived from hyperlipidemic serum may play an important part in the deranged metabolism and death of these cells, which could be responsible for the development of the necrotic cholesterol-rich center of the advanced atheroma.

Low Density Lipoproteins from Hyperlipidemic Serum and the Accumulation of Lipid in the Atherosclerotic Plaque

Studies of atherosclerotic lesions of human subjects have yielded much of the evidence that LDL fractions and apolipoprotein B gain entrance to the arterial wall and accumulate there. This evidence is derived from studies of extracts of the artery wall (28, 29), including work by Tracy et al. in this laboratory (30), from

immunohistochemical studies by Harvey Watts (31), from research in
this laboratory (14, 15) and from more recent studies by Walton et
al. (32) and by Hoff et al. (33).   There is also increasing semi-
quantitative evidence emerging from studies by Smith (9, 34) and
from tracer studies in moribund human subjects (35, 36) supporting
this view and suggesting that a substantial part of the lipid in
some types of plaques may still include the apolipoprotein B as a
marker.

Recent studies of Goldstein and Brown (37-39) indicate that
there is specific binding of apolipoprotein B on the surface of human fibroblasts.   There are now additional results indicating that
arterial smooth muscle cells have this same mechanism of binding of
LDL apo B (40).   Furthermore, there is increasing evidence that GAGs
from atherosclerotic plaques bind LDL (41, 42).   This relationship
had been suggested by early studies of Tracy et al. (43) in this
laboratory.

Many of the dynamic relationships of LDL molecules, arterial
smooth muscle cells, including their intracellular lipid metabolic
functions and the binding capacities of the extracellular products
of the smooth muscle cell, still need to be worked out.   Nevertheless it is becoming increasingly clear that almost all of the cholesterol in the advancing atherosclerotic plaque originates with the
LDL molecules that gain entrance to the artery wall from the blood
and become sequestered in the plaque.

Endothelial Integrity and the Development of
the Atherosclerotic Plaque

Accelerated and often severe atherogenesis has been observed in
studies in which experimental injury of the arterial intima has been
combined with hyperlipidemia (44-48).   Some of this effect, however,
may be due to the fact that platelets with their growth promoting
factor come in close proximity to the arterial medial smooth muscle
cells under these conditions.   Since most studies indicate that the
platelet stimulation of smooth muscle cell proliferation in vivo is
not sustained unless there is also hyperlipidemia, this effect of
damaged intima seems to be a function of both elevated LDL levels
and the loss of the endothelial integrity.   A simple diagram of
these relationships is given in Figure 3.

Some of the conditions under which arterial endothelial injury
might contribute to accelerated atherogenesis in human subjects is
given in Table 1.   It is evident that there are many such conditions
and that the prevention or regression of atherosclerosis will probably require special attention not only to blood lipid levels but
also to conditions promoting endothelial health.

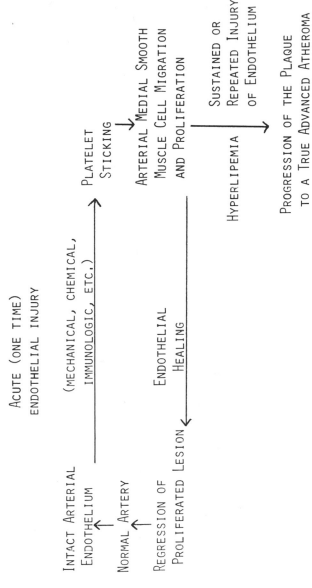

Figure 3.   The Interaction of Hyperlipemia and Sustained (or Repeated) Endothelial
Injury to Produce Advanced Atherosclerosis

Table 1. Factors Which Have Been Shown to Injure Arterial Endothelium and to Produce Increased
Permeability to Macromolecules, Including Lipoproteins

SUBSTANCE OR PHYSICAL CONDITION	MECHANISM INVOLVED	CLINICAL CONDITION
Hemodynamic forces: tension, stretching, shearing, eddy currents	Separation or damage to endothelial cells, increased permeability, platelet sticking, stimulation of smooth muscle cell proliferation	Hypertension
Angiotensin II	"Trap-door" effect	Hypertension
Carbon monoxide or decreased O_2 saturation	Destruction of endothelial cells	Cigarette smoking
Catecholamines (epinephrine, norepinephrine, serotonin, bradykinin)	Hypercontraction, swelling and loss of endothelial cells, platelet agglutination	Stress, cigarette smoking
Endotoxins and other similar bacterial products	Endothelial cell destruction, platelet sticking	Acute bacterial infections
Ag-Ab complexes	Platelet agglutination	Serum sickness, transplant rejection, immune complex diseases
Virus diseases	Endothelial cell infection, necrosis	Viremias
Mechanical trauma to endothelium	Platelet sticking, increased local permeability	Catheter injury
Hyperlipemia with increase in circulating lipoproteins (cholesterol, triglycerides, phospholipids) and free fatty acids	Platelet agglutination in areas of usual hemodynamic damage, over "fatty streaks"	Chronic nutritional imbalance (high fat and cholesterol diets), familial hypercholesterolemia, diabetes, nephrosis, hypothyroidism

Special Stimulatory Properties of Hyperlipidemic Serum
or the LDL Derived from It

LDL derived from hyperlipidemic serum appears to stimulate unusual proliferation of monkey arterial medial smooth muscle cells in
vitro after they have grown to a stationary phase (22, 25, 49-51).
This effect is not dependent on the cholesterol level in the serum
(52-54) and appears to be associated with a very narrow cut of LDL_2
(55). This effect has been confirmed using subcultured rabbit arterial smooth muscle cells and rabbit LDL (21, 24, 25) and using
human arterial smooth muscle cells and human LDL (56, 57). Estrogen
in small amounts appears to block this effect (58) and so does normal high density lipoprotein (59). Work is now underway to elucidate
the mechanism that underlies this response.

Although the number of "factors" that have been recently implicated in the proliferation of mesenchymal cells is mind-boggling
(22, 25, 49-55, 60-65), it is tempting to try to sort them out and
to try to find common denominators that may be helpful in understanding general biological principles. We have recently called attention
to a considerable body of evidence which makes it seem reasonable to
suppose that many of these factors may in some way be related to
lysosomal products emanating from a number of cell types (66).

It should be noted that numerous reports indicate that progressive arterial smooth muscle cell proliferation does not occur, even
following rather extensive endothelial damage, unless there is concomitant hyperlipidemia (67-71). It appears that sustained elevations in LDL of at least moderate degree may be necessary to promote
the progressive cell proliferation that appears necessary for an
advanced atherosclerotic plaque to develop. Exceptions to this may
be noted from time to time if very severe endothelial injury is sustained long enough.

Platelet Factor Stimulation of Arterial Smooth
Muscle Cell Proliferation

Ross and coworkers (62, 71, 73) have published a number of reports recently indicating that platelets stimulate arterial smooth
muscle cells to proliferate both in vitro and in vivo.

These reports suggest that a number of experimental and clinical
conditions will accelerate atherosclerosis at a given level of lipoprotein in the circulation if accompanied by constant exposure of
the smooth muscle cells to platelets or platelet products (Figure
4). Other recent studies both in Dr. Ross's laboratory (74, 75) and
elsewhere (76) indicate that the converse is also true. In other
words endothelial damage without exposure of the underlying arterial

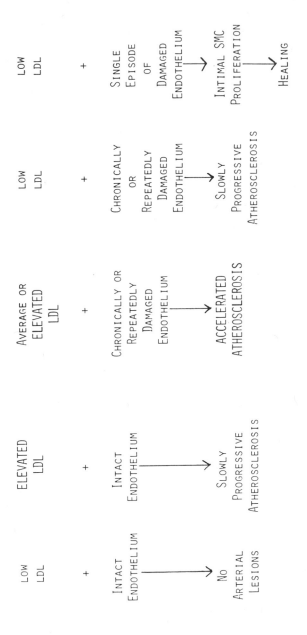

Figure 4. The Spectrum of Interactions of Low Density Lipoproteins with the Inner Surface of the Artery under Conditions of Varying Arterial Endothelial Injury

components to circulating platelets will not sustain a progressive proliferation of arterial smooth muscle cells or atherogenesis.

These investigations suggest that a low molecular weight polypeptide from platelets is responsible for this effect and that arterial smooth muscle cells cannot proliferate in the absence of this factor.

THE EMERGING PATHOBIOLOGY OF ATHEROGENESIS

Studies of the factors responsible for cell proliferation and lipid accumulation in the atherosclerotic plaque and the in vitro systems being used for these investigations form the basis of an emerging group of approaches that are being used by many scientists who are studying the artery wall.

Several of these in vitro methods are diagrammed in Figure 5. They include the study of small fragments of arterial medial tissue, either free floating or on a grid; the use of outgrowths from primary explants of artery wall; the use of subcultures of arterial medial cells or endothelial cells, and the study of plaques using carefully monitored microdissections of various areas of the plaque.

Highlights of a few of the studies using these in vitro approaches are presented diagrammatically in Figure 6. It is evident that they cover a wide range of approaches, varying from enzyme genetic methods used by Benditt (77) and by the Johns Hopkins and the Albany groups (78, 79), to the exquisite enzyme studies of LDL-cell interaction as pioneered by Goldstein and Brown (38). They also include excellent chemical, cell kinetic and ultrastructural studies by Ross, Glomset and their coworkers (62) and by Fischer-Dzoga, Scanu and myself (55), as well as the microchemical approaches used to study lipid metabolism by Rothblat, St. Clair, Bates, Chen and others (21, 24-27, 80-82). They also involve the cell fractionation approaches and lysosomal studies of DeDuve and Wolinsky and the use of cell extracts for immunochemical studies as developed by Elspeth Smith and coworkers (9, 34, 83-85).

This must only be the beginning of an intensive consideration of the artery wall cells, including endothelium, arterial smooth muscle cells, platelets, monocytes, adventitial fibroblasts, lipoproteins and several other substances. It appears to be a field of endeavor that is likely to enrich our understanding of the fundamental processes involved in atherogenesis. It may also help us understand the mechanisms responsible for regression of the advanced atherosclerotic plaque.

ORGAN CULTURE

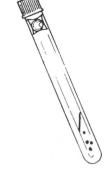

FREE FLOATING EXPLANTS OF MEDIA
(Jarmolych, Daoud, Fritz)

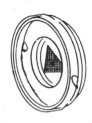

SEGMENT OF ARTERY CULTURED ON GRID
(St. Clair)

CELL CULTURE

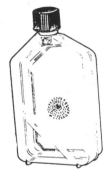

OUTGROWTH OF CELLS FROM PRIMARY EXPLANTS
OF MEDIA, ENDOTHELIUM AND ADVENTITIA,
PLAQUE CELLS AND FIBROBLASTS
(Fischer-Dzoga and Wissler)

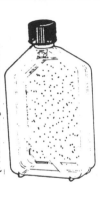

SUBCULTURES OF AORTIC CELLS,
ENDOTHELIAL, MEDIAL CELLS,
FIBROBLASTS AND PLAQUE CELLS
(Lazzarini-Robertson, Ross, Chen,
Bates, Lewis, Stein, etc.)

MICRODISSECTION OF PLAQUES

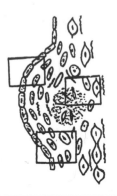

G6PD ISOENZYMES QUANTITATION AND
LDL IMMUNOCHEMICAL QUANTITATION
STUDIES ON LYSOSOMES
(Benditt, E. Smith, DeDuve, Wolinsky)

Figure 5.   Methods in Use to Study Artery Wall Cells and Plaque Cells in vitro

THE CONTRIBUTION OF ANIMAL MODELS

The last two decades have been marked by the rapid development of the new models of advanced atherosclerosis which have many of the features of the advanced plaques in human subjects (86, 87, 88). Although many of these studies have utilized nonhuman primates and have been reviewed from different viewpoints recently (89-91), there are also examples of highly useful new developments in the use of rabbit (46), swine (92, 93), and pigeon (94) models.

Those studies of more humanoid animal models have been particularly useful in documenting that animal models can be expected to have many of the complications that are seen in human atherosclerosis (95-97). They have also contributed to our understanding of some of the factors that are likely to contribute to progression of atherosclerotic plaques in people (44, 46, 98, 99).

One of the most promising ways of using some of these new models of advanced atherosclerosis has been to study regression of these advanced plaques (100).

PLAQUE REGRESSION STUDIES

There is increasing evidence that atherosclerosis is a substantially reversible process. This comes from numerous studies in experimental animals, from retrospective and prospective epidemiologic studies in humans--some of which have utilized evaluation of the severity of the disease process at autopsy--and, more recently, from intervention studies which have evaluated cardiovascular function and/or the size of plaques before and after therapy (7, 101).

Plaque Regression in Experimental Animals

The documented results in those experimental regression studies that have been most significant, in our opinion, have recently been summarized (Table 2) (102). Though not all have actually dealt with advanced plaques, all have made important contributions to the increasing understanding of regression.

The initial studies of Armstrong, Warner and Connor (103) pioneered the reversal of severe diet-induced disease in hypercholesterolemic rhesus monkeys, using increase in lumen size in the coronary arteries as one of their main criteria of regression. They illustrated their articles with photomicrographs showing severe coronary artery lesions with all of the components of advanced human plaques, as well as pictures of regression lesions which appeared to be much smaller, much poorer in lipid with more condensed and re-

Table 2. Major Findings Reported from Recent Studies of Regression of Advanced Atherosclerosis in Macaques and Swine

A. ARMSTRONG, WARNER, CONNOR, ET AL., UNIVERSITY OF IOWA (RHESUS AND CYNOMOLGUS)
    1. LESIONS IN CORONARY ARTERIES AND OTHER ARTERIES DECREASE IN SIZE (DEGREE OF LUMEN NARROWING).
    2. BOTH CHOLESTEROL AND CHOLESTEROL ESTERS DECREASE.
    3. COLLAGEN AND ELASTIN DECREASE PER ANATOMICAL UNIT.

B. VESSELINOVITCH, WISSLER, ET AL., UNIVERSITY OF CHICAGO (RHESUS)
    1. LESIONS IN CORONARY ARTERIES AND OTHER ARTERIES INCREASE USING MORPHOMETRIC MEASUREMENTS.
        A. LIPID AND CONNECTIVE TISSUE ANALYSES ALSO DECREASE.
    2. NECROTIC CENTER REDUCED AND REMAINING LIPID MOSTLY RELATED TO INTERNAL ELASTIC MEMBRANE.
    3. PRELABELED LESIONS INDICATE INCREASED TURNOVER OF CHOLESTEROL AND ITS ESTERS DURING REGRESSION.
    4. CHOLESTYRAMINE INCREASES DIET EFFECTIVENESS.

C. DAOUD, FRITZ, LEE, THOMAS, ET AL., ALBANY (SWINE)
    1. LESION SIZE AND COMPLEXITY DECREASES REMARKABLY.
    2. CELLULARITY AND CELL PROLIFERATION DECREASE.
    3. CALCIUM DECREASES.

D. WAGNER, BOND, BULLOCK, CLARKSON, ET AL., BOWMAN-GRAY (RHESUS)
    1. SOME REGRESSION WITH SERUM CHOLESTEROL LEVELS OF 200 MG%.
    2. REGRESSION DIRECTLY PROPORTIONAL TO SERUM CHOLESTEROL LOWERING.

E. STARY, STRONG, EGGEN, ET AL., LOUISIANA STATE UNIVERSITY (RHESUS)
    1. LYSOSOMAL ACTIVITY INCREASES AS LESIONS BEGIN TO REGRESS.
    2. FATTY LESIONS REGRESS ALMOST COMPLETELY IN 10 MONTHS.

modeled connective tissue. They quickly followed this report with
published evidence of substantial decrease in cholesterol and lipid
in the diseased arteries (104), and more recently reported rather
striking evidence of a definite, if rather slow, decrease in collagen and elastin in these experimental lesions (101, 105, 106).

In our initial studies of regression of advanced lesions in
rhesus monkeys (107), we used a shorter period of therapy (18 months
instead of 40) and achieved large decreases of these sizeable lesions, many of which had necrotic centers and fibrous caps. They
were apparently converted to much smaller and simpler plaques. The
little lipid remaining seemed to be localized in or on the internal
elastic membrane, a histopathological pattern we have come to associate with regression.

It is noteworthy that in both of these studies in rhesus monkeys (103, 107) promising results were obtained under conditions in
which the serum cholesterol levels were lowered by dietary means to
levels that approximated the basal level in this species, i.e., 150
mg% or below.

More recently we have completed three consecutive rhesus monkey regression experiments in which cholestyramine was added to the
diets of two groups of atherosclerotic monkeys, one of which was
also receiving a low fat, low cholesterol ration, while the other
received cholestyramine in addition to continuation of the atherogenic ration. The results of one of these have been reported briefly (108). In general, the results of each of these experiments
have been very similar to the results shown in Table 3. In all
three of these experiments, feeding a low fat, low cholesterol ration for a period of approximately 12 months following a similar
period of induction has resulted in consistent and definite regression of lesions. However, addition of cholestyramine to this ration
has not produced much increased evidence of regression.

Paradoxically, the addition of cholestyramine to the atherogenic ration (the same ration used to produce the lesions), consistently resulted in evidence of substantial regression, even though
the serum cholesterol levels did not return to normal or baseline
levels. This finding suggests that cholestyramine has some effect
on lipids and the artery wall that does not depend solely on the
serum cholesterol (LDL) levels. Thus far, our attempts to elucidate
the mechanism of this unexpected effect of cholestyramine have not
been successful.

In all three of these experiments, the gross and microscopic
study of the other parts of the arterial tree have shown results
similar to those in the aorta. There is definite evidence of regression of lesions in the coronary, iliac, carotid and femoral
arteries of the animals treated with diet and/or cholestyramine.

Table 3. Aortic Gross and Microscopic Lesions from Second Diet and Drug Regression Experiment in Rhesus Monkeys

Group	Treatment	No. of Animals	Group % of Intimal Surface Involved	Microscopic	
				Frequency	Severity
I	Atherogenic Diet (12 months)	5	62 ± 14.2	100 ± 0.0	1.6 ± 0.2
II	Atherogenic Diet (24 months)	4	84 ± 6.9	100 ± 0.0	2.1 ± 0.2
III	Low-fat, Low-cholesterol Diet	5	23 ± 9.9*	50 ± 10.0*	0.2 ± 0.1*
IV	Low-fat, Low-cholesterol Diet + Cholestyramine	5	10 ± 5.6*	48 ± 11.1*	0.2 ± 0.1*
V	Atherogenic Diet + Cholestyramine	5	31 ± 8.2*	55 ± 11.1*	0.3 ± 0.1*

* Different from groups I and II at P 0.01

$\pm$ Standard error, P based on Behrens-Fisher Test

Additional facets of these more recent studies have been the aortic chemical analyses aimed at quantitating the cholesterol and cholesterol esters in the arteries. In general, these have confirmed and extended our gross and microscopic results (108). Isotopic studies, which have involved loading the lesions and all the other pools with radioactive cholesterol during the induction period and then studying the specific activity of the cholesterol in each pool 12 months later, at the end of the regression period, have also yielded valuable data (109). Thus far these very useful results have indicated that both the cholesterol and cholesterol esters in the lesions are fairly labile, both mvoing in as well as out of the artery under the conditions of therapy (110).

Further facets of these studies including the analyses of collagen and elastin and their potential to turnover will be reported soon.

Dr. Giorgio Weber, in collaboration with us, has conducted scanning electron microscopic studies on the endothelial surfaces of standardized aortic samples from some of these animals (111). In general, scanning electron microscopy of the aorta prior to regression shows areas of endothelial defects in the most advanced plaques. After one year of the regression regimen the aortic samples showed little or no evidence of endothelial cell damage.

Daoud, Fritz and coworkers (112, 113) at Albany Medical College have reported on regression studies in swine whose abdominal aortas were made severely atherosclerotic by means of balloon catheter injury combined with an atherogenic diet and metabolic manipulation. Their studies show that the size, severity, complexity and cholesterol content of these advanced lesions are reduced by treatment with a low fat, low cholesterol ration. They also show that the number of cells, as well as the rate of cell division in the plaques is reduced and that the deposits of calcium seemed to shrink (111).

Evidence of Plaque Regression from Human Studies

Many retrospective epidemiologic studies show a decrease in heart attacks or a lower mortality rate from heart diesase during periods when supplies of saturated fats, cholesterol or calories were severely limited (5). In this review, we will consider only a few of the studies, mostly prospective, which were primarily concerned with either severity of atherosclerosis as judged at autopsy or peripheral vascular and circulatory function (Table 4). Most of these studies involved direct comparisons of severity of atherosclerosis or arterial function, in age- and sex-matched groups of individuals, who were and were not subjected to the dietary deprivation or other therapies being compared (7). As the methods of mea-

Table 4. List of Studies with Evidence of Regression of Atherosclerotic Lesions in Man

PRINCIPAL INVESTIGATOR (YEAR)	CONDITIONS OF REGRESSION	EVIDENCE OF REGRESSION
ASCHOFF (1924)	POST WORLD WAR I--SEMISTARVATION	AORTIC ATHEROSCLEROSIS IS REDUCED
VARTIAINEN (1946)	POST WORLD WAR II--MALNUTRITION	LESS ATHEROSCLEROSIS, ESPECIALLY IN THE 30-49 YEAR AGE GROUP
WILENS (1947)	WASTING DISEASE--40-60 YEAR OLDS	LESS SEVERE ATHEROSCLEROSIS CORRELATED WITH WEIGHT LOSS
RIVIN (1954)	CARCINOMA OF THE PROSTATE AND BREAST, ESTROGEN TREATED	DIMUNITION OF CORONARY ATHEROSCLEROSIS
LONDON (1961)	METASTATIC CARCINOMA OF PROSTATE TREATED WITH ESTROGEN	LESS SEVERE ATHEROSCLEROSIS
BUCHWALD (1967)	ILEAL BYPASS OPERATION	MANY CLINICAL SIGNS OF IMPROVED CIRCULATION
ZELIS (1970)	HYPERLIPOPROTEINEMIAS, CLOFIBRATE TREATED	IMPROVEMENT OF PERIPHERAL CIRCULATION

suring the severity of atherosclerosis become more exact and reliable, this approach should be applicable to some of the primary and
secondary intervention trials now being carried out.

Two recent and continuing studies in which sequential and quan-
titatively evaluated arteriography is being employed (115, 116) are
worthy of mention. It is obvious that much more work along this
line needs to be done. The methods being developed will make it
possible to evaluate the potential and the time table for regression
in human atherosclerosis at various ages and in response to various
types of therapy.

Dr. David Blankenhorn and his colleagues at the University of
Southern California have reported decreases in plaque size in one
year (117). More recently they have published evidence indicating
that plaques are more likely to shrink in those patients who show
a decrease in serum cholesterol during a therapeutic trial (88).

Dr. Henry Buchwald has also presented data indicating that the
large and sustained decreases in serum cholesterol he is able to
produce in hyperlipidemic patients with partial ileal bypass will
half progression of coronary atherosclerotic plaques or produce
definite regression in 80% of the treated patients (118). Progression is usually the rule in about 60% of the untreated patients
studied by sequential arteriography (119). In some of the patients
he has studied, the evidence of regression in a two-year period has
been quite impressive. This method of evaluating the effects of
therapy by means of sequential arteriography, when it is perfected,
should greatly simplify the process of documenting and quantitating
regression. Significant results may be possible in relatively small
groups of patients.

Mechanisms of Plaque Regression

The major changes in a plaque that occur during regression, and
which should make it safer for the individual, are shown in the next
diagram (Figure 7). It is evident from the regressed plaques illustrated in both experimental animals and humans that the major changes
which occur can be described as regression (decrease in lipid, cells,
fiber proteins and calcium), remodeling (condensation and reorienta-
tion of collagen and elastin), and healing (decrease in evidence of
endothelial damage, increased cell proliferation, etc.).

If one thinks of these mechanisms of atherogenesis in this way,
then one can also visualize how the reduction of serum cholesterol
(LDL) to a low level could block many of these pathogenetic reactions (Figure 8).

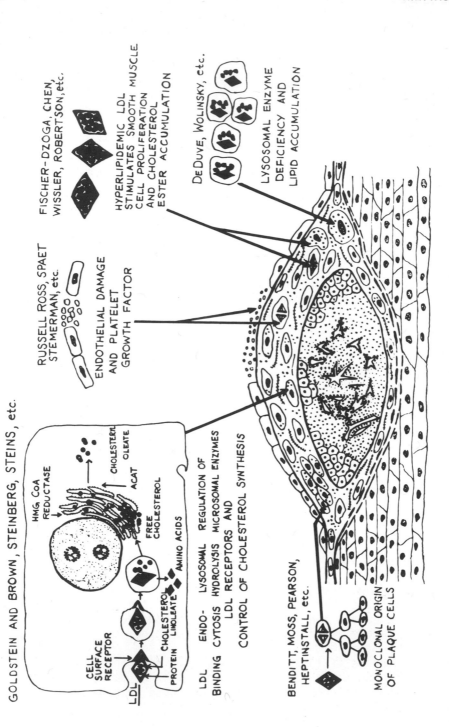

Figure 6.   The Emerging Pathobiology of Atherogenesis (Recent *in vitro* Observations)

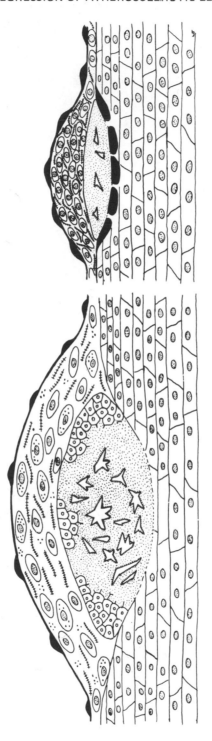

Figure 7. Does the Regressed Plaque Represent a Less Dangerous Lesion?

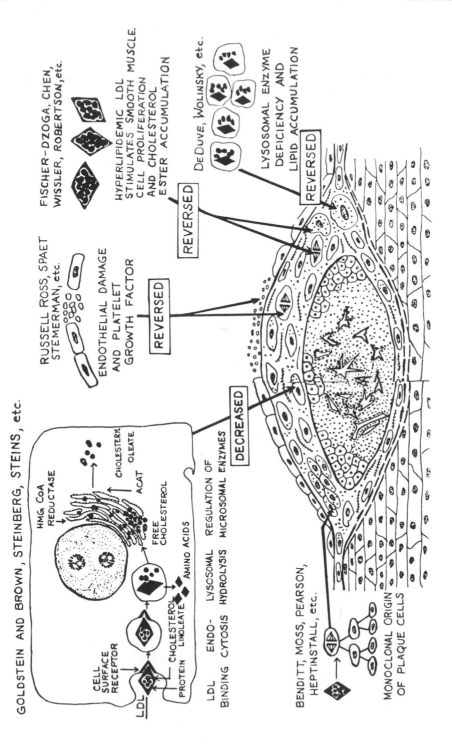

Figure 8.   The Emerging Pathobiology of Regression

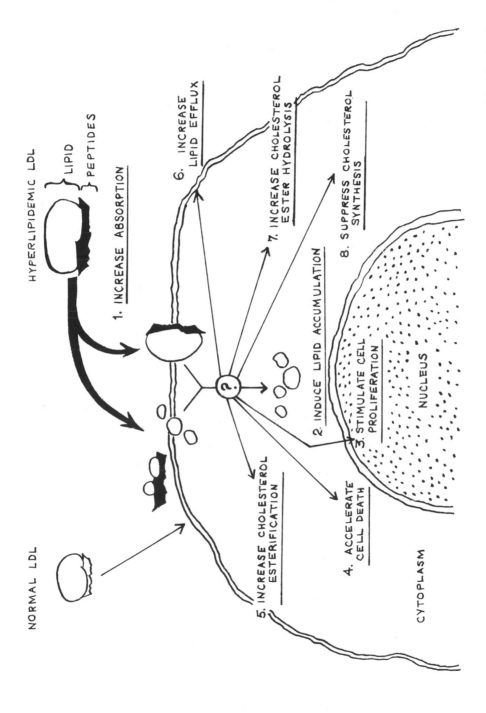

Figure 9. Reactions of Aortic Medial Cells to Low Density Lipoproteins from Hyperlipidemic Serum

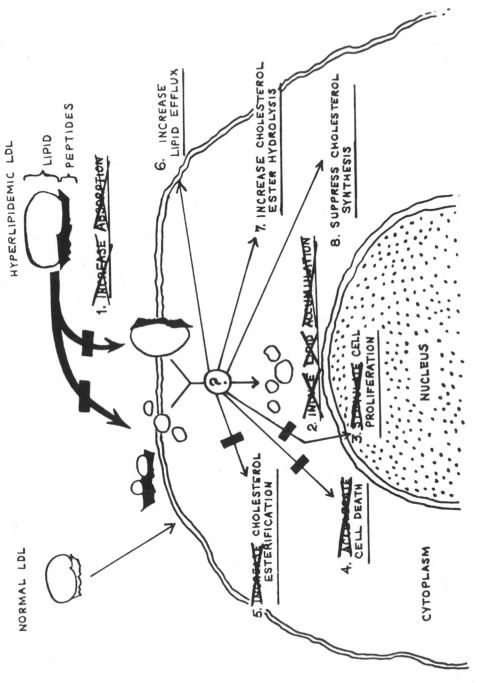

Figure 10. What Happens to Aortic Medial Cells during Regression?

Similarly, if the atherogenic and protective forces, as proposed by Chen (120), are considered in relation to the smooth muscle cell and low density lipoproteins, then those toward the left of the diagram (Figure 9) are largely atherogenic and those to the right can be expected to be protective. Here, again, it is possible to modify the diagram (Figure 10) so that it can be used to visualize the protective (or regressive) mechanisms as becoming predominant under conditions in which the LDL molecules are reduced to low levels.

Obviously, much more needs to be done to understand fully the mechanisms of regression. In general, however, it appears that the spectrum of intervention relative to both prevention and regression of atherosclerosis may be much wider than previously appreciated. In fact, there is reason to believe that vigorous efforts to lower serum lipids (cholesterol) to the levels commonly found in the majority of the world's adult population (150 mg% or below) will likely yield very worthwhile results.

ACKNOWLEDGMENTS

The author would like to express his thanks to Dr. Draga Vesselinovitch, Dr. Godfrey Getz, Dr. Jayme Borensztajn, Dr. Katti Fischer-Dzoga, Dr. Robert Chen, Dr. Thomas Schaffner, Dr. Sandra Bates and Mr. Randolph Hughes and his many other associates for their help with the research in this laboratory referred to in this manuscript. He would also like to thank Mr. Robert Pisciotta, Ms. Judy D. Johnson and Mr. William Johnson for their assistance in the preparation of the paper.

REFERENCES

1. Getz, G.S., Vesselinovitch, D., and Wissler, R.W. (1969) Amer. J. Med. 46, 657-673.

2. Wissler, R.W. (1974) in The Myocardium: Failure and Infarction, (Braunwald, E., Ed.), H.P. Publishing Co., New York, pp. 155-166.

3. Wissler, R.W. (1974) in Comparative Pathology of the Heart (Adv. Cardiol., vol. 13) (Homberger, F., Ed.), S. Karger, Basel, pp. 10-13.

4. Wissler, R.W., Vesselinovitch, D., and Getz, G.S. (1976) Prog. Cardiovas. Dis. 18, 341-369.

5. Wissler, R.W., and Vesselinovitch, D. (1974) in Atherosclerosis III (Proc. 3rd Intl. Symp.) (Schettler, G. and Weizel, A., Eds.), Springer-Verlag, Berlin/Heidelberg/New York, pp. 747-750.

6. Wissler, R.W., and Vesselinovitch, D. (1975) in Verh. deuts. Ges. inn. Med., J.F. Bergmann, Munich, pp. 857-865.

7. Wissler, R.W., and Vesselinovitch, D. (1976) Ann. N.Y. Acad. Sci. 275, 363-378.

8. Wissler, R.W. (1977) in Brain and Heart Infarct, (Zulch, K.J., Ed.), Springer-Verlag, Berlin/Heidelberg/New York, pp. 206-255.

9. Smith, E.B. (1977) Am. J. Pathol. 86, 665-674.

10. Haust, M.D., More, R.H., and Movat, H.Z. (1960) Am. J. Pathol. 37, 377-389.

11. Geer, J.C., McGill, H.C., Jr., and Strong, J.P. (1961) Am. J. Pathol. 38, 263-287.

12. McGill, H.C., and Geer, J.C. (1963) in Evolution of the Athero-sclerotic Plaque (Jones, R.J., Ed.), University of Chicago Press, Chicago, pp. 65-76.

13. Geer, J.C., and Haust, M.D. (1972) Smooth Muscle Cells in Athe-rosclerosis, Vol. 2, S. Karger, Basel.

14. Kao, V.C.Y., and Wissler, R.W. (1965) Exp. Mol. Pathol. 4, 465-479.

15. Knieriem, H.J., Kao, V.C.Y., and Wissler, R.W. (1967) Arch. Pathol. 84, 118-129.

16. Wissler, R.W. (1968) J. Atheroscl. Res. 8, 201-213.

17. Ross, R., and Klebanoff, S.J. (1971) J. Cell Biol. 50, 159-171.

18. Ross, R. (1971) J. Cell Biol. 50, 172-186.

19. Fischer-Dzoga, K., Jones, R.M., Vesselinovitch, D., and Wissler, R.W. (1973) Exp. Mol. Pathol. 18, 162-176.

20. Chen, R., Dzoga, K., Borensztajn, J., and Wissler, R.W. (1972) Circulation 46 (Suppl. II), 253.

21. Chen, R. (1973) Ph.D. Thesis, University of Chicago.

22. Fischer-Dzoga, K., Chen, R., and Wissler, R.W. (1974) in Arterial Mesenchyme and Arteriosclerosis (Wagner, W.D. and Clarkson, T.B., Eds.), Plenum Press, New York, pp. 299-311.

23. Bates, S.R. (1976) Fed. Proc. 35, 7a.

24. Chen, R.M., Getz, G.S., Fischer-Dzoga, K., and Wissler, R.W. (1974) Fed. Proc. 33, 623a.

25. Chen, R.M., Getz, G.S., Fischer-Dzoga, K., and Wissler, R.W. (1977) Exp. Mol. Pathol. 26, 359-374.

26. Chen, R.M., Fischer-Dzoga, K., and Wissler, R.W. (1977) in Atherosclerosis IV (Proc. 4th Intl. Symp.), (Schettler, G., Klose, G., Hata, Y. and Goto, Y., Eds.), Springer-Verlag, Berlin/Heidelberg/New York. In press.

27. Chen, R.M., and Fischer-Dzoga, K. (1977) Atherosclerosis. In press.

28. Hanig, M., Shainoff, J.R., and Lowry, A.D. (1956) Science 124, 176-178.

29. Gero, S., Gergely, J., Jakab, L., Szekely, J., and Virag, S. (1961) J. Atheroscl. Res. 1, 88-91.

30. Tracy, R.E., Merchant, E.B., and Kao, V. (1961) Circ. Res. 9, 472-478.

31. Watts, H.F. (1963) in Evolution of the Atherosclerotic Plaque (Jones, R.J., Ed.), University of Chicago Press, Chicago, pp. 117-132.

32. Walton, K.W., and Williamson, N. (1968) J. Atheroscl. Res. 8, 599-624.

33. Hoff, H.F., Lie, J.T., Titus, J.L., Bayardo, R.J., Jackson, R.,
     L., DeBakey, M.E., and Gotto, A.M., Jr. (1975) Arch. Pathol.
     99, 253-258.

34. Smith, E.B., Slater, R.S., and Crothers, D.C. (1974) in Athero-
     sclerosis III (Proc. 3rd Intl. Symp.), (Schettler, G. and
     Weizel, A., Eds.), Springer-Verlag, Berlin/Heidelberg/New York,
     pp. 96-99.

35. Hollander, W., Kramsch, D.M., and Inoune, G. (1968) in Progress
     in Biochemical Pharmacology, vol. 4 (Miras, C.J., Howard, A.N.
     and Paoletti, R., Eds.), S. Karger, Basel, pp. 270-279.

36. Scott, P.J., and Hurley, P.J. (1970) Atherosclerosis 11, 77-
     103.

37. Brown, M.S., and Goldstein, J.L. (1974) Proc. Nat. Acad. Sci.
     USA 71, 788-790.

38. Brown, M.S., and Goldstein, J.L. (1976) Science 191, 150-154.

39. Goldstein, J.L., and Brown, M.S. (1977) Ann. Rev. Biochem. 46,
     897-930.

40. Weinstein, D.B., Carew, T.E., and Steinberg, D. (1976) Biochim.
     Biophys. Acta 424, 404-421.

41. Iverius, P.H. (1972) J. Biol. Chem. 247, 2607-2613.

42. Berenson, G.S., Srinivasan, S.R., Radhakrishnamurthy, B., and
     Dalferes, E.R., Jr. (1974) in Arterial Mesenchyme and Arterio-
     sclerosis (Wagner, W.D. and Clarkson, T.B., Eds.), Plenum
     Press, New York, pp. 141-159.

43. Tracy, R.E., Dzoga, K., and Wissler, R.W. (1965) Proc. Soc.
     Exp. Biol. Med. 118, 1095-1098.

44. Constantinides, P. (1965) Experimental Atherosclerosis, Else-
     vier, Amsterdam.

45. Bondjers, G., and Bjorkerud, S. (1972) Atherosclerosis 15,
     273-284.

46. Minick, C.R., and Murphy, G.E. (1973) Am. J. Pathol. 73, 265-
     300.

47. Astrup, P., Kjeldsen, K., and Wanstrup, J. (1967) J. Atheroscl.
     Res. 7, 343-354.

48. Ross, R., and Harker, L.B. (1977) N. Engl. J. Med. In press.

49. Kao, V.C.Y., Wissler, R.W., and Dzoga, K. (1968) Circulation 38, (Suppl. IV) 12.

50. Dzoga, K., Vesselinovitch, D., Fraser, R., and Wissler, R.W. (1971) Am. J. Pathol. 62, 32a.

51. Fischer-Dzoga, K., Jones, R.M., Vesselinovitch, D., and Wissler, R.W. (1974) in Atherosclerosis III (Proc. 3rd Intl. Symp.), (Schettler, G. and Weizel, A., Eds.), Springer-Verlag, Berlin/Heidelberg/New York, pp. 193-195.

52. Fischer-Dzoga, K., Wissler, R.W., and Scanu, A.M. (1974) Circulation 50 (Suppl. III), 263.

53. Fischer-Dzoga, K., and Wissler, R.W. (1976) Atherosclerosis 24, 515-525.

54. Fischer-Dzoga, K., Fraser, R., and Wissler, R.W. (1976) Exp. Mol. Pathol. 24, 346-359.

55. Fischer-Dzoga, K., Wissler, R.W., and Scanu, A.M. (1977) in Atherosclerosis: Metabolic, Morphologic and Clinical Aspects (Adv. Exp. Biol. Med., vol. 82), (Manning, G.W. and Haust, M.D., Eds.), Plenum Press, New York, pp. 915-920.

56. Robertson, A.L. (1974) Am. J. Pathol. 74, 94a.

57. Robertson, A.L. (1974) in Atherosclerosis III (Proc. 3rd Intl. Symp.), (Schettler, G. and Weizel, A., Eds.), Springer-Verlag, Berlin/Heidelberg/New York, pp. 175-184.

58. Fischer-Dzoga, K., Vesselinovitch, D., and Wissler, R.W. (1974) Am. J. Pathol. 74, 52a.

59. Yoshida, Y., Fischer-Dzoga, K., and Wissler, R.W. (1977) Circulation. In press.

60. Gospodarowicz, D., and Moran, J.S. (1975) J. Cell Biol. 66, 451-457.

61. Antoniades, H.N., Strathkos, D., and Scher, C.D. (1975) Proc. Nat. Acad. Sci. USA 72, 2635-2639.

62. Ross, R., Glomset, J., Kariya, B., and Harker, L.B. (1974) Proc. Nat. Acad. Sci. USA 71, 1027-1210.

63. Van Wyk, J.J., and Underwood, L.E. (1975) <u>Ann. Rev. Med.</u> 26, 427-441.

64. Ledet, T., Fischer-Dzoga, K., and Wissler, R.W. (1976) <u>Diabetes</u> 25, 207-215.

65. Fischer-Dzoga, K., Pick, R., and Kuo, Y-F. (1977) <u>Circulation.</u> In press.

66. Wissler, R.W. (1977) in <u>Biochemistry of Atherosclerosis</u> (Scanu, A.M., Ed.), Marcel Dekker, New York. In press.

67. Fishman, J.A., Ryan, G.B., and Karnovsky, M.J. (1975) <u>Lab. Invest.</u> 32, 339-351.

68. Bjorkerud, S., and Bondjers, G. (1971) <u>Atherosclerosis</u> 14, 259-276.

69. Bjorkerud, S., and Bondjers, G. (1973) <u>Atherosclerosis</u> 18, 235-255.

70. Glagov, S., and Ts'ao, C.H. (1975) <u>Am. J. Pathol.</u> 79, 7-30.

71. Ross, R., and Harker, L. (1976) <u>Science</u> 193, 1094-1100.

72. Ross, R., and Glomset, J. (1973) <u>Science</u> 180, 1332-1339.

73. Ross, R., and Glomset, J. (1974) in <u>Arterial Mesenchyme and Arteriosclerosis</u> (Wagner, W.D. and Clarkson, T.B., Eds.), Plenum Press, New York, pp. 265-279.

74. Harker, L., Slichter, S.J., Scott, C.R., and Ross, R. (1974) <u>N. Engl. J. Med.</u> 291, 537-543.

75. Harker, L.A., Ross, R., Slichter, S.J., and Scott, C.R. (1976) <u>J. Clin. Invest.</u> 58, 731-741.

76. Moore, S., Friedman, R.J., Singal, D.P., Gauldie, J., and Blajchman, M. (1976) <u>Thromb. Diathes. Haemorrh.</u> 35, 70-81.

77. Benditt, E.P., and Benditt, J.M. (1973) <u>Proc. Nat. Acad. Sci. USA</u> 70, 1753-1756.

78. Pearson, T.A., Wang, A., Solez, K., and Heptinstall, R.H. (1975) <u>Am. J. Pathol.</u> 81, 379-388.

79. Thomas, W.A., Janakidevi, K., Reiner, J.M., and Lee, K.T. (1976) <u>Circulation</u> 54 (Suppl. II), 137.

80. Rothblat, G.H. (1973) in Growth, Nutrition and Metabolism of Cells in Culture, vol. 1, (Rothblat, G.H. and Cristofalo, V., Eds.), Academic Press, New York, pp. 297-325.

81. St. Clair, R.W., Lofland, H.B., Jr., Prichard, R.W., and Clarkson, T.B. (1968) Exp. Mol. Pathol. 8, 201-215.

82. Bates, S.R., and Wissler, R.W. (1976) Biochim. Biophys. Acta 450, 78-88.

83. Peters, T.J., Takano, T., and DeDuve, C. (1973) in Atherogenesis: Initiating Factors (Ciba Found. Symp. 12), Elsevier, Amsterdam, pp. 197-214.

84. Goldfischer, S., Daly, M.M., Kasak, L.E., and Coltoff-Schiller, B. (1975) Circ. Res. 36, 553-561.

85. Smith, E.B., and Slater, R.J. (1973) in Atherogenesis: Initiating Factors (Ciba Found. Symp. 12), Elsevier, Amsterdam, pp. 39-52.

86. Wissler, R.W., and Vesselinovitch, D. (1968) Ann. N.Y. Acad. Sci. 149, 907-922.

87. Wissler, R.W., and Vesselinovitch, D. (1974) in Atherosclerosis III (Proc. 3rd Intl. Symp.), (Schettler, G. and Weizel, A., Eds.), Springer-Verlag, Berlin/Heidelberg/New York, pp. 319-325.

88. Vesslinovitch, D., and Wissler, R.W. (1977) in Atherosclerosis: Metabolic, Morphologic and Clinical Aspects (Adv. Exp. Biol. Med., vol. 82), (Manning, G.W. and Haust, M.D., Eds.), Plenum Press, New York, pp. 614-622.

89. Strong, J.P., Ed. (1976) Atherosclerosis in Primates (Prim. in Med., vol. 9), S. Karger, Basel.

90. Gresham, G.A. (1976) Primate Atherosclerosis, S. Karger, Basel.

91. Wissler, R.W., and Vesselinovitch, D. (1977) Advances in Veterinary Science and Comparative Medicine, Vol. 21, (Simpson, C. F., Ed.), pp. 351-420.

92. Florentin, R.A., and Nam, S.C. (1968) Exp. Mol. Pathol. 8, 263-301.

93. Thomas, W.A., Florentin, R.A., Nam, S.C., Kim, D.N., Jones, R. M., and Lee, K.T. (1968) Arch. Pathol. 86, 621-643.

94. Prichard, R.W., Clarkson, T.B., Goodman, H.O., and Lofland, H. B. (1966) Arch. Pathol. 81, 292-301.

95. Taylor, C.B., Patton, D.E., and Cox, G.E. (1963) A.M.A. Arch. Pathol. 76, 404-412.

96. Taylor, C.B., Manalo-Estrella, P., and Cox, G.E. (1963) A.M.A. Arch. Pathol. 76, 239-249.

97. Kramsch, D.M., and Hollander, W. (1968) Exp. Mol. Pathol. 9, 1-22.

98. Vesselinovitch, D., Getz, G.S., Hughes, R.H., and Wissler, R.W. (1974) Atherosclerosis 20, 303-321.

99. Wissler, R.W., Vesselinovitch, D., Borensztajn, J., Schaffner, T., and Hughes, R. (1976) Fed. Proc. 35, 294.

100. Wissler, R.W., and Vesselinovitch, D. (1977) in Atherosclerosis IV (Proc. 4th Intl. Symp.), (Schettler, G., Klose, G., Hata, Y. and Goto, Y., Eds.), Springer-Verlag, Berlin/Heidelberg/New York. In press.

101. Armstrong, M.L. (1976) Atherosclerosis Reviews 1, 137-182.

102. Wissler, R.W. (1977) in Proceedings of the First Joint Meeting of the German, Swiss and Austrian Societies for Angiology, Springer-Verlag, Berlin/Heidelberg/New York. In press.

103. Armstrong, M.L., Warner, E.D., and Connor, W.E. (1970) Circ. Res. 27, 59-67.

104. Armstrong, M.L., and Megan, M.B. (1972) Circ. Res. 30, 675-680.

105. Armstrong, M.L., and Megan, M.B. (1975) Circ. Res. 36, 256-261.

106. Armstrong, M.L. (1977) in Atherosclerosis IV (Proc. 4th Intl. Symp.), (Schettler, G., Klose, G., Hata, Y. and Goto, Y., Eds.), Springer-Verlag, Berlin/Heidelberg/New York. In press.

107. Vesselinovitch, D., Wissler, R.W., Hughes, R., and Borensztajn, J. (1976) Atherosclerosis 23, 155-176.

108. Wissler, R.W., Vesselinovitch, D., Borensztajn, J., and Hughes, R. (1975) Circulation 52 (Suppl. II), 16.

109. Borensztajn, J., Foreman, K., Wissler, R.W., van Zutphen, H., Vesselinovitch, D., and Hughes, R. (1975) Circulation 52 (Suppl. II), 269.

110. Borensztajn, J. Personal communication.

111. Weber, G., Fabbrini, P., Resi, L., Jones, R., Vesselinovitch, D., and Wissler, R.W. (1977) Atherosclerosis 26, 535-547.

112. Daoud, A.S., Jarmolych, J., Augustyn, J.M., Fritz, K.E., Singh, K.E., and Lee, K.T. (1976) Arch. Pathol. Lab. Med. 100, 372-379.

113. Fritz, K.E., Augustyn, J.M., Jarmolych, J., Daoud, A.S., and Lee, K.T. (1976) Arch. Pathol. Lab. Med. 100, 380-385.

114. Blankenhorn, D.H., Brooks, S.H., Selzer, R.H., Crawford, D.W., and Chin, H.P. (1974) Proc. Soc. Exp. Biol. Med. 145, 1298-1300.

115. Crawford, D.W., Beckenback, E.S., Blankenhorn, D.H., Selzer, R.H., and Brooks, S.H. (1974) Atherosclerosis 19, 231-241.

116. Barndt, R., Jr., Blankenhorn, D.H., Crawford, D.W., and Brooks, S.H. (1977) Ann. Int. Med. 86, 139-146.

117. Blankenhorn, D. (1977) in Atherosclerosis: Metabolic, Morphologic and Clinical Aspects (Adv. Exp. Biol. Med., vol. 82), (Manning, G.W. and Haust, M.D., Eds.), Plenum Press, New York, pp. 453-458.

118. Buchwald, H., Moore, R.B., and Varco, R.L. (1975) in Lipids, Lipoproteins and Drugs (Adv. Exp. Biol. Med., vol. 63), (Kritchevsky, D., Paoletti, R. and Holmes, W.L., Eds.), Plenum Press, New York, pp. 221-230.

119. Buchwald, H., Amplatz, K., and Varco, R.L. (1977) in Proceedings of the International Symposium State of Prevention and Therapy in Human Arteriosclerosis and in Animal Models, Springer-Verlag, Berlin/Heidelberg/New York. In press.

120. Chen, R.M. (1975) Presented in a paper which won the Young Investigator's Award of the American College of Cardiology.

CLINICAL AND PATHOLOGICAL ASPECTS OF ARTERIAL

THROMBOSIS AND THROMBOEMBOLISM

Colin J. Schwartz, A. Bleakley Chandler,
Ross G. Gerrity and Herbert K. Naito

The Cleveland Clinic Foundation, Cleveland, Ohio
The Department of Pathology, Medical College of
Georgia, Augusta, Georgia

Although over one hundred years have elapsed since the succinct mid-19th century descriptions of thrombosis and thrombogenesis were published (1-5), widespread recognition of the clinical importance of thrombosis and thromboembolism in a variety of disease states is largely a phenomenon of the 20th century. It was, for example, not until early in this century that the first authoritative clinical descriptions of coronary thrombosis and myocardial infarction were provided (6, 7), even though William Herberden had, with meticulous accuracy described the features of angina pectoris in 1772 (8), and Hammer in 1878 (9) had correctly diagnosed coronary thrombosis during life.

Arterial thromboembolism was described in 1684 by Dr. William Gould of Oxford (10), who noted that particles of a "polypus" in the left ventrical of the heart could be broken off by the bloodstream and impacted into the carotid arteries. Another seminal account of arterial thromboembolism was that of Kirkes (11), a physician at St. Bartholomew's Hospital, London. In his paper entitled "On Some of the Principal Effects Resulting from the Detachment of Fibrinous Deposits From the Interior of the Heart, and Their Mixture with the Circulating Blood" published in 1852, he described embolism associated with probable bacterial endocarditis, and also emboli to the lower extremity complicating an abdominal aortic aneurysm. While the pathological basis for, and effects of, large thromboemboli are well known, microembolic disease is assuming a greater degree of clinical and pathological importance, largely as a result of the landmark observations of Russell in 1961 (12) on retinal artery microembolism and the subsequent study of Gunning and his colleagues in 1964 on retinal and cerebral ischemia (13).

PATHOGENESIS OF ARTERIAL THROMBOSIS

Thrombi form from flowing blood in both arteries and veins. In arteries, in situ mixed thrombi usually develop at the site of an underlying intimal injury. The basic structure of mixed thrombi, which are composed of platelet-fibrin units bordered by leucocytes and variable numbers of entrapped red blood cells, is similar at any site of formation. In general, the site of formation and local conditions of blood flow influence structure. Thrombi that form in fast-moving pulsatile arterial blood are apt to contain more platelets and fewer entrapped red cells and to be more compact than thrombi that have formed in slower currents of veins (14).

By far, the most frequent arterial lesions associated with thrombi are those of atherosclerotic origin. Benson in 1926 (15) noted that coronary thrombi customarily develop in narrowed and sclerotic arteries in which the luminal or plaque surface is physically disrupted. There remains little doubt that disruption of the plaque surface, variously described as intimal tears or ulcerations, plaque fissures, or plaque ruptures, is associated with a significant number of arterial thrombi (13, 16-20). Despite the early awareness of these ulcerative lesions, little is still known of their pathogenesis. Intramural or plaque hemorrhage, a suction Venturi effect, and failure of endothelium to regenerate have been cited as factors in the genesis and perpetuation of these lesions (21). Whatever the cause, rupture or ulceration of an atherosclerotic plaque clearly exposes to the lumen thrombogenic elements within the arterial wall. Exposed connective tissue fibers promote platelet adhesion and aggregation, while both collagen and tissue thromboplastin activate the coagulation system to generate thrombin.

In reviewing these aspects of the pathogenesis of arterial thrombosis, it should be recognized that the association between plaque rupture and thrombosis, although impressive, is not universal. Arterial thrombi may develop over minor intimal breaks of largely fibrous plaques in the absence of underlying hemorrhage or rupture of a necrotic atheroma (22, 23). Hemodynamic factors also may interact with acute arterial injury to promote thrombosis. The separation of platelets from blood and their deposition at sites of injury is enhanced in zones of slowed or turbulent flow, and the removal of thrombogenic substances generated in the blood or released from an injured vessel wall may be retarded. Lastly, it is possible that changes in the thrombogenic potential of the blood itself may be as important in thrombogenesis as the influence of localized arterial lesions.

Once a mural thrombus has formed, it may provide a nidus for its own subsequent growth. Many thrombi have layers of differing age, which suggests that they were formed episodically over a period of time. Though recurrent thrombosis is commonly observed, the mechanisms governing this form of growth remain unexplained. It has been proposed that the older thrombus may absorb and accumulate on its surface thrombogenic substances from the blood until a critical level initiates another episode of thrombosis (14). Repeated thrombotic deposits may be important in the progressive build-up of a stenotic lumen in a process that may extend over months or years until ultimate occlusion of the artery (24).

Recent thrombotic occlusion of some arteries, notably the carotid, coronary, and iliac arteries is associated with a greater degree of adventitial lymphocytic infiltration than would be anticipated on the basis of plaque severity alone (25). This observation may indicate that thrombosis induces an adventitial lymphocytosis, or alternatively that an immune mechanism reflected by the lymphocytic infiltration, is in some way associated with thrombogenesis.

THROMBOSIS IN THE CORONARY CIRCULATION

The frequency and role of occlusive coronary thrombi in myocardial infarction have been the subject of sporadic and oft-times vigorous debate. A number of investigators have reported a relatively low frequency of occlusive thrombi and some have concluded that the thrombi are younger than the associated infarcts (26). As a result, it has been argued that coronary arterial thrombosis is a consequence rather than a cause of acute infarction. One step toward clarification of this issue has been the recognition that only one form of acute myocardial infarction is usually associated with coronary thrombosis. Thrombotic occlusion is frequently found in regional transmural infarction, but is infrequent in subendocardial infarction. These data are included in Table 1, where the frequency of coronary thrombosis is considered according to both clinical and pathological categories (27-34).

The incorporation of ^{125}I-fibrinogen into coronary arterial thrombi after the onset of typical ischemic chest pain and electrocardiographic changes of recent anteroseptal infarction was interpreted by Erhardt et al. (35) as evidence that thrombosis occurs after infarction. However, it was recognized at the time that a pre-existing thrombus could incorporate radiofibrinogen by subsequent propagation (35). Furthermore, Moschos et al. (36) have demonstrated that radiofibrinogen can penetrate experimental coronary arterial thrombi after their formation. Subsequently, Erhardt et al. (37) modified their earlier views to suggest that the major part of the thrombus may form after the onset of necrosis. Fulton and

Sumner (38) have corroborated the findings of Erhardt et al. (37) in similar studies that have shown by means of more detailed correlative morphologic appraisals that the central occlusive portion of a thrombus subtending an infarct is characteristically radionegative, which would indicate formation of the thrombus before administration of radiofibrinogen and antecedent to infarction.

The pathologists who hold that coronary thrombi cause infarcts point out that the thrombi are consistently located at a proximal position in the artery supplying the infarcted myocardium and that the thrombi, in most cases, are found to arise at specific sites of rupture or ulceration of atherosclerotic plaques (26). The striking and consistent spatial relationships between occlusive thrombi and myocardial infarcts, in conjunction with the high frequency of thrombi in transmural infarction together provide strong evidence that prior thrombosis is critical to the development of transmural myocardial infarcts. In marked contrast to transmural infarction, subendocardial infarction is only infrequently associated with occlusive coronary thrombi (27, 34). It is likely that anomalies in regional myocardial perfusion plus severe coronary stenosis rather than acute thrombotic occlusion of the epicardial arteries are major factors in the development of so-called subendocardial infarction.

Not all occlusive coronary thrombi, of course, are associated with myocardial infarction. If the collateral circulation is adequate, an infarct may not develop following an acute thrombotic occlusion (17, 39). At times, acute thrombi are present in patients who die suddenly, before an infarct has had time to develop. This phenomenon may occur in coronary embolism or in cases of severe coronary atherosclerosis with acute coronary thrombosis. The immediate fatal event in these cases is probably a cardiac arrythmia (40). It should be emphasized that coronary thrombosis is by no means found in all cases of sudden cardiac death occurring in the presence of advanced coronary sclerosis (41). Coronary thrombosis occurs in about one-third of the cases in patients dying within 10 mintues to two hours of the onset of the fatal illness and in even fewer cases in those patients who die instantaneously (Table 1). Clearly, explanations in addition to coronary thrombosis must be sought for precipitating causes of lethal arrythmias in sudden cardiac death.

These observations on the interrelationships of coronary thrombosis, myocardial infarction, and sudden cardiac death derived from autopsy studies are in good agreement with an important clinical study recently reported by Cobb et al. (42). In a unique population of patients in Seattle, Washington, only a small number of those who were successfully resuscitated after prehospital ven-

Table 1. Frequency of Coronary Arterial Thrombosis in Various Categories of Recent Myocardial Infarction and Sudden Cardiac Death.

Category & Reference	No. of Cases	Frequency of Coronary Thrombosis
Transmural Infarction		
Miller et al.[27]	93	90%
Workshop Report; Chandler, et al.[32]	597	54 - 96.5%*
Davies et al.[34]	469	95%
Subendocardial Infarction		
Miller et al.[27]	50	20%
Davies et al.[34]	31	13%
Sudden Cardiac Death (within time of onset)		
Friedman et al.[31] (within 30 seconds)	25	4%
Haerem[33] (within 10 minutes)	47	30%
Spain and Bradess[29] (within 1 hour)	303	16%
Scott and Briggs[30] (within 1 hour)	183	30%
Adelson and Hoffman[28] (within 2 hours)	560	33%

*Report of 5 studies: Roberts 40/74, cases 54%; Schwartz 18/21, 86%; Spain 45/50, 90%; Chapman 257/282, 91%; Sinapius 164/170, 96.5%.

tricular fibrillation subsequently developed evidence of transmural
infarction. Specifically, pathological Q waves, indicative of
transmural infarction were observed in 16%, and elevated myocardial
serum isoenzyme levels were observed in only 45% of the patients
surviving resuscitation. Elevated isoenzyme levels alone in some
of the surviving patients would suggest the presence of myocardial
necrosis that may or may not be associated with thrombi in the coronary circulation. In this population, only a small proportion
of the patients subsequently developed transmural infarction, a
finding that is compatible with the low frequency of coronary
thrombosis in autopsy studies of sudden cardiac death.

ARTERIAL THROMBOEMBOLISM AND MICROEMBOLISM

Emboli may arise from thrombi on the valvular endocardium,
the mural endocardium, usually in association with infarction, and
from ulcerated plaques or aneurysms of the aorta and great vessels.
Emboli arising from the mitral or aortic valves, or from mural
thrombi in the left ventricle most frequently produce clinical
manifestations by obstruction of the circulation in the cerebral,
mesenteric, renal, splenic, and lower limb arteries. Indeed, acute
arterial thromboembolism is not an infrequent presentation of an
hitherto unrecognized or silent myocardial infarction. Mural aortic thrombosis not infrequently gives rise to renal artery thromboembolism, which may be important in the genesis of some instances
of renal disease and hypertension (43). Similarly, aortic emboli
of either thrombotic or atheromatous material may contribute to
ischemia in some cases of chronic mesenteric or peripheral vascular
insufficiency.

Thrombotic microemboli, like their larger counterparts, are
derived from mural thrombi, from valvular endocarditis, and during
cardiopulmonary bypass procedures. In the latter, the small platelet-fibrin plugs, frequent in the microcirculation within the first
24 hours, have largely disappeared by 48 hours (44). Such observations emphasize the transient nature of many microemboli, and
the possibility that their frequency in the microcirculation is
likely to be considerably underestimated.

Although many platelet microthrombi and emboli originate in
the blood-vascular interface, it is important to recognize that
embolic microthrombi may also form within the circulation without
any apparent contact with the arterial wall. For example, in both
the rat (45) and the pig (46) infused platelet aggregants such as
adenosine diphosphate result in the production of transient intravascular microthrombi of aggregated platelets. In the pig, intra-
coronary artery infusions of adenosine diphosphate are associated
with transient platelet aggregation in the myocardial microcirculation and a high frequency of lethal arrhythmias, which may be

induced by ischemia of the conduction system, possibly in conjunction with the release of platelet constituents (46). The constituents released by platelets may have profound effects not only on
the structure and function of the arterial wall but also on the
development of lethal cardiac arrythmias. The dense granules have
been shown to contain serotonin, adenosine diphosphate and triphos-
phate, and antiplasmin, while the alpha-granules have a number of
lysosomal enzymes (47).

The role of platelet microthrombi and microemboli in the pathogenesis of some cases of sudden cardiac death has been the subject
of increasing interest. Haerem (48, 49) and Jørgensen et al. (50)
have observed platelet microthrombi and emboli in the coronary vasculature in a number of cases of sudden cardiac death occurring
instantaneously or within a few minutes of the onset of the fatal
illness. Coronary microemboli may arise from thrombi in the coronary arteries, the heart, the ascending aorta, or alternatively
may form within the circulation itself. At least some intramyocardial microthrombi may have arisen by embolization from mural thrombi in the more proximal segments of the coronary arteries (33).

Apart from the potential role of platelet microemboli in the
genesis of some cases of sudden cardiac death, there appears to be
little doubt that microthromboemboli are important in the pathogenesis of transient monocular blindness and cerebral ischemia (12,
13). Nevertheless, the probable short-lived and reversible nature
of these small emboli make it desirable to exercise caution in
evaluating their significance in the production of ischemia in
these and other areas of the body (41).

POTENTIAL RISK FACTORS FOR ARTERIAL THROMBOSIS

Inasmuch as thrombosis and atherosclerosis are so closely
associated, risk factors for clinical arterial disease usually do
not differentiate between atherogenesis and thrombogenesis. Clinical manifestations that reflect such secondary events as infarction
are generally unreliable markers for specifically detecting thrombosis. There is an increasing body of both experimental and human
data, however, linking certain risk factors for arterial disease
such as disturbed lipid metabolism with altered blood coagulation,
platelet function, and thrombosis (51-60). Recent studies have
shown abnormal in vitro platelet function in patients with Type II
hyperlipoproteinemia (61, 62) and an increased frequency of thrombotic events has been reported in this disorder (63). Whether such
findings of abnormal platelet reactivity reflect differences in
platelet membrane structure, the fatty acid composition of membrane
phospholipids and subsequent prostaglandin synthesis, or some other
mechanism, has yet to be established.

Cigarette smoking, like dietary and plasma lipids, may enhance the risk for clinical coronary disease through a thrombogenic mechanism. Mustard and Murphy (64) have established that smoking reduces platelet survival in man. Whether a shortened platelet survival is secondary to endothelial injury or to intrinsic platelet alterations has yet to be established (65). In a large scale and comprehensive prospective study of hemostatic variables in ischemic heart disease now underway in England, it has been found that smoking in males is associated with increased plasma levels of fibrinogen and lowered fibrinolytic activity (66). It is anticipated that this study will give further insight into the complex interrelationships between hemostatic variables, thrombosis, and atherosclerosis.

There seems little doubt that both venous thromboembolism and arterial thrombosis occur more frequently in women taking oral contraceptives. Mann and Inman (67) concluded that the risk of fatal myocardial infarction was greatest in the older age groups. Other studies have come to essentially similar conclusions, with respect to both myocardial infarction and cerebrovascular disease (68, 69). The mechanisms by which oral contraceptives influence thrombosis are incompletely known. Elevated plasma lipids have been reported, the most estrogenic of the pills resulting in the highest triglyceride levels, and the most progestational giving the highest cholesterol levels (70). Wessler et al. (71) have demonstrated that estrogenic-containing contraceptives significantly retard factor Xa inhibitory activity. Meade et al. (72) found fibrinogen levels elevated and fibrinolytic activity increased. Smoking abolished the effect on fibrinolytic activity in these subjects, whereas fibrinogen levels significantly increased with age.

THROMBOSIS AND ATHEROGENESIS

In his "Manual of Pathological Anatomy" (73), the celebrated pathologist Carl von Rokitansky first postulated what has become widely known as the thrombogenic or encrustation hypothesis of atherosclerosis. Rokitansky proposed that the disease is the result of an excessive intimal deposition of blood components, including fibrin. In recent years, it has been demonstrated conclusively that the organization of experimental thrombi may result in atheromatous plaques, both in the pulmonary arteries (74-84), and in the systemic circulation (85-94). Indeed, it has been found that fibrofatty atherosclerotic plaques can form from experimental platelet-rich thrombi or thromboemboli in the absence of any dietary manipulation that might produce hyperlipemia (79, 80, 91, 93). Cellular elements of thrombi, especially platelets, which are rich in lipids, and entrapped or absorbed plasma lipids may contribute to the fat content of thrombic plaques (95-97), while fibrin seems to actively stimulate the production of collagen (98, 99).

All of the experimental studies cited support the pathological observations in man that indicate that plaque growth may be greatly dependent upon the organization and incorporation of mural thrombi (18, 24, 73, 98-106). The laminated structure of many atheromatous lesions suggests they were formed by repeated deposits of thrombi (18, 24, 100, 103). The true extent of the thrombotic contribution to plaque growth in a given case, however, is difficult to ascertain, for, in time, the resolution and conversion of residual thrombi to plaque tissue may obscure the thrombotic origin of the lesion. For this reason, any estimate of the frequency of thrombi incorporated in plaques is apt to be an underestimation. Although there is only limited evidence that incorporation of thrombi is a factor in the inception of atherosclerosis, it seems clear that this mechanism is a major factor in the growth and progression of atherosclerotic lesions (107).

Of the three important mechanisms relating the processes of thrombosis and atherogenesis, the least controversial concerns organization and incorporation of mural thrombi. This mechanism is examined in depth in Dr. Woolf's chapter. The remaining two mechanisms relate to the role of platelets and platelet constituents in the initiation or enhancement of endothelial and arterial injury, and secondly, to a mitogen derived from platelets that is considered to influence the proliferation of smooth muscle cells in atherogenesis. Jørgensen et al. (108) have demonstrated deposition of formed elements of the blood in areas of spontaneously-enhanced aortic endothelial permeability to proteins (109-111). They have suggested that both platelets and leucocytes may cause focal vascular injury in areas of abnormal or altered blood flow (108). Such foci are characterized by the uptake of the protein-binding azo dye, Evans Blue, and are considered to represent sites destined to develop atheromatous lesions subsequently (108, 109, 112, 113). The complex nature of platelet-vascular interactions, the platelet mitogen described by Ross et al. (114), and the pathological implications of the platelet secretory-release reaction in atherogenesis are discussed in detail in other presentations and workshops of these proceedings.

REFERENCES

1. Wharton-Jones, T. (1852) Phil. Trans. 142, 131-136.

2. Virchow, R. (1860) Cellular Pathology, 7th American Ed., R.M. Dewitt, New York, pp. 230-245.

3. Bizzozero, J. (1882) Virchows Arch. Path. Anat. 90, 261-332.

4. Eberth, C.J., and Schimmelbusch, C. (1888) Die Thrombose nach Versuchen und Leichenbefunden, Ferdinand Enke, Stuttgart, p. 144.

5. Welch, W.H. (1899) in A System of Medicine (Allbutt, T.C., Ed.), MacMillan and Co., Ltd., London, Volume 6, pp. 155-285.

6. Obrastov, W.P., and Straschko, N.D. (1910) Z. Klein Med. 71, 116-132.

7. Herrick, J. (1912) JAMA 59, 2015-2020.

8. Herberden, W. (1772) Trans. Coll. Physns. Lond. 2, 59-67.

9. Hammer, A. (1878) Wien. Med. Wschr. 28, 97-102.

10. Gould, W. (1684) Phil. Trans. 14, 537-548, reprinted 1963.

11. Kirkes, W.S. (1852) Med. Chirurg. Trans. 35, 281-324.

12. Russell, R.W.R. (1961) Lancet 2, 1422-1428.

13. Gunning, A.J., Pickering, G.W., Robb-Smith, A.H.T., and Russell, R.W.R. (1964) Quart. J. Med. 33, 155-195.

14. Chandler, A.B. (1969) in Thrombosis (Sherry, S., Brinkhaus, K.M., Genton, E. and Stengle, J.M., Eds.), Natl. Acad. Sci., Washington, pp. 279-299.

15. Benson, R.L. (1926) Arch. Pathol. 2, 870-916.

16. Leary, T. (1934) Arch. Pathol. 17, 453-492.

17. Saphir, O., Priest, W.S., Hamburger, W.W., and Katz, L.N. (1935) Am. Heart J. 10, 567-595; 762-792.

18. Clark, E., Graef, I., and Chasis, H. (1936) Arch. Pathol. 22, 183-212.

19. Chapman, I. (1965) Arch. Pathol. 256-261.

20. Constantinides, P. (1966) J. Atheroscler. Res. 6, 1-17.

21. Chandler, A.B. (1974) Thrombosis Research 4, Suppl. 1, 3-23.

22. Fischer, S. (1964) J. Atheroscler. Res. 4, 230-238.

23. Jørgensen, L., Chandler, A.B. and Borchgrevink, C.F. (1971) Atherosclerosis 13, 21-44.

24. Crawford, T. (1963) in Evolution of the Atherosclerotic Plaque (Jones, R.J. Ed.), University of Chicago Press, Chicago, pp. 279-290.

25. Schwartz, C.J., and Mitchell, J.R.A. (1962) Circulation 36, 73-78.

26. Chandler, A.B. (1975) Mod. Concepts Cardiovasc. Dis. 44, 1-5.

27. Miller, R.D., Burchell, H.B., and Edwards, J.E. (1951) Arch. Int. Med. 88, 597-604.

28. Adelson, L., and Hoffman, W. (1961) JAMA 176, 129-135.

29. Spain, D.M., and Bradess, V.A. (1960) Am. J. Med. Sci. 240, 701-710.

30. Scott, R.F., and Briggs, T.S. (1972) Am. J. Cardiol. 29, 782-787.

31. Friedman, M., Manwaring, J.H., Rosenman, R.H., Donlon, G., Ortega, P., and Grube, S.M. (1973) JAMA 225, 1319-1328.

32. Chandler, A.B., Chapman, I., Erhardt, L.R., Roberts, W.C., Schwartz, C.J., Sinapius, D., Spain, D.M., Sherry, S., Ness, P.M., and Simons, T.L. (1974) Am. J. Cardiol. 34, 823-833.

33. Haerem, J.W. (1974) Atherosclerosis 19, 529-541.

34. Davies, M.J., Woolf, N., and Robertson, W.B. (1976) Br. Heart J. 38, 659-664.

35. Erhardt, L.R., Lundman, T., and Mellstedt, H. (1973) Lancet 1, 387-390.

36. Moschos, C.B., Oldewurtel, H.A., Haider, B., and Regan, T.J. (1976) Circulation 54, 653-656.

37. Erhardt, L.R., Unge, G., and Boman, G. (1976) Am. Heart J. 91, 592-598.

38. Fulton, W.F.M., and Sumner, D.J. (1977) Am. J. Cardiol. 39, 322.

39. Blumgart, H.L., Schlesinger, M.J. and Davis, D. (1940) Am. Heart J. 19, 1-91.

40. Romo, M. (1972) Acta Med. Scand. Suppl. 547, 1-92.

41. Schwartz, C.J., and Gerrity, R.G. (1975) Circulation, 51 and 52, Suppl. III, 18-26.

42. Cobb, L.A., Baum, R.S., Alvarez, H., and Schaffer, W.A. (1975) Circulation 51 and 52, Suppl. III, 223-228.

43. Moore, S., and Mersereau, W.A. (1968) Arch. Pathol. 85, 623-630.

44. Schwartz, C.J., Korns, M.E., Edwards, J.E., and Lillehei, C.W. (1970) Arch. Pathol. 89, 56-64.

45. Nordøy, A., and Chandler, A.B. (1964) Scand. J. Haematol. 1, 16-25.

46. Jørgensen, L., Rowsell, H.C., Hovig, T., Glynn, M.F., and Mustard, J.F. (1967) Lab. Invest. 17, 616-644.

47. Holmsen, H. (1975) in Biochemistry and Pharmacology of Platelets (Born, G.V.R., Ed.), Ciba Found. Symp. 35, Elsevier, Amsterdam, pp. 175-196.

48. Haerem, J.W. (1971) Atherosclerosis 14, 417-432.

49. Haerem, J.W. (1972) Atherosclerosis 15, 199-213.

50. Jørgensen, L., Haerem, J.W., Chandler, A.B., and Borchgrevink, C.F. (1968) Acta. Anaesth. Scand. Suppl. 29, 193-199.

51. Poole, J.C.F. (1955) Brit. J. Exp. Path. 36, 248-253.

52. Greig, H.B.W., and Runde, I.A. (1957) Lancet 2, 461-464.

53. Mustard, J.F., and Murphy, E.A. (1962) Br. Med. J. 1, 1651-1655.

54. Mustard, J.F., Rowsell, H.C., Murphy, E.A., and Downie, H.S. (1963) J. Clin. Invest. 42, 1783-1789.

55. Ardlie, N.G., Kinlough, R.L., Glew, G., and Schwartz, C.J. (1966) Aust. J. Exp. Biol. Med. Sci. 44, 105-110.

56. Conner, W.E., Hoak, J.C., and Warner, E.D. (1969) in Thrombosis (Sherry, S., Brinkhous, K.M., Genton, E. and Stengle, J.M., Eds.), Natl. Acad. Sci., Washington, pp. 355-373.

57. Renaud, S., Kinlough, R.L., and Mustard, J.F. (1970) Lab. Invest. 22, 339-343.

58. Hornstra, G. (1973-74) Haemostasis 2, 21-53.

59. Hornstra, G., and Lussenburg, R.N. (1975) Atherosclerosis 22, 499-516.

60. Nordøy, A. (1976) Thrombos. Haemostas. 35, 32-48.

61. Carvalho, A.C.A., Colman, R.W., and Lees, R.S. (1974) Circulation 50, 570-574.

62. Carvalho, A.C.A., Colman, R.W., and Lees, R.S. (1974) N. Engl. J. Med. 290, 434-438.

63. Carvalho, A.C.A., Lees, R.S., Vaillancourt, R.A., and Colman, R.W. (1977) Circulation 56, 114-118.

64. Mustard, J.F., and Murphy, E.A. (1963) Br. Med. J. 1, 846-849.

65. Murphy, E.A., and Mustard, J.F. (1966) Am. J. Public Health 56, 1061-1073.

66. Meade, T.W., and North, W.R.S. (1977) Br. Med. Bull. 33, 283-288.

67. Mann, J.I., and Inman, W.H.W. (1975) Br. Med. J. 2, 245-248.

68. Mann, J.I., Vessey, M.P., Thorogood, M., and Doll, R. (1975) Br. Med. J. 2, 241-245.

69. Masi, A.T., and Dugdale, M. (1970) Ann. Int. Med. 72, 111-121.

70. Stokes, T., and Wynn, V. (1972) Lancet 2, 677-680.

71. Wessler, S., Gitel, S.N., Wan, L.S., and Pasternack, B.S. (1976) JAMA 236, 2179-2182.

72. Meade, T.W., Borzovic, M., Chakrabarti, R., Howarth, D.J., North, W.R.S., and Stirling, Y. (1976) Br. J. Haematol. 34, 353-364.

73. Rokitansky, C.A. (1855) Manual of Pathological Anatomy, (Swaine, W.E., Sieveking, E., Moore, C.H. and Day, G.E., translators), Blanchard and Lea, Philadelphia, Vol. 4, pp. 198-207.

74. Harrison, C.V. (1948) J. Path. Bact. 60, 289-293.

75. Heard, B.E. (1952) J. Path. Bact. 64, 13-19.

76. McLetchie, N.G.B. (1952) Am. J. Pathol. 28, 413-435.

77. Barnard, P.J. (1953) J. Path. Bact. 65, 129-136.

78. Thomas, W.A., O'Neal, R.M., and Lee, K.T. (1956) Arch. Pathol. 61, 380-389.

79. Hand, R.A., and Chandler, A.B. (1962) Am. J. Pathol. 40, 469-486.

80. Ardlie, N.G., and Schwartz, C.J. (1968) J. Path. Bact. 95, 1-18.

81. Ardlie, N.G., and Schwartz, C.J. (1968) J. Path. Bact. 95, 19-29.

82. Craig, I.H., and Schwartz, C.J. (1972) Pathol. 4, 303-306.

83. Craig, I.H., Bell, F.P., Goldsmith, C.H., and Schwartz, C.J. (1973) Atherosclerosis 18, 277-300.

84. Craig, I.H., Bell, F.P., and Schwartz, C.J. (1973) Exp. Molec. Path. 18, 290-304.

85. Williams, G. (1955) J. Path. Bact. 69, 199-206.

86. Friedman, M., and Byers, S.O. (1961) J. Clin. Invest. 40, 1139-1152.

87. Mitchell, J.R.A. (1964) in Biological Aspects of Occlusive Vascular Disease, (Chalfmer, D.G. and Gresham, G.A., Eds.), Cambridge University Press, Cambridge, pp. 185-190.

88. Jørgensen, L., Rowsell, H.C., Hovig, T., and Mustard, J.L. (1967) Am. J. Pathol. 51, 681-719.

89. Woolf, N., Bradley, J.W.P., Crawford, T., and Carstairs, C. (1968) Br. J. Exp. Path. 49, 257-264.

90. Crawford, T., and Woolf, N. (1970) Thromb. Diath. Haemorrh. Suppl. 40, 289-295.

91, Moore, S. (1973) Lab. Invest. 29, 478-487.

92. Prathhap, K. (1973) J. Pathol. 110, 145-151, and 203-212.

93. Sumiyoshi, A., Moore, R.H., and Weignesberg, B.I. (1973) Atherosclerosis 18, 43-57.

94. Pope, J.T., Chandler, A.B., Asokan, S.K., and Pollard, D. (1973) Circulation 48, Suppl. 4, 204.

95. Chandler, A.B., and Hand, R.A. (1961) Science 134, 946-947.

96. Woolf, N., Pilkington, T.R.E., and Carstairs, K.C. (1966) J. Path. Bact. 91, 383.

97. Weigensberg, B.I., and More, R.H. (1977) in Atherosclerosis (Manning, G.W. and Haust, M.D., Eds.) Plenum Press, New York, pp. 552-557.

98. Mallory, F.B. (1912-13) in The Harvey Lectures, J.B. Lippincott Co., Philadelphia, pp. 150-166.

99. Haust, M.D., Movat, H.Z., and More, R.H. (1956) Circulation 14, 483.

100. Duguid, J.B. (1946) J. Path. Bact. 58, 207-212.

101. Heard, B.E. (1949) J. Path. Bact. 61, 635-637.

102. Crawford, T., and Levene, C.I. (1952) J. Path. Bact. 64, 523-528.

103. Morgan, A.D. (1956) The Pathogenesis of Coronary Occlusion, Blackwell Scientific Publication, Oxford, p. 171.

104. Haust, M.D., More, R.H., and Movat, H.Z. (1959) Am. J. Pathol. 35, 265-273.

105. Mitchell, J.R.A., and Schwartz, C.J. (1965) Arterial Disease, Blackwell Scientific Publication, Oxford, pp. 283-325.

106. Woolf, N., and Carstairs, K.C. (1967) Am. J. Pathol. 51, 373-386.

107. Chandler, A.B., and Pope, J.T. (1975) in Blood and Arterial Wall in Atherogenesis and Arterial Thrombosis (Hautvast, J.G. A.J., Hermus, R.J.J. and Van Der Haar, R., Eds.) E.J. Brill, Leiden, Netherlands, pp. 110-118.

108. Jørgensen, L., Packham, M.A., Rowsell, H.C., and Mustard, J.F. (1972) Lab Invest. 27, 341-350.

109. Packham, M.A., Rowsell, H.C., Jørgensen, L., and Mustard, J.F. (1967) Exp. Molec. Path. 7, 214-232.

110. Bell, F.P., Adamson, I.L., and Schwartz, C.J. (1974) Exp. Molec. Path. 20, 57-68.

111. Bell, F.P., Gallus, A., and Schwartz, C.J. (1974) Exp. Molec. Path. 20, 281-292.

112. McGill, H.C., Geer, J.C., and Holman, R.L. (1957) Arch. Path.
     64, 303-311.

113. Schwartz, C.J., Somer, J.B., and Gerrity, R.G. (1978) in Very
     Early Recognition of Coronary Heart Disease, (McDonald, L., Ed.),
     Excerpta Medica, Amsterdam. In press.

114. Ross, R., Glomset, J., Kariya, B., and Harker, L. (1974) Proc.
     Natl. Acad. Sci. USA 71, 1207-1210.

PLATELETS, THROMBOSIS AND ATHEROSCLEROSIS

J.F. Mustard, M.A. Packham, R. Kinlough-Rathbone
Faculty of Health Sciences, McMaster University, Hamilton
Faculty of Medicine, University of Toronto,
Toronto, Ontario, Canada

Injury to the endothelium plays an important part in the development of atherosclerosis and its thromboembolic complications. The constituents of the blood that interact at the injury site are platelets, blood coagulation factors, white blood cells, and plasma lipoproteins. Hemodynamic forces also influence the process. Materials released or formed from platelets can affect the endothelium and the smooth muscle cells in the vessel wall. In addition, substances formed by the vessel wall at the injury site (such as prostaglandins and proteoglycans) influence the formation of thrombi and the development of atherosclerotic lesions.

VESSEL INJURY

Injury to the endothelium causes migration of smooth muscle cells into the intima and their proliferation (1-3). This response has been shown to occur in rats (4), rabbits (2, 3), pigs (5), monkeys (1), and man (6), when the endothelium is removed. The methods used to produce experimental endothelial injury include indwelling cannulae (3), balloon catheters (2), antibodies (7), air drying of the endothelium (4), infusion of homocystine (8), and hypercholesterolemia (1).

A number of factors have been shown to be, or are suspected of being injurious to the endothelium. These include bacteria and products such as endotoxin (9), viruses (10), products associated with smoking such as carbon monoxide (11), and antigen-antibody complexes (12). Hemodynamic forces (13) also contribute to vessel wall injury. The frequency and sites of endothelial injury in young humans (14) and normal animals (15) have been studied. The principal sites appear to be around vessel orifices and branches, and regions of the vessel wall where there is a major bend in the vessel.

Morphological examination of the sites of predilection for athe-rosclerosis in young humans killed in accidents (14) showed intimal edema, accumulation of white cells, platelets and platelet-fibrin thrombi, and some loss of endothelium. This morphological evidence is compatible with the conclusion that there are focal sites of ⌐do-thelial injury and inflammation in the human aorta. Similar patterns of focal endothelial injury have been found in pigs (14-17), and rab-bits (15). These sites correspond to the regions where atheroscle-rosis develops in the vessels of these animals. Because these sites are associated with vessel branches and orifices, hemodynamic forces may contribute to the alteration of the endothelium (18).

Altered flow patterns may concentrate substances in the blood at certain sites; these substances may include ones that are injuri-ous to the endothelium (19). In addition, regions of disturbed flow play an important part in causing extensive formed element deposition (20, 21). A number of factors can influence the endothe-lium, such as bradykinin (22), angiotensin (23), cationic protein from white blood cells (24) and platelets (25), and thrombin. Re-cently it has been shown that when endothelial cells are appropri-ately stimulated they can synthesize prostaglandins, in particular PGI_2, which causes relaxation of some smooth muscle, such as in arteries, and inhibits platelet aggregation (26). It is of some interest that exposure of the endothelium to thrombin changes its surface characteristics so that it becomes attractive to platelets (27) and the endothelium may be injured in sites of local thrombin generation (28). Thrombin formation on the surface of the normal endothelium could lead to platelet adherence to the endothelium and the release of factors that could damage it.

EFFECT OF BLOOD CONSTITUENTS

There are a number of components of the blood that may modify the response of the vessel to endothelial injury. These include hormones such as insulin, vasoactive peptides, substances released by formed elements such as platelets and white blood cells, products derived from blood coagulation, and plasma lipoproteins. Of prin-cipal interest at the present moment are the effects of products released by platelets and the effects of plasma lipoproteins.

When platelets are stimulated to undergo the release reaction they release a polypeptide or polypeptides of molecular weight about 13,000 to 23,000 that is mitogenic for smooth muscle cells (29, 30). This factor does not appear to be present in plasma in any signifi-cant amounts, unless the platelets have undergone the release reac-

tion (29). Thus the localized release of this material when platelets adhere to the vessel wall could be an important factor in
localized smooth muscle cell migration into the intima and proliferation in response to endothelial injury. Platelets adhere to subendothelial structures, and collagen in the subendothelium can induce the release reaction (31).

Proof that the platelets are involved in this response comes
from experiments in which animals have been made thrombocytopenic
before endothelial injury was induced. Using an indwelling cannula,
Moore and his colleagues (32) showed that the atherosclerosis caused
by repeated injury of the vessel wall by the cannula could be prevented if the animals were made thrombocytopenic before introduction
of the cannula. More recently, Friedman and colleagues (33) found
that the smooth muscle cell proliferation observed when the endothelium was removed by a single balloon catheter injury could also be
prevented if the animals were made thrombocytopenic before the balloon injury was induced. However, if the animals were made thrombocytopenic following the balloon injury, there was apparently no
protection against the smooth muscle cell proliferation (Friedman,
R.J., personal communication).

Less direct evidence comes from the studies of Harker, Ross
and their colleagues who found that dipyridamole (a drug that causes
some inhibition of platelet adherence to the vessel wall) inhibits
intimal thickening in animals infused with homocystine (34).

The platelet is probably not the only source of mitogens that
can cause smooth muscle cell proliferation. It has been reported
that a mitogen can be obtained from macrophages (Ross, R., personal
communication).

The role of blood coagulation in the response of the vessel
wall to injury has not been well defined. Since some of the constituents of the sub-endothelium, such as collagen, can activate
the coagulation process (35) and when the endothelium is injured
tissue thromboplastin becomes available (36), one would expect local
thrombin generation at an injury site. All of the available evidence indicates that thrombin does not stimulate smooth muscle cell
proliferation (29, 36), although thrombin has been reported to be
mitogenic for other cells in culture (37). Clowes and Karnovsky
(38) found that the smooth muscle cell proliferation following
endothelial injury of the carotid artery of rats could be prevented
by treating the animals with heparin. It is not known whether
the heparin blocks thrombin formation which may modify the platelet
response to the vessel wall, or whether the heparin blocks the
effect of the mitogen on the smooth muscle cells.

Low density lipoproteins (LDL) and very low density lipoproteins interact with specific receptors on fibroblasts and smooth
muscle cells (39). There is evidence from tissue culture studies
that when the LDL receptor regulatory system is bypassed and smooth
muscle cells take up LDL in excess of their cholesterol need, they
accumulate massive amounts of cholesteryl ester (40). Cholesterol
and cholesteryl esters tend to accumulate at sites of endothelial
injury (41). Lipoproteins, particularly low density lipoproteins,
have been shown to bind to the connective tissue in the wall, particularly to the proteoglycans (42). This may be a mechanism that
leads to trapping of the lipoproteins in the vessel wall (43).
Finally, low density lipoprotein may enhance the response of smooth
muscle cells to the mitogens (44).

ENDOTHELIAL INJURY

A number of mechanisms appear to be potentially important as
causes of endothelial injury (45-48): mechanical - in an intact
animal this probably consists of hemodynamic and blood pressure
effects (13); microbiological - some viruses, bacteria and bacterial products such as endotoxin (9, 10); metabolic - some serum
lipids or lipoproteins and metabolic products such as homocystine
(1, 8, 34); smoking (11) and immune injury (12, 48).

The localization of the early vessel wall change in atherosclerosis around vessel branches and orifices lends support to the
concept that alterations in flow contribute to these changes (16,
45, 49-51). It is perhaps important to appreciate that the hemodynamic factors might operate by localizing the accumulation of
substances in the blood and facilitating their interaction with
the wall (19, 50). Where there is flow separation, the formed
elements such as platelets may accumulate on the wall of the aorta
(14, 45, 49, 51-54).

Homocystine infusions have been shown to cause loss of endothelium in baboons (8) and humans with homocystinemia show an increased susceptibility to vascular disease and thrombosis (34, 55).
Hypercholesterolemia produced by the feeding of egg yolk and corn
oil to monkeys was associated with endothelial injury (1) and in
pigs there is indirect evidence that dietary fat can damage the endothelium (56). Indirect evidence of the effect of dietary fat
on the endothelium in man comes from the observations that diets
rich in saturated fat shorten platelet survival, whereas diets low
in fat or diets rich in vegetable fat lengthen platelet survival
(57). Since vessel wall injury appears to be a major factor influencing platelet survival (8, 58), these diet-induced changes in
platelet survival in man may reflect alterations in the endothelium.

There is some evidence that smoking may damage the endothelium through the effects of carbon monoxide (11). It has been reported recently that some cigarette smokers become sensitized to a glycoprotein from tobacco (59). If this leads to the episodic formation of circulating immune complexes, this process could cause the formation of atherosclerotic lesions because in serum sickness it has been shown that the intravascular antigen-antibody complexes damage the endothelium and cause atherosclerosis (12, 48). Smoking in man shortens platelet survival and increases platelet turnover (60). Since platelet survival may reflect endothelial injury (1, 8, 58), it may be that smoking does damage the endothelium. This may account for the observation that cessation of smoking significantly reduces the risk of the individual dying from coronary artery disease (61).

INTERACTIONS BETWEEN PLATELETS AND THE VESSEL WALL

In view of the effect of the platelet mitogen on smooth muscle cell proliferation, knowledge of factors influencing the interaction of platelets with the subendothelium is of some importance. Of the subendothelial constituents exposed when the endothelium is lost, collagen (31, 62) is important in causing platelet aggregation, the platelet release reaction and activation of coagulation (35). Although platelets can adhere to the basement membrane and microfibrils, these structures do not appear to induce the release reaction (31, 62). Platelet adherence to collagen and the release reaction of platelets adherent to collagen is independent of the arachidonate:cyclo-oxygenase pathway (27, 63). Thus, non-steroidal, anti-inflammatory drugs such as aspirin or indomethacin do not inhibit the release reaction of platelets adherent to collagen. Their major effect is on the formation of thromboxane A_2 by the platelets adherent to the collagen thereby preventing the effect of thromboxane A_2 on the platelets not in contact with collagen. In both rats (4) and rabbits (64) aspirin was not found to inhibit smooth muscle cell proliferation following endothelial injury. Sulphinpyrazone, which also does not block the release reaction of platelets adherent to collagen, does not inhibit smooth muscle cell proliferation following endothelial injury (Moore, S., personal communication).

Studies in rabbits of platelet turnover on the surface of the damaged aorta have shown that immediately following removal of the endothelium, there is a rapid accumulation of a platelet monolayer on the subendothelium. Once this initial layer is formed there is very little turnover of the platelets on the surface (65). After a period of four to five days the denuded surface has few platelets

on it and is non-reactive as far as circulating platelets are concerned (64, 65). These observations are in keeping with the observation that if rabbits are made thrombocytopenic four hours after
balloon injury, smooth muscle cell proliferation is not prevented
(Friedman, R.J., personal communication). The rabbits must be made
thrombocytopenic before balloon injury in order to prevent smooth
muscle cell proliferation (32, 33) (Friedman, R.J., personal communication).

The mechanisms involved in the formation of a thrombus have
been extensively reviewed elsewhere (45, 66, 67). Three of the
main findings concerning the formation of thrombi involve the role
of thrombin, the influence of dietary lipids, and the formation of
prostacyclin by the vessel wall.

(i) Thrombin can mediate platelet aggregation through pathways
which are independent of the release of ADP or the formation of
endoperoxides and thromboxane A_2 (68, 69). ADP induces aggregation
through a mechanism which does not, in the presence of normal
concentrations of calcium, lead to activation of phospholipase A_2
and the formation of endoperoxides and thromboxane A_2 (70, 71).
Thus, neither thrombin- nor ADP-induced aggregation will be significantly influenced by the non-steroidal anti-inflammatory drugs
such as aspirin. In the case of collagen, the non-steroidal anti-
inflammatory drugs do inhibit collagen-induced aggregation, particularly to low concentrations of collagen (72). However, aspirin
does not inhibit platelet adherence to the subendothelium or collagen although indomethacin has a slight inhibitory effect (27, 63).
Neither drug inhibits the release reaction of platelets adherent
to collagen (27, 63). It appears that the major effect of the
drugs is to block the formation of thromboxane A_2 and thereby prevent the aggregation and release effect on the platelets that are
not adherent to the collagen. Platelet adherence to collagen and
the release reaction of the adherent platelets is obviously not
dependent upon the platelet cyclo-oxygenase. Thus, the non-steroidal
anti-inflammatory drugs are not likely to be potent inhibitors of
arterial thrombus formation. In animal experiments, drugs such as
aspirin have not been found to be strong inhibitors of thrombus
formation (73).

(ii) Modification of the platelet fatty acids could be expected
to alter platelet function. There is some evidence that di-homo-
γ-linolenic acid may substitute for arachidonic acid in the platelet membrane phospholipids (74, 75). Di-homo-γ-linolenic acid is
a precursor of PGE_1 which is a potent inhibitor of platelet adhesion to collagen and platelet aggregation. When animals or humans
are fed di-homo-γ-linolenic acid, their platelets are less sensitive to aggregating agents and are less adherent to collagen (74-
76). In contrast, arachidonic acid is a precursor of PGH_2, PGG_2

and thromboxane A_2 which are potent stimulators of platelet aggregation and the platelet release reaction (66, 67, 77, 78). Dietary linoleic acid has been reported to make platelets less sensitive to aggregating agents and reduce susceptibility to thrombosis in rats (79-81). Platelets from humans fed increased amounts of arachidonic acid are more sensitive to aggregating agents than platelets from control subjects given a normal diet (77). There are animal experiments showing that feeding saturated fat to animals and man, particularly butterfat, makes platelets more sensitive to agents such as thrombin (81-84) and makes animals more sensitive to thrombosis induced by substances such as endotoxin (82, 84).

(iii) Demonstration that the vessel wall can produce prostacyclin (PGI_2) from PGG_2 and PGH_2 (26, 85, 86) has led to considerable interest in the possible role of PGI_2 in preventing platelet adherence to the vessel wall and thrombosis. Whether smooth muscle cells can produce PGI_2 is not settled but endothelial cells have been shown to form PGI_2 (26). However, treatment of de-endothelialized aorta with aspirin increases platelet adherence to the subendothelium (27). Since compounds like PGE_1 that increase platelet cyclic AMP levels inhibit platelet adherence to the vessel wall (27), this may mean that the smooth muscle cells can form PGI_2 and inhibition of its formation by aspirin gives increased platelet adherence to the subendothelium. Treatment of a normal aorta segment (intact endothelium) with aspirin does not cause platelets to adhere to the endothelium (27) indicating that PGI_2 formation by endothelium is probably not the mechanism by which platelets are prevented from adhering to it. Weksler and associates could not detect PGI_2 formation by unstimulated endothelial cells in tissue culture (26). It seems unlikely that the unstimulated, intact vessel wall and platelets release arachidonic acid form endoperoxides necessary for the formation of PGI_2. Thus, prevention of platelet adherence to the intact endothelium is probably related to other factors such as membrane glycoproteins (46).

Another important effect of PGI_2 is on vessel tone and there is evidence that it causes arterial wall relaxation (87). This may be important in view of the fact that thromboxane A_2 released from platelets can cause arterial contraction (88). The net effect of the products of arachidonic acid metabolism on vessel tone in the microcirculation may have a bearing on the effect of platelet-fibrin emboli in the microcirculation. Thus, non-steroidal anti-inflammatory drugs might prevent vasoconstriction induced by thromboxane A_2 formed from platelets in the embolus. PGI_2 formed from platelet endoperoxides could also inhibit vasoconstriction induced by thromboxane A_2. This might reduce the duration that the emboli are trapped in the microcirculation. There is evidence from animal experiments that mural thrombi induced in the coronary artery of dogs cause extensive accumulation of platelet fibrin emboli in the microcirculation and that the administration of aspirin diminishes this (89).

Study of hemostasis in thrombocytopenic rabbits has shown the importance of vessel tone in hemostasis (Hirsh, J., personal communication). If a puncture wound is made in the jugular vein there is prolonged bleeding that can be arrested by the infusion of normal platelets. However, the bleeding can also be stopped by applying aspirin, indomethacin, hydrocortisone or methylprednisolone to the vessel wall. The non-steroidal anti-inflammatory drugs would block PGI_2 formation by the damaged vessel wall by inhibiting the cyclo-oxygenase (90). The steroids will inhibit by preventing the splitting of arachidonic acid from the membrane phospholipids by phospholipase A_2 (91). The arrest of bleeding produced by the steroids can be reversed by adding arachidonic acid to the vessel wall. The arachidonic acid, of course, does not overcome the inhibition produced by the non-steroidal anti-inflammatory drugs. These observations are in keeping with the hypothesis that when the vessel wall is injured, PGI_2 is formed from arachidonic acid released by the injured cells in the vein wall. This prevents contractions of the wall and blood loss continues through the patent puncture wound in the thrombocytopenic animals. If PGI_2 formation is blocked, the injured wall can contract, closing the puncture site and thereby preventing blood loss.

THROMBOSIS AND THE EVOLUTION OF ATHEROSCLEROTIC PLAQUES

Evidence (92-96) derived from human studies and experimental studies in animals has confirmed Duguid's observation (97) that organization of mural thrombi is a significant factor in the evolution of thickened atherosclerotic plaques. In advanced atherosclerosis this may be the important mechanism causing severe narrowing of the lumen of vessels such as the coronary arteries (94). The severe narrowing of arteries to the heart and brain is a major factor contributing to the clinical complications of atherosclerosis.

LIPIDS, VESSEL INJURY, THROMBOSIS AND ATHEROSCLEROSIS

The relationship among these factors in the development of atherosclerosis is much clearer now than it was several decades ago when the tendency was to consider the various theories of atherosclerosis as independent of each other (98). Proponents of the thrombotic and lipid theories of atherosclerosis now have a great deal of common ground that is centered on endothelial injury and smooth muscle cell proliferation and upon which mechanisms involved in the development of atherosclerotic lesions can be explored.

Endothelial injury is a key factor in the localization of atherosclerotic lesions, in the initiation of platelet vessel wall interaction and thrombus formation and in determining sites of increased
vessel permeability. The transfer of unesterified cholesterol and
cholesteryl ester from blood to the vessel wall is less in the
parts of the aorta with intact endothelium than in tissues with
defective endothlium (41). Bjorkerud and Bondjers (99, 100) observed that when the serum lipoproteins are increased in rabbits,
the lipid accumulation in the aorta with damaged endothelium is
greater than in the parts of the aorta with intact endothelium.
The increase was proportional in both the damaged and undamaged
vessel wall to the serum lipoprotein level. They concluded that
endothelial injury has a greater effect on the development of atherosclerosis than the level of serum cholesterol (99, 100). This
raises the question of the value of decreasing serum cholesterol
levels without reducing endothelial injury. Theoretically inter-
ventions which decreased serum LDL and reduced endothelial injury
would have a greater effect than just decreasing the serum LDL
level. It is of some significance that elevation of serum cholesterol by dietary means is associated with evidence of endothelial
injury in monkeys (1) and pigs (56). Thus it may be possible to
reduce serum LDL levels and reduce the extent of endothelial injury
by changing the lipid composition of diets.

   Repeated endothelial injury appears to produce changes in the
vessel wall that modify the response of blood to vessel wall injury.
In rabbits the subendothelium has been found to be more thrombogenic
following a second endothelial injury (101). Moore has found that
repeated injury to the endothelium in rabbits maintained on low fat
diets with normal serum cholesterol levels, produced raised lipid-
rich atherosclerotic plaques (3, 102, 103). Originally it was
thought that the sites where the endothelium is lost and does not
regenerate would be the sites continuously exposed to plasma constituents and platelets and thereby the most affected. However, the
maximum lipid accumulation has been observed at the sites where the
endothelium regenerates between the injuries and is then lost with
each repeated injury (103, 104). This may mean that at these sites
there is decreased clearance or metabolism of the lipid that accumulates. Recently it has been observed that material with the histological characteristics of proteoglycans accumulated at sites of repeated endothelial injury (43). The binding of low density lipoproteins to the proteoglycans that accumulate may be a part of the
mechanism whereby the low density lipoproteins are trapped in the
vessel wall at injury sites.

   Vessel injury in association with hyperlipidemia can lead to
more extensive atherosclerosis than either stimulus alone (48).
In rabbits it was observed that serum sickness in animals fed a
hypercholesterolemic diet produced more extensive atherosclerosis

(105, 106). In rats, however, hypercholesterolemia was not found
to have much effect on the vessel wall thickening following extensive endothelial injury (107). However, the finding that the sites
in rabbits where there is most lipid accumulation are areas where
there is intermittent loss of endothelium rather than chronic endothelial loss (102, 103) may be an explanation for the difference
between the rat and rabbit experiments. It seems possible that the
injury in the rat experiments could have produced a chronic endothelial loss.

RISK FACTORS, VESSEL INJURY, THROMBOSIS
LIPIDS AND ATHEROSCLEROSIS

The increased understanding of how the factors that have been
discussed can influence the development of atherosclerosis gives
further support to the importance of some of the identified risk
factors for death from the complications of atherosclerosis. Thus,
dietary fat and elevation of serum low density lipoprotein can
contribute to injury to the endothelium and the response of the
smooth muscle cells to endothelial injury. Furthermore, the fatty
acid composition of the diet appears to influence platelet interaction with the subendothelium and thrombosis following endothelial injury. The observation that populations consuming large
quantities of butterfat have a greater incidence of cardiovascular
deaths than subjects eating diets rich in vegetable fat (108) is
in keeping with the evidence derived from the experimental studies.

There is a high risk of myocardial infarction in subjects who
smoke cigarettes (61, 109). The experimental evidence suggests
that, at least in some subjects, smoking may injure the vessel
wall. If so, then the incidence of clinical complications of
atherosclerosis could be expected to fall in those who stop smoking.

High blood pressure may contribute to the problem because of
its effects on the vessel wall and the endothelium (110). High
blood pressure is known to enhance the development of experimental
atherosclerosis (111).

The benefits to be derived from changing these risk factors
in a population are hard to establish. It may be virtually impossible to do controlled trials of the effects of changes in these
risk factors by modifying human behavior. There is some evidence
that drugs which influence factors such as serum cholesterol do
not have much effect in the complications of atherosclerosis (112).
However, the mistake must not be made of interpreting the effect
of drugs on serum cholesterol as similar to the effect of any modification of diet on serum cholesterol levels and the response of the
endothelium to injury. The decline in the age-specific coronary

mortality in the United States since 1963 by more than 25% for subjects under age 55 (113) has been associated with a change in the dietary and smoking habits of Americans. This change in recorded deaths from coronary artery disease was associated with a 22.4% decline in the per capita consumption of tobacco, a 31.9% decline in the per capita consumption of butter, a 56.7% decline in the per capita use of animal fats and oils, and a 41.1% increase in the per capita consumption of vegetable fats and oils. Although this does not establish a cause and effect relationship, the observations are all compatible with our increased understanding of the mechanisms that produce atherosclerosis and thrombosis as a result of injury to the endothelium.

REFERENCES

1. Ross, R., and Harker, L.A. (1976) Science 193, 1094-1100.

2. Stemerman, M.B., and Ross, R. (1972) J. Exp. Med. 136, 769-789.

3. Moore, S. (1973) Lab. Invest. 29, 478-487.

4. Clowes, A.W., and Karnovsky, M.J. (1977) Lab. Invest. 36, 452-464.

5. Nam, S.C., Lee, W.M., Jarmolych, J., Lee, K.T., and Thomas, W.A. (1973) Exp. Molec. Pathol. 18, 369-379.

6. Tyson, J.E., deSa, D.J., and Moore, S. (1976) Arch. Dis. Childhood 51, 744-754.

7. Friedman, R.J., Moore, S., and Singal, D.P. (1975) Lab. Invest. 30, 404-415.

8. Harker, L.A., Slichter, S.J., Scott, R., and Ross, R. (1974) N. Engl. J. Med. 291, 537-543.

9. Gaynor, E., Bouvier, C.A., and Spaet, T.H. (1968) Clin. Res. 16, 535.

10. Turpie, A.G.G., Chernesky, M.A., Larke, R.P.B., Moore, S., Regoeczi, E., and Mustard, J.F. (1972) Proc. III Congr. Int. Soc. Thromb. Haemostasis, Washington, p. 344.

11. Thomsen, H.K. (1974) Atherosclerosis 20, 233-240.

12. Kniker, W.T., and Cochrane, C.G. (1968) J. Exp. Med. 127, 119-135.

13. Fry, D.L. (1973) in Atherogenesis: Initiating Factors, Ciba Foundation Symposium 12 (new series). Elsevier Excerpta Medica, North-Holland. Associated Scientific Publishers, New York, pp. 93-125.

14. Jørgensen, L., Packham, M.A., Rowsell, H.C., and Mustard, J. F. (1972) Lab. Invest. 27, 341-350.

15. Packham, M.A., Rowsell, H.C., Jørgensen, L., and Mustard, J. F. (1967) Exp. Molec. Pathol. 7, 214-232.

16. Gutstein, W.H., Farrell, G.A., and Armellini, C. (1973) Lab. Invest. 29, 134-149.

17. Caplan, B.A., Gerrity, R.G., and Schwartz, C.J. (1974) Exp. Molec. Pathol. 21, 102-117.

18. Fry, D.L. (1968) Circ. Res. 22, 165-197.

19. Caro, C.G., and Nerem, R.M. (1973) Circ. Res. 32, 187-205.

20. Goldsmith, H.L. (1972) in Progress in Hemostasis and Thrombosis, Vol. 1 (Spaet, T.H., Ed.), Grune and Stratton, New York, pp. 97-139.

21. Stein, P.D., and Sabbah, H.N. (1974) Circ. Res. 35, 608-614.

22. Rocha e Silva, M., Beraldo, W.T., and Rosenfeld, G. (1949) Am. J. Physiol. 156, 261-273.

23. Ryan, U.S., Ryan, J.W., Smith, D.S., and Winkler, H. (1975) Tissue Cell 7, 181-190.

24. Movat, H.Z., Uriuhara, T., Macmorine, D.R.L., and Burke, J.S. (1964) Life Sci. 3, 1025-1032.

25. Nachman, R.L., Weksler, B., and Ferris, B. (1972) J. Clin. Invest. 51, 549-556.

26. Weksler, B.B., Marcus, A.J., and Jaffe, E.A. (1977) Proc. Natl. Acad. Sci. USA 74, 3922-3926.

27. Cazenave, J.-P., Packham, M.A., Kinlough-Rathbone, R.L., and Mustard, J.F. (1977). Workshop on Animal and Human Models for Thrombosis Research, Brook Lodge, Oct. 1977. In press.

28. Lough, J., and Moore, S. (1975) Lab. Invest. 33, 130-135.

29. Rutherford, R.B., and Ross, R. (1976) J. Cell Biol. 69, 196-203.

30. Antoniades, H.N., and Scher, C.D. (1977) Proc. Natl. Acad. Sci. USA 74, 1973-1977.

31. Baumgartner, H.R., Muggli, R., Tschopp, T.B., and Turitto, V.T. (1976) Thrombos. Haemostas. 35, 124-138.

32. Moore, S., Friedman, R.J., Singal, D.P., Gauldie, J., Blajch-man, M.A., and Roberts, R.S. (1976) Thrombos. Haemostas. 35, 70-81.

33. Friedman, R.J., Stemerman, M.B., Wenz, B., Moore, S., Gauldie, J., Gent, M., Tiell, M.L., and Spaet, T.H. J. Clin. Invest. In press.

34. Harker, L.A., Ross, R., Slichter, S.J., and Scott, C.R. (1976) J. Clin. Invest. 58, 731-741.

35. Niewiarowski, S., Stuart, R.K., and Thomas, D.P. (1966) Proc. Soc. Fxp. Biol. Med. 123, 196-200.

36. Nemerson, Y., and Pitlick, F.A. (19720 in Progress in Hemo-stasis and Thrombosis, Vol. 1 (Spaet, T.H., Ed.) Grune and Stratton, New York, pp. 1-37.

37. Chen, L.B., and Buchanan, J.M. (1975) Proc. Natl. Acad. Sci. USA 72, 131-135.

38. Clowes, A.W., and Karnowsky, M. (1977) Nature 265, 625-626.

39. Brown, M.S., and Goldstein, J.L. (1976) Science 191, 150-154.

40. Goldstein, J.L., Anderson, R.G.W., Buja, L.M., Basu, S.K., and Brown, M.S. (1977) J. Clin. Invest. 59, 1196-1202.

41. Bondjers, G., and Bjorkerud, S. (1973) Atherosclerosis 17, 71-83.

42. Hollander, V. (1976) Exp. Molec. Pathol. 25, 106-120.

43. Minick, C.R., Alonso, D.R., Litrenta, M., Silane, M.F., and Stemerman, M.B. (1977) Circulation 56, Part II: 144.

44. Ross, R., and Glomset, J.A. (1973) Science 180, 1332-1339.

45. Mustard, J.F., and Packham, M.A. (1975) Thromb. Diath. Hae-morrh. 33, 444-456.

46. Mason, R.G., Sharp, D., Chuang, H.Y.K., and Mohammad, S.F. (1977) Arch. Pathol. & Lab. Med. 101, 61-64.

47. Schwartz, S.M., and Benditt, E.P. (1977) Circ. Res. 41, 248-255.

48. Alonso, D.R., Starek, P.K., and Minick, C.R. (1977) Am. J. Pathol. 87, 415-442.

49. Fry, D.L. (1976) in Cerebrovascular Dis. (Scheinberg P., Ed.) Raven Press, New York, pp. 77-95.

50. Goldsmith, H.L. (1972) in Progress in Hemostasis and Thrombosis, Vol. 1 (Spaet, T.H., Ed.) Grune and Stratton, New York, pp. 97-139.

51. Murphy, E.A., Rowsell, H.C., Downie, H.G., Robinson, G.A., and Mustard, J.F. (1962) Can. Med. Assoc. J. 87, 259-274.

52. Geissinger, H.D., Mustard, J.F., and Rowsell, H.C. (1962) Can. Med. Assoc. J. 87, 405-408.

53. Lewis, J.C., and Kottke, B.A. (1977) Science 196, 1007-1009.

54. Svendsen, E., and Jørgensen, L. (1977) Acta Path. Microbiol. Scand. Sect. A. 85, 25-32.

55. McCully, K.S. (1969) Am. J. Pathol. 56, 111-128.

56. Florentin, R.A., Nam, S.C., Lee, K.T., and Thomas, W.A. (1969) Exp. Molec. Pathol. 10, 250-255.

57. Mustard, J.F., and Murphy, E.A. (1962) Br. Med. J. 1, 1651-1655.

58. Mustard, J.F., Packham, M.A., and Kinlough-Rathbone, R.L. (1976) in The Significance of Platelet Function Tests in the Evaluation of Hemostatic and Thrombotic Tendencies, Workshop on Platelets. (Day, H.J., Zucker, M.B. and Holmsen, H., Eds.) Philadelphia 1976. U.S. Govt. Printing Office. In press.

59. Becker, C.G., Dubin, T., and Wiedemann, H.P. (1976) Proc. Natl. Acad. Sci. USA 73, 1712-1716.

60. Mustard, J.F., and Murphy, E.A. (1963) Br. Med. J. 1, 846-849.

61. Doll, R., and Peto, R. (1976) Br. Med. J. 2, 1525-1536.

62. Baumgartner, H.R. (1977) Thrombos. Haemostas. 37, 1-16.

63. Packham, M.A., Cazenave, J.-P., Kinlough-Rathbone, R.L., and Mustard, J.F. Adv. Exp. Med. Biol. In press.

64. Baumgartner, H.R., and Studer, A. (1976). Workshop on Thrombosis and Atherosclerosis, IVth International Symposium on Atherosclerosis, Tokyo.

65. Groves, H.M., Kinlough-Rathbone, R.L., Richardson, M., and Mustard, J.F. Blood. In press.

66. Mustard, J.F. (1976) Trans. Am. Clin. Climatol. Assoc. 87, 104-127.

67. Mustard, J.F., Moore, S., Packham, M.A., and Kinlough-Rathbone, R.L. in Proceedings of the First International Atherosclerosis Conference, Progress in Biochemical Pharmacology. Karger, Basel. In press.

68. Packham, M.A., Kinlough-Rathbone, R.L., Reimers, H.-J., Scott, S., and Mustard, J.F. (1977) in Prostaglandins in Hematology (Silver, M.J., Smith, J.B. and Kocsis, J.J., Eds.) New York, Spectrum Publications, Inc. pp. 247-276.

69. Kinlough-Rathbone, R.L., Packham, M.A., Reimers, H.-J., Cazenave, J.-P., and Mustard, J.F. (1977) J. Lab. Clin. Med. 90, 707-719.

70. Mustard, J.F., Perry, D.W., Kinlough-Rathbone, R.L., and Packham, M.A. (1975) Am. J. Physiol. 228, 1757-1765.

71. Macfarlane, D.E., Walsh, P.N., Mills, D.C.B., Holmsen, H., and Day, H.J. (1975) Br. J. Haematol. 30, 457-463.

72. Packham, M.A., Warrior, E.S., Glynn, M.F., Senyi, A.S., and Mustard, J.F. (1967) J. Exp. Med. 126, 171-188.

73. Danese, C.A., Voleti, C.D., and Weiss, H.J. (1971) Thromb. Diath. Haemorrh. 25, 288-296.

74. Willis, A.L., Stone, K.J., Hart, M., Gibson, V., Marples, P., Botfield, E., Comai, K., and Kuhn, D.C. (1977) in Prostaglandins in Hematology (Silver, M.J., Smith, J.B. and Kocsis, J.J., Eds.) New York, Spectrum Publications, Inc. pp. 371-410.

75. Kernoff, P.B.A., Davies, J.A., McNicol, G.P., Willis, A.L., and Stone, K.J. (1977) Thrombos. Haemostas. 38, 194.

76. Sim, A.K., and McCraw, A.P. (1977) Thrombosis Research 10, 385-397.

77. Seyberth, H.W., Oelz, O., Kennedy, T., Sweetman, B.J., Danon, A., Frolich, J.C., Heimberg, M., and Oates, J.A. (1975) Clin. Parmacol. Therap. 18, 521-529.

78. Smith, J.B., Ingerman, C.M., and Silver, M.J. (1977) in Prostaglandins in Hematology (Silver, M.J., Smith, J.B. and Kocsis, J.J., Eds.) New York, Spectrum Publications, Inc. pp. 277-292.

79. Hornstra, G., Chait, A., Karvonen, M.J., Lewis, B., Turpeinen, O., and Vergroesen, A.J. (1973) Lancet 1, 1155-1157.

80. Fleischman, A.I., Justice, D., Bierenbaum, M.L., Stier, A., and Sullivan, A. (1975) J. Nutrition 105, 1286-1290.

81. Hornstra, G., and Lussenburg, R.N. (1975) Atherosclerosis 22, 499-516.

82. Renaud, S., Kinlough, R.L., and Mustard, J.F. (1970) Lab. Invest 22, 339-343.

83. O'Brien, J.R., Etherington, M.D., and Jamieson, S. (1976) Lancet 2, 995-996.

84. Renaud, S., and Lecompte, F. (1970) Circ. Res. 27, 1003-1011.

85. Moncada, S., Gryglewski, R., Bunting, S., and Vane, J.R. (1976) Nature 263, 663-665.

86. Moncada, S., Herman, A.G., Higgs, E.A., and Vane, J.R. (1977) Thromb. Res. 11, 323-344.

87. Blumberg, A.L., Denny, S.E., Marshall, G.R., and Needleman, P. (1977) Am. J. Physiol. 232, H305-H310.

88. Needleman, P., Kulkarni, P.S., and Raz, A. (1977) Science 195, 409-412.

89. Moschos, C.B., Lahiri, K., Lyons, M.M., Weisse, A.B., Oldewurtel, H.A., and Regan, T.J. (1973) Am. Heart J. 86, 61-68.

90. Roth, G.J., and Majerus, P.W. (1975) J. Clin. Invest. 56, 624-632.

91. Hong, S.-C.L., and Levine, L. (1976) Proc. Natl. Acad. Sci. USA 73, 1730-1734.

92. Hand, R.A., and Chandler, A.B. (1962) Am. J. Pathol. 40, 469-486.

93. Woolf, N., Bradley, J.W.P., Crawford, T., and Carstairs, K.C. (1968) Br. J. Exp. Pathol. 49, 257-264.

94. Mitchell, J.R.A., and Schwartz, C.J. (1963) Br. Heart J. 25, 1-24.

95. Moore, R.H., and Haust, M.D. (1961) Am. J. Pathol. 38, 527-537.

96. Jørgensen, L., Rowsell, H.C., Hovig, T., and Mustard, J.F. (1967) Am. J. Pathol. 51, 681-719.

97. Duguid, J.B. (1948) J. Pathol. Bact. 60, 57-61.

98. Davignon, J. (1977) Current Views on the Etiology and Pathogenesis of Atherosclerosis in Hypertension. Physiopathology and Treatment. (Genest, J., Koin, E. and Kuchel, O., Eds.) McGraw-Hill, Inc., New York.

99. Bjorkerud, S., and Bondjers, G. (1976) Ann. N.Y. Acad. Sci. 275, 180-198.

100. Bondjers, G., Brattsand, R., Hansson, G.K., and Bjorkerud, S. 6th International Symposium on Drugs Affecting Lipid Metabolism. Adv. in Exp. Med. Biol. In press.

101. Stemerman, M.B. (1973) Am. J. Pathol. 73, 7-26.

102. Friedman, R.J., Moore, S., and Singal, D.P. (1975) Lab. Invest 30, 404-415.

103. Moore, S., and Ihnatowycz, I.O. in Animal and Human Models in Thrombosis Research. In press.

104. Minick, C.R., Stemerman, M.B. and Insull, W., Jr. (1977) Proc. Natl. Acad. Sci. USA 74, 1724-1728.

105. Minick, C.R., Murphy, G.E., and Campbell, W.G., Jr. (1966) J. Exp. Med. 124, 635-652.

106. Minick, C.R., and Murphy, G.E. (19730 Am. J. Pathol. 73, 265-300.

107. Clowes, A.W., Ryan, G.B., Breslow, J.L., and Karnovsky, M.J. (1976) Lab. Invest. 35, 6-17.

108. Joossens, J.V.K., Vuylsteek, E., Brems-Heyns et al. (1977)
     Lancet 1, 1069-1072.

109. Doyle, J.T., Dawber, T.R., Kannel, W.B., Kinch, S.H., and
     Kahn, H.A. (1964) JAMA 190, 886-890.

110. Lazzarini-Robertson, A., Jr. (1968) in Renal Hypertension
     (Page, I.H. and McGubbin, J.W., Eds.) Year Book Medical Pub-
     lishers, Inc., Chicago, Ill., pp. 372-390.

111. Bronte-Stewart, B., and Heptinstall, R.H. (1954) J. Pathol.
     Bact. 68, 407-417.

112. Coronary Drug Project Research Group: Clofibrate and niacin
     in coronary heart disease. (1975) JAMA 231, 360-381.

113. Walker, W.J. (1977) N. Engl. J. Med. 297, 163-165.

THROMBOSIS AND ATHEROSCLEROSIS

Neville Woolf

Department of Histopathology
The Middlesex Hospital Medical School
London, England

From the clinical point of view the most important end results
of atherosclerosis are stenosis and occlusion of the affected artery. A prerequisite for this is a degree of plaque growth sufficient to encroach significantly on the integrity of the vessel
lumen. It is clear that in the earlier phases of the natural history of an atherosclerotic plaque, this growth is mediated via
the proliferation of modified smooth muscle cells in the affected
area of the arterial intima and by the elaboration of extra-cellu-
lar connective tissue elements such as collagen, elastin and gly-
coso-amino-glycans of which these cells are capable (1, 2, 3).
Experimental data now exist which suggest that one of the factors
stimulating this form of localized connective tissue proliferation is platelet adhesion and aggregation and the evidence for
this will be reviewed briefly in a later section of this paper.
Of equal, perhaps greater importance, is the proposition that
mural thrombi occur in relation to established atherosclerotic
plaques and that the thrombi may become incorporated into the substances of the arterial wall with a subsequent increase in plaque
thickness.

Much of the comparatively recent interest in the putative
role of mural thrombi as a contributor to plaque growth stems
from the studies of J.B. Duguid (4, 5, 6), who stated that many
of the lesions we now classify as atherosclerosis are arterial
thrombi which, by the ordinary processes of organization, have
been transformed into fibrous thickenings. This view as Duguid
pointed out represents a partial return to the "encrustation hypothesis" enunciated by Rokitansky (7) a century before. Rokitansky
ascribed all the features of atherosclerosis to "recurrent deposition of elements derived from the blood mass". However, those

views were regarded as completely unacceptable by Rokitansky's
contemporaries, notably Virchow, the chief grounds for rejection
being that the intimal thickenings were sub-endothelial and hence
could not be derived from surface deposits (8). This essentially
static view of structural pathology led to a long period of ne-
glect of any possible relationship between thrombosis and plaque
buildup, despite the fact that morphological features suggestive
of a thrombotic component within certain atherosclerotic plaques
were recognized and described by a number of workers in the earlier part of this century (9, 10, 11).

Assessment of the role of mural thrombosis in plaque growth
and genesis can be carried out in a number of ways. In human
material the presence of residua of thrombus can be searched for
both in atherosclerotic lesions and lesion free areas, and it may
be possible to identify transition from obvious thrombus to equally obvious atherosclerotic plaque (4). A complementary approach
lies in the study of the natural history of experimentally induced
thrombi with particular reference to the possibility that their
presence may elicit connective tissue responses similar to those
found in spontaneously occurring atherosclerosis.

1. The Identification of Mural Thrombi and Their Residua in Atherosclerotic Plaques

In many instances it is possible to identify transitions
between obvious mural thrombi and sub-endothelial deposits, or the
remains of previously incorporated mural thrombi by the use of
the simplest and most conventional histological techniques which,
of course, were the basis for the observations mentioned in the
introduction (Fig. 1). Duguid's description of the natural history of aortic mural thrombi is so masterly that it is worth recalling in extenso: "Most aortic thrombi are composed of fibrin
which when newly formed is loose in texture and somewhat ragged
but later becomes more compact. At first the fibrin is exposed
to the blood stream but soon a layer of endothelium grows over
its surface and this is followed by the formation of a layer of
fibrous tissue in the sub-endothelial zone making the thrombus
appear as if it were part of the intima. Two forms of change then
follow, both of them tending to accentuate this effect. The first
consists of a condensation of fibrin whereby it comes to resemble
fibrous tissue; the second is true organization.

"The first change is best seen in parts, where as frequently
happens, there has been recurring thrombosis with one deposit on
top of another. Whereas the newly formed fibrin appears reticular
and somewhat flocculated, older deposits are compact and almost
homogeneous, but often with a laminated structure which in sec-

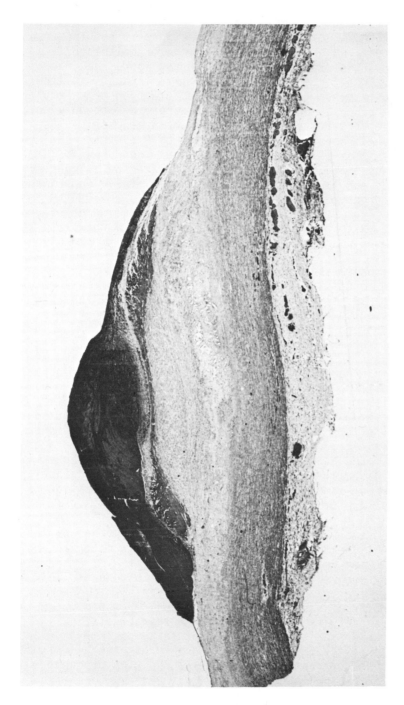

Figure 1. Aortic atherosclerotic plaque. The plaque is overlaid by a large recent but endothelialized thrombus. Separated from this and lying more deeply within the connective tissue cap of the plaque is a darkly stained band which represents the residuum of a previous mural thrombus (picro-Mallory x 14).

tion gives a coarse fibrous appearance. In the older deposits
the fibrin may lose its specific staining characters and stains
a variable yellow with picrofuchsin and brown with phosphotungstic
acid haemotoxylin, so that in paraffin sections it has the appearance of hyaline fibrous tissue. Thus before organization is far
advanced many of the older deposits no longer look like thrombi
and may be mistaken for degenerate connective tissue. In the
aorta, thrombosis tends to recur with the formation of multiple
deposits and the appearances are varied, depending not only on
the size of the deposits but on the time which elapses between
their formation. When one follows quickly on the other, the new
layer of fibrin lies directly on the old, but when a sufficient
interval elapses the older deposit may be covered by a layer of
fibrous tissue, and thus alternating strata of fibrin and fibrous
tissue may be produced. Not infrequently, deeply embedded within
the structure of a 'fibrous' plaque, layers of hyaline of 'fibrin-
oid' substance, with nothing in their appearance to show that they
originated as surface deposits, may be present."

     Duguid's observations were confirmed within a short time by
Heard (11) who found similar appearances in stenosed renal arteries, and by Morgan (12) who published a beautifully illustrated
study of stenosed coronary arteries, unhappily no longer in print.
In 1952 Crawford and Levene (13) carried out a study of the incidence of mural thrombi in the aorta which is of particular interest in that in selecting blocks for study these workers avoided
atherosclerotic plaques and instead chose areas of macroscopically
normal aorta, which, when examined with a hand lens, showed some
slight irregularity of the intima. Of ninety-nine such areas
examined, nineteen showed surface encrustations, ten showed superficial but definitely sub-endothelial deposits and twenty-four
showed fibrin situated deeply within the intima. Crawford and
Levene's work found strong support in a long series of papers by
Movat and his associates (14-18) in which they make the important
point that the cells most active in the surface organization of
surface thrombi are smooth muscle cells.

     All these studies depend essentially on the demonstration of
fibrin on or within the arterial intima. While it is true that
fibrin can be demonstrated successfully in paraffin-embedded tissue sections by such methods as Mallory's phosphotungstic acid
haemotoxylin or the picro-Mallory technique (19) it is, from the
histological point of view, a most capricious substance which
fairly rapidly loses its specific staining characteristics.
Failure to demonstrate its presence within atherosclerotic plaques
by conventional histological methods probably has little validity
and has led to an underestimate of its frequency in plaques.

The need for a more sensitive and reliable method for the identification of fibrin in the artery wall is largely met by the Coons' fluorescent antibody technique (20). The use of anti-human fibrin sera prepared in rabbits has shown fibrin or fibrinogen (which are immunohistologically indistinguishable) to be present even in aortic fatty streaks (21). When a wide range of atherosclerotic lesions is examined for the presence of immunologically identifiable fibrin or fibrinogen it becomes obvious that the anti-fibrin binding antigen is present within the thickened intima in two principal morphological forms. In the first of these the antigen is diffusely distributed in the form of minute fluorescent flecks (Fig. 2). In the second, the antigen appears in the form of brilliantly fluorescent coarse aggregates of material which may form encrustations on the surface of the vessel wall, or, more frequently, lie at different levels within the plaque substance roughly parallel to the luminal surface (Figs. 3 and 4). Woolf (22) suggested that these widely disparate distribution patterns of the anti-fibrin binding antigen represented two possible pathogenetic mechanisms: infiltration and holdup of fibrinogen from the plasma and incorporation of mural thrombus. These immuno-histological demonstrations of fibrin and/or fibrinogen have been confirmed by a number of other workers (23-26) but in at least one study, the demonstration of fibrin within the artery wall is not regarded as representing the residuum of mural thrombus (27).

2. Platelet Antigens in Atherosclerotic Plaques

The presence of fibrin within the arterial wall has been accepted by some as constituting prima facie evidence in favor of a role for mural thrombosis in plaque growth. However, Adams (23) rightly points out that the crucial question arising from these data is whether the fibrin is derived from incorporated mural thrombus or from an infiltrating stream of plasma. While the point is well taken insofar as the presence of fibrin is concerned, it loses much of its validity in the case of aggregated masses of platelets, the presence of which within the arterial intima cannot reasonably be ascribed to any mechanism other than the incorporation of mural thrombus. The presence of platelet masses within atherosclerotic plaques was first demonstrated by Carstairs (29) using a highly specific anti-human platelet serum and, interestingly enough, he also showed that fibrin and platelets in recent thrombi could be distinguished from each other in paraffin sections by means of a modified picro-Mallory technique. It is also of some interest to note that the anti-platelet serum used by Carstairs does not cross-react with fibrin though anti-fibrin sera do cross-react with platelets (30).

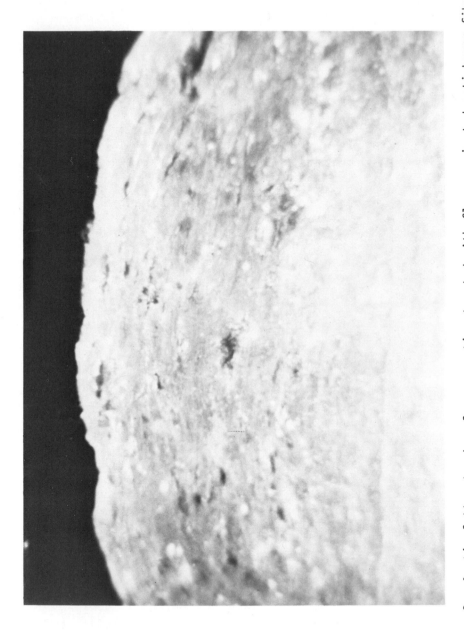

Figure 2. Aortic fatty streak: frozen section treated with fluoresceinated anti-human fibrin serum. The thickened intima shows diffuse fluorescence with occasional brighter flecks. No fluorescence found when sequential section treated with anti-human platelet serum. (UVL x 300).

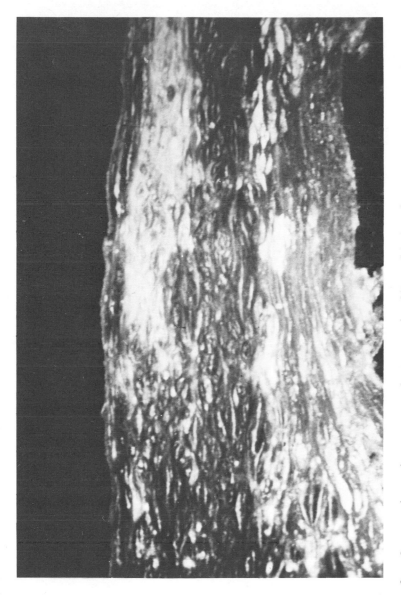

Figure 3. Connective tissue cap of an aortic fibro-lipid plaque. Frozen section treated with fluoresceinated anti-human fibrin serum. The thickened intima shows discrete bands of brilliantly fluorescent material lying roughly parallel to the luminal surface. (UVL x 500).

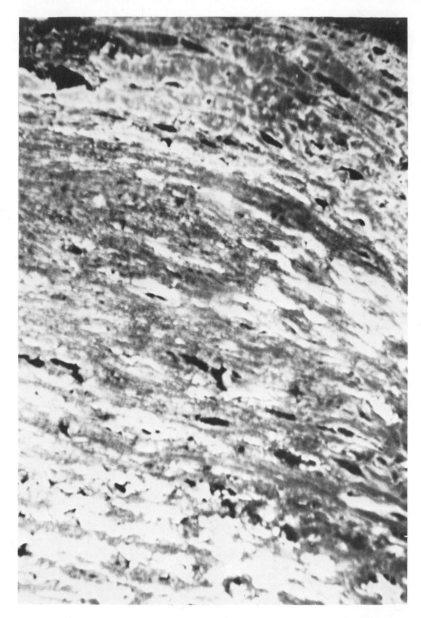

Figure 4. Aortic fibro-lipid plaque. Frozen section treated with fluoresceinated anti-human fibrin serum. The thickened intima shows very numerous layers of brilliantly fluorescent material lying roughly parallel to the luminal surface. (UVL x 300).

3. Platelet Antigens in Atherosclerotic Plaques and Patterns of Anti-Fibrin Binding

As mentioned earlier, binding of fluorescein coupled anti-human fibrin sera occurs in two basic distribution patterns which gave rise to the suggestion that both infiltration and mural thrombus may account for the presence of this antigen in athero-sclerotic lesions. However, the presence of platelet masses gives unequivocal evidence of incorporated thrombus. With these considerations in mind (31) Woolf and Carstairs studied sequential frozen sections of atherosclerotic lesions of different macroscopic appearances with both anti-fibrin and anti-platelet sera. Their objective was to assess the relative frequency of the different patterns of anti-fibrin binding in relation to the various macroscopic types of lesion, and the correlation, if any, which exists between these patterns and the presence of platelet antigens. Fatty streaks and small lipid plaques showed a uniformly diffuse pattern of anti-fibrin binding suggesting the presence of fibrinogen derived from infiltration. No platelet antigens could be demonstrated in these lesions. In contrast, advanced fibro-lipid plaques showed the presence of the localized banded pattern of anti-fibrin binding suggesting the presence of polymerized fibrin in 38/56 lesions. Platelet antigens were present in just under half of the lesions showing this pattern (Figs. 5 and 6). These workers infer that the presence of fibrin in discrete, band-like masses within fibro-lipid plaques strongly suggests that these accumulations represent the residuum of buried thrombus. Similar results have been obtained by others (32). The fact that platelet antigens are only identifiable in approximately half the lesions to which incorporation of thrombus is deemed to have made a contribution, raises various possibilities. The absence of platelets from any individual plaque could mean that platelets were never present in that lesion. Alternatively, platelets might have been present earlier in the natural history of the lesion but no longer be identifiable at the time of the patient's death. It is impossible to determine which of these hypotheses is valid from a study of human lesions, but some useful information on this point has accrued from an experimental study in which mural thrombi were induced by light abrasion of the luminal surface of the pig aorta (33). Within 30 days of the thrombi being produced, fibro-muscular plaques were present. Sampling of the lesions at different times after operation showed that while platelets were easily identifiable during the first three weeks after that the number of lesions in which immunological identification of platelets was possible fell off sharply, so that by six months platelets were found in only three of thirty plaques.

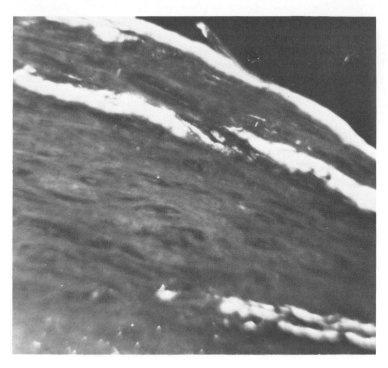

Figure 5. Aortic fibro-lipid plaque. Frozen section treated
with anti-human platelet serum. The connective tissue cap shows
discrete bands of fluorescent material at different levels within
the thickened intima. (UVL x 1200).

4. The Frequency of Incorporated Thrombus
in Relation to Atherosclerotic Plaques

        The frequency with which morphological features (either his-
tological or immuno-histochemical) suggesting the presence of
buried thrombus, within atherosclerotic plaques occur, has been
reviewed recently (34). In the aorta there is a fair degree of
uniformity as far as the proportion of all plaques is concerned
(41-45%) though there is a considerable degree of scatter when
the proportion of cases in which buried thrombus can be found is
considered. Studies were carried out (35, 36) which attempted
to relate the frequency with which "thrombotic" plaques could be
found in a single vessel to the presence or absence of occlusive
arterial disease in that patient. In the first of these studies
all the uncomplicated fibro-lipid plaques in the aortae of 53
patients aged 36-80 were examined for the presence of the "banded"

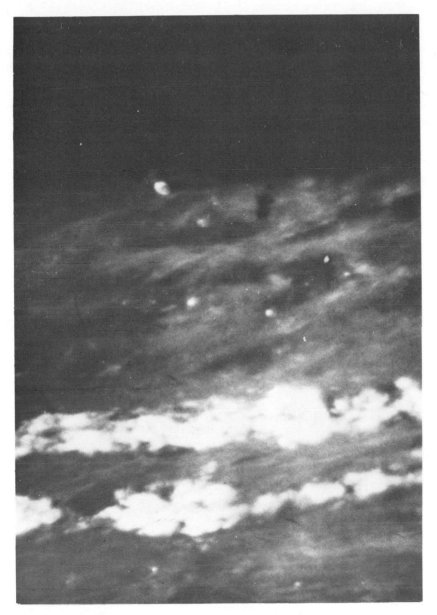

Figure 6. Connective tissue cap of aortic fibro-lipid plaque.
Frozen section treated with anti-human fibrin serum. Note presence of two discrete bands of brilliantly fluorescent material
lying deep within the thickened intima. (UVL x 1200).

or post-thrombotic pattern of anti-fibrin binding. The 53 patients
were divided into three groups: 1) those with no stenosis of the
coronary arteries; 2) those with recent occlusion of the coronary
arteries; 3) those with old occlusion of the coronary arteries.

The proportion of lesions, expressed as a percentage of the
number of plaques examined from each patient, showing the localized pattern of anti-fibrin banding, is shown in Fig. 7. A fairly
wide scatter is present in each of the three groups. Despite this
scatter a definite relationship is seen to exist between the presence of coronary artery occlusion, whether recent or old, and a
high incidence of aortic atherosclerotic plaques which show the
banded pattern of anti-fibrin binding. When the raw data were
analyzed, using a method appropriate to a situation where sample
sizes are different (37-39), the differences observed between the
"occlusion" and "no stenosis" groups were found to be highly
significant ($p < 0.001$). Similar results were obtained (36) in a
larger number of cases. In this study, plaques in the coronary
arteries, as well as those in the aorta, were examined for the
presence both of fibrin and platelet antigens. In the coronary
artery plaques, evidence of what is deemed by us to represent incorporated thrombus was found in 71% of the patients with coronary
artery occlusion. It should be emphasized that the sections examined did not include the occluded segments. Only 28% of the
patients without coronary artery occlusion of significant degrees
of stenosis showed any evidence of buried thrombus.

The association between the localized or "banded" pattern
of fibrin distribution in fibro-lipid, aortic plaques and the presence of occlusive coronary artery disease may be interpreted in
a variety of ways. It may be that in patients dying with a recent
coronary artery occlusion, the final episode is preceded by a
period in which there is an increased thrombotic tendency throughout the arterial tree. It is possible that such a period could
be of relatively short duration since animal studies (40) have
shown that incorporation of thrombus can occur quite rapidly.
An alternative explanation may result in possible impairment of
the thrombolytic mechanisms. For the present both of these must
remain speculative.

5. Experimental Mural Thrombosis and Its Relation to Plaque Formation

Nearly all the foregoing sections deal with the identification of incorporated thrombus within the substance of pre-existing
fibro-lipid plaques. The evidence derived from these and similar
studies cannot be adduced as having any bearing on the question
as to whether plaques can arise as a result of the occurrence of

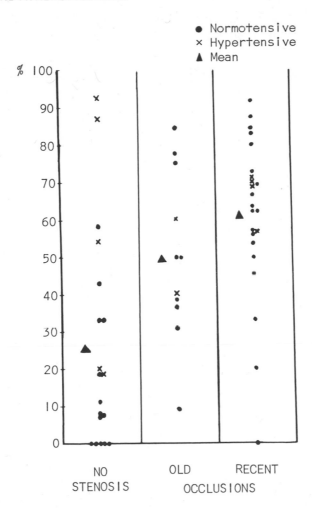

Figure 7. Diagram of the proportion of aortic plaques from each
case which shows the "banded pattern" of anti-fibrin binding and,
hence, by implication, the proportion of plaques containing incorporated thrombus. Each dot or cross represents one patient, and
the proportions are expressed as a percentage of the plaques
examined in each vessel. The cases have been divided into three
groups: those with no stenosis; those with a recent coronary
artery occlusion; and those with an old coronary artery occlusion.

Figures 1, 5, and 7 have been reproduced from "The Pathology of
the Heart," edited by Pomerance and Davies, by kind permission
of Blackwell Scientific Publications.

mural thrombi in previously lesion-free areas of the arterial
intima. It is true that small mural thrombi have been described
as occurring in portions of the arterial intima which are macroscopically normal (13, 41, 42), both in man and in the pig, but
no data exist as to the fate of such thrombi.

For these reasons numerous experimental models have been devised to study the natural history of arterial thrombus with particular reference to the reactions of the subjacent arterial wall.

The earliest reports relate to experimental pulmonary embolism produced either by using fibrin clots (43-46) or artificial
"thrombi" formed in a rotating loop as described (47-50).

Hand and Chandler (48) studied the natural history of platelet rich pulmonary emboli in rabbits fed a normal stock diet. The
time elapsing between embolization and killing ranged from 1 1/2
hours to one year. On light microscopic examination some evidence
of endothelial covering of the retracted emboli was apparent by
the third day and deemed to be nearing completion by one week.
Lesions seen at the end of three weeks were complex, fibro-fatty
plaques with a dense connective tissue cap overlying a basal pool
of intracellular lipid. The presence of lipid was attributed to
phagocytosis and digestion of platelets by monocytes within the
thrombi. Ardlie and Schwartz (50) noted in a similar study that
the amount of lipid in the lesions was increased when animals
were rendered hyperlipidemic by a diet high in fat.

As a model system, pulmonary embolization has certain built-in
weaknesses. Chief among these are the facts that at some stage
in their natural history the emboli must, of necessity, be occlusive rather than mural and that the hemodynamics in the pulmonary
vascular bed differ considerably from those obtaining in systemic
arteries. The logical correlate of this position is a need for
a system for the production of mural thrombi in systemic arteries.
Many methods have been employed with this end in view (51). These
include intimal abrasions under direct vision (40), the use of
balloon catheters to denude the intima of its endothelial covering
(52) and the use of indwelling cannulae which probably produce
repeated injuries of the intima (53). All these methods produce
a significant degree of mural thrombosis. Within a few days of
such endothelial injury in the pig aorta light microscopic evidence of re-endothelialization can be seen (54, 55) and ten days
after the production of the thrombus, it can be seen to be incorporated into the substance of the vessel wall (Fig. 8). However,
it is possible that the time required for complete restoration
of the endothelium to normal may be somewhat longer. Recent studies of the end results of endothelial denudation in the rabbit
aorta produced by the insertion of a Fogarty catheter show that
even after five weeks the new endothelium has an abnormal pattern

and that small raw areas and craters can be seen around which macrophages and a small number of platelets adhere (Fig. 9).

Within ten days of endothelial abrasion in the aorta of a large animal like the pig, active cell proliferation can be seen. The ultrastructural changes occurring in these organizing thrombi have been described (49, 56, 57). Davies et al. (56) found that the early stages of organization of experimentally induced mural thrombi were characterized by the presence of two distinct cell populations. One of these was clearly made up of mononuclear phagocytes. The second population comprised cells lying on the luminal surface of the thrombus and cells with identical ultra-structural features lying more deeply within the substance of the thrombus. within a short time the relatively simple cell populations are replaced by cells which show morphological evidence related to the acquisition of more specialized functions, notably those associated with differentiation towards smooth muscle. At the same time new vascular channels develop which connect the depths of the thrombus with the arterial lumen. However, before this linking up of the main arterial lumen and the substance of the thrombus occurs, capillary spaces appear within the center of some of the clumps of cells within the thrombus and these come to be lined by endothelial cells in no way different from those which appear on the surface of the thrombus. Other members of the original cell population within the depths of the thrombus show peripheral condensation of their cytoplasmic filaments, develop fusiform dense bodies and may become bound by a basement membrane substance. This, in short, represents a degree of differentiation towards smooth muscle.

Within three weeks after intimal abrasion and the formation of the thrombus there is a large population of easily recognizable smooth muscle cells concentrated in layers beneath and parallel to the new endothelial covering (Fig. 10). Mature smooth muscle cells derived from the media are not seen invading the thrombus from the abluminal aspect and the new population of SMC is not, in my view, derived in this way. At this stage, therefore, the operation site shows the presence of a fibro-muscular plaque in which a fair amount of largely intracellular lipid can be identified. Some of these lesions contain a central core in which foam cells and cholesterol clefts can be seen. Such fibro-fatty plaques in systemic arteries, following on the induction of mural thrombosis, can occur even in the presence of normal plasma lipid levels (58). The presence of platelets in these lesions can be confirmed by the use of fluoresceinated anti-platelet sera. Platelets are abundant for the first three weeks following intimal abrasion but thereafter the frequency with which platelet antigens can be detected falls sharply and in lesions which are six months old they can be detected in only a very small proportion of the lesions (33).

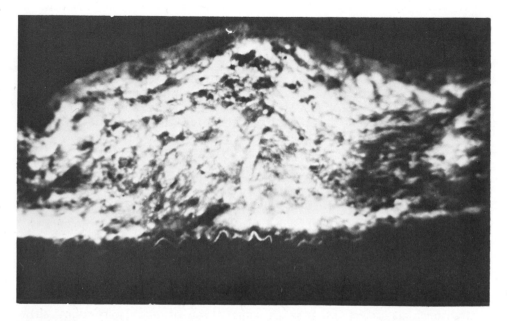

Figure 8. Site of intimal abrasion of pig aorta ten days previously.
Frozen section treated with fluoresceinated anti-pig platelet serum.
Intima shows the presence of abundant fluorescent material which
is clearly separated from the lumina by a narrow band of tissue
which shows auto-fluorescence only. (UVL x 700). Reproduced by
permission of the editors of the Journal of Pathology.

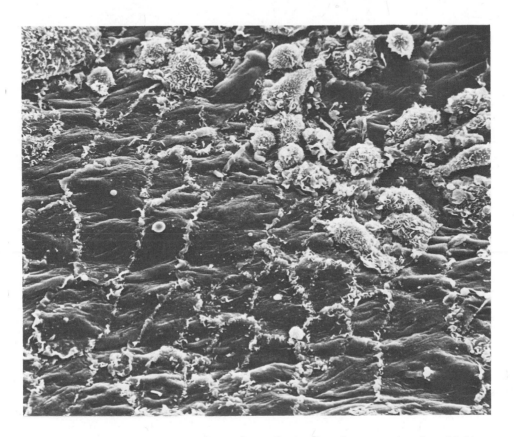

Figure 9. Rabbit aorta. Scanning electron micrograph of rabbit
aorta four weeks after a single injury produced by a Fogarty
catheter. The normal streamlining of endothelial cells is lost
and the new endothelium appears as irregular pavement-like covering. In some areas the endothelial covering appears incomplete,
and numerous macrophages and a moderate number of platelets can
be seen adhering to the intimal surface. (SEM x 936).

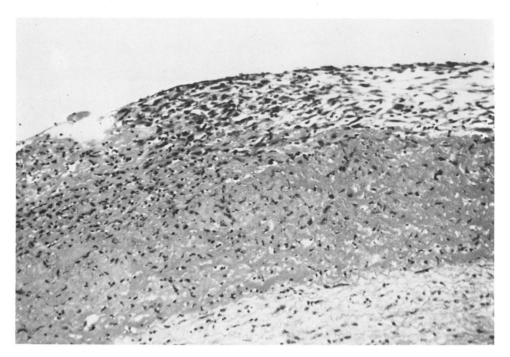

Figure 10. Site of intimal abrasion of pig aorta three weeks previously. Section shows the residuum of a large thrombus which abuts on the media. The thrombus is covered by layers of spindle-shaped cells which, on ultra-structural examination, show some of the features of smooth muscle. (H & E x 75).

6. Are Platelets Essential for Intimal Hyperplasia Following Loss of Endothelium

It could be said that the intimal hyperplasia described in the preceding section is the direct consequence of the traumatic injury to the artery wall and that the presence of mural thrombus is merely incidental in the natural history of the lesion. However, some simple morphological observations suggest that this is not so, and that the presence of adherent and aggregated platelets is causally related to the arterial wall reaction. Pulmonary embolization by "artificial" thrombi results, as noted in a preceding section, in the occurrence of fibro-fatty plaques. In systemic arteries the whole sequence of fibro-muscular formation has been seen in the iliac arteries of the pig where propagated thrombus has occurred following an abrasion of the aorta. It is clear therefore, that direct trauma to the endothelium is not necessary for the formation of these experimentally induced fibro-muscular plaques.

Moore (59) shows the production of raised lesions in the rabbit aorta following an intimal injury caused by an indwelling cannula was inhibited to a considerable extent by the prior administration of anti-platelet serum. Harker (60) states that in baboons made chronically homocystinemic (which produced marked loss of endothelium) the administration of the platelet inhibits dypridamole a diminution of the fibro-muscular proliferation which normally follows endothelial injury. Other workers (61) however, using a rat model, have been able to confirm these results.

7. Interaction between Platelets and Smooth Muscle Cells

Some interesting studies which may relate to the effect of platelets in sub-endothelial connective tissue elements have been carried out by Ross et al. (62, 63). These workers have shown that arterial smooth muscle cell cultures grown in media containing homologous cell-free, plasma derived serum, remain for the most part quiescent, only 3% of the cells synthesizing DNA and going on to divide. However, if serum derived from whole blood which has been allowed to clot is added to the cultures, the smooth muscle cells begin to proliferate. The "trigger" to proliferation has been found to be a factor released from platelets during clotting. The nature of this platelet release factor has not yet been fully established. It is non-dialysable, relatively soluble and appears to be a low molecular weight (13,500) basic protein. It is suggested (64) that this substance has the capacity to recruit smooth muscle cells that are in GO to enter GI phase and, thus, the reproductive cycle. These workers put forward the view that intimal smooth muscle cells in vivo are normally in the same quiescent state as those cultured in the plasma-derived serum. The removal of endothelial cells and the subsequent exposure of sub-endothelial tissues might lead to platelet adhesion, aggregation and release with a consequent increase in the turnover of smooth muscle cells.

These experimental data do not, of course, necessarily constitute the homologue of what occurs in the initiation of spontaneous human atherosclerotic plaques and this reservation is particularly apropos in view of the reports (65, 66) that the smooth muscle cell proliferation in aortic fibrous plaques is monoclonal in type. However, it is clear from the experiments briefly outlined here that incorporation of mural thrombus can and does take place rapidly and that this is associated with a considerable degree of intimal hyperplasia.

REFERENCES

1. Ross, R. (1973) Proc. Sigrid Juselius Foundation Symposium,
    Turku, Finland, E. Kulonen, Ed. Academic Press, London,
    623-636.

2. Narayanan, A.S., Sandberg, L.B., Ross, R., and Layman, D.L.
    (1976) J. Cell Biol. 68, 411-419.

3. Wight, T.N., and Ross, R. (1975) J. Cell Biol. 67, 675-686.

4. Duguid, J.B. (1946) J. Pathol. Bact. 58, 207-212.

5. Duguid, J.B. (1948) J. Pathol. Bact. 60, 57.

6. Duguid, J.B. (1976) The Dynamics of Atherosclerosis, Aberdeen
    Univ. Press, pp. 1-75.

7. Rokitansky, K. von. (1844) in Handbuch der Pathologischen
    Anatomie, 2, Braunmuller & Seidel, Vienna.

8. Long, E.R. (1933) in Arteriosclerosis (Cowdrey, E.V., Ed.)
    MacMillan, New York, p. 19.

9. Mallory, F.B. (1912) in The Harvey Lectures, J.B. Lippincott
    Co., Philadelphia, p. 150.

10. Clark, E., Graef, I., and Chasis, H. (1936) Archives of Pathol-
    ogy, 22, 183-212.

11. Heard, B.E. (1949) J. Pathol. Bact. 61, 635-637.

12. Morgan, A.D. (1956) Blackwell, Oxford.

13. Crawford, R., and Levene, C.I. (1952) J. Pathol. Bact. 64,
    523-528.

14. Movat, H.Z., and More, R.H. (1957) Am. J. Clin. Pathol. 28,
    331-353.

15. More, R.H., and Haust, D. (1957) Archives of Pathol. 63, 612-
    620.

16. Movat, H.Z., Haust, M.D., and More, R.H. (1959) Am. J. Pathol.
    35, 93-101.

17. Haust, M.D., More, R.H., and Movat, H.Z. (1959) Am. J. Pathol.
    37, 377.

18. Haust, M.D., More, R.H., and Movat, H.Z. (1960) Am. J. Pathol. 37, 377.

19. Lendrum, A.C. (1949) J. Pathol. Bact. 61, 443.

20. Coons, A.H., Leduc, E.H., and Kaplan, M.H. (1951) J. Exp. Med. 93, 173-188.

21. Woolf, N., and Crawford, T. (1960) J. Pathol. Bact. 80, 405-408.

22. Woolf, N. (1961) Am. J. Pathol. 39, 521-532.

23. Wyllie, J.C., More, R.H., and Haust, M.D. (1964) J. Pathol. Bact. 88, 335-338.

24. Haust, M.D., Wyllie, J.C., and More, R.H. (1964) Am. J. Pathol. 44, 255-267.

25. Haust, M.D., Wyllie, J.C., and More, R.H. (1965) Exp. Molec. Path. 4, 205-216.

26. Walton, K.W., and Williamson, N. (1968) J. Ather. Res. 8, 599-624.

27. Kao, V.C.Y., and Wissler, R.W. (1965) Exp. Molec. Pathol. 4, 465-479.

28. Adams, C.W.M. (1967) in Vascular Histochemistry, London, Lloyd-Luke.

29. Carstairs, K.C. (1965) J. Pathol. Bact. 90, 225-231.

30. Carstairs, K.C., Woolf, N., and Crawford, T. (1964) J. Pathol. Bact. 88, 537-540.

31. Woolf, N., and Carstairs, K.C. (1967) Am. J. Pathol. 51, 373-386.

32. Hudson, J., and McCaughey, W.T.E. (1974) Atherosclerosis 19, 543-553.

33. Woolf, N., and Carstairs, K.C. (1969) J. Pathol. 97, 595-601.

34. Chandler, A.B., and Pope, J.T. (1975) in Blood and Arterial Wall in Atherogenesis and Arterial Thrombosis. IFMA Scientific Symposia. No. 4. (Hautvast, J.G.A.J., Hermus, R.J.J. and van der Haap, F., Eds.) E.J. Brill, Leiden, 111-118.

35. Woolf, N., Sacks, M.I., and Davies, M.J. (1969) Am. J.
     Pathol. 57, 187.

36. Cottam, D. (1971) Thesis for the Ph.D. degree, University of
     London.

37. Dyke, C.V., and Patterson, H.D. (1952) Biometrics 8, 1-12.

38. Walker, S.H., and Duncan, D.B. (1967) Biometrika, 54, 167-179.

39. Naylor, A.S. (1964) Ann. Hum. Genet. (London) 27, 241-246.

40. Woolf, N., Bradley, J.P.W., Crawford, T., and Carstairs, K.C.
     (1968) Brit. J. Exper. Pathol. 49, 257-264.

41. Geissinger, H.D., Mustard, J.F., and Rowsell, H.C. Can. Med.
     Assoc. J. 87, 405-408.

42. Campbell, R.S.F. (1965) J. Ather. Res. 5, 483.

43. Harrison, C.V. (1948) J. Pathol. Bact. 60, 289-293.

44. Heard, B.E. (1952) J. Pathol. Bact. 64, 13-19.

45. Thomas, W.A., O'Neal, R.M., and Lee, K.T. (1956) Archives of
     Pathology 61, 380-389.

46. Heptinstall, R.H. (1957) Brit. J. Exp. Pathol. 38, 438-445.

47. Chandler, A.B. (1958) Lab. Invest. 7, 110-114.

48. Hand, R.A., and Chandler, A.B. (1962) Am. J. Pathol. 40,
     469-482.

49. Still, W.J.S. (1966) Lab. Invest. 15, 1492-1507.

50. Ardlie, N.G., and Schwartz, C.J. (1968) J. Pathol. Bact. 95,
     19-29.

51. Henry, R.L. (1962) Angiology 13, 554-557.

52. Stemerman, M.B., and Ross, R. (1972) J. Exp. Med.. 136, 769-
     789.

53. Moore, S. (1973) Lab. Invest. 29, 478-487.

54. Crawford, T., and Woolf, N. (1968) in Colloques Internationaux
     du Centre National de la Recherche Scientifique, No. 169,
     597-604.

55. Davies, M.J., Woolf, N., and Bradley, J.P.W. (1969) J. Pathol. 97, 589-594.

56. Jørgensen, L., Rowsell, H.C., Hovig, T., and Mustard, J.F. (1967) Am. J. Pathol. 51, 681-719.

57. Davies, M.J., Ballantine, S.J., Robertson, W.B., and Woolf, N. (1975) J. Pathol. 117, 75-81.

58. Sumiyoshi, A., More, R.H., and Weigensberg, B.I. (1973) Athero-sclerosis 18, 43-57.

59. Moore, S., Friedman, R.J., Singal, D.P., Gauldie, J., and Blajchman, M. (1976) Thrombosis et Diathesis Haemorrhageia 35, 70-81.

60. Harker, L., Ross, R., Schlichter, S., and Scott, C. (1976) J. Chem. Invest. 58, 731-741.

61. Clowes, A.W., and Karnovsky, M.J. (1977) Lab. Invest. 36, 452-464.

62. Ross, R., and Glomset, J.A. (1976) N. Engl. J. Med. 295, 369-377.

63. Rutherford, R.B., and Ross, R. (1976) J. Cell. Biol. 69, 196-203.

64. Ross, R., Glomset, J., and Harker, L. (1977) Am. J. Pathol. 86, 675-684.

65. Benditt, E.P., and Benditt, J.M. (1973) Proc. Nat. Acad. Sci. USA 70, 1753-1756.

66. Benditt, E.P. (1977) Am. J. Pathol. 86, 693-702.

ENDOTHELIUM 1977: A REVIEW

Guido Majno and Isabelle Joris

Department of Pathology
University of Massachusetts Medical School
Worcester, Massachusetts

This paper is conceived as a short update of the review published in 1965 (1). It is based on a set of 2,476 references assembled through a MEDLARS search limited to the single word endothelium (January 1966 - June 1977; a few references were added up to the end of 1977). Much to our regret, we were obliged to omit from our search the word capillary, which would have yielded an unmanageable number of additional papers. About 5% of the MEDLARS titles referred to corneal endothelium and were eliminated. This decision, which was based on limitations of space, may well have discarded relevant data: vascular and corneal endothelium are both mesodermal structures, and although the corneal endothelium has some attributes which appear to be distinctive, such as a water pump (2), other properties are similar (3). In limiting the number of references to about 500, arbitrary choices had to be made; papers obviously belonging under the headings of inflammation, atherosclerosis, or thrombosis were not included and will be found in other portions of this volume. Some of the inevitable gaps will be filled by the bibliography of the papers quoted herein, by other reviews (4-15), and by the proceedings of the A. Benzon Symposium of 1969 (16).

The abbreviations used in this paper are TEM and SEM - transmission and scanning electron microscopy. The bibliography appears as Appendix A, pages 481-526.

1. VARIABILITY OF THE ENDOTHELIAL LINING

One of the main themes of this review is about as old as the
first electron micrographs of capillaries: it has become more
and more obvious that endothelia differ in structure, function
and metabolic properties not only in different organs, but in
different parts of the same organ and even in different segments
of a single microcirculatory loop. It is impossible to make generalized statements concerning "the endothelium" or "the capillaries" without further specifications. We cannot overemphasize
the importance of this obvious truth, which is still not foremost
in the minds of all concerned. We shall mention later, within the
microcirculation, differences in reactivity without a morphologic
counterpart. In large vessels, the "normal" intima is not necessarily uniform: areas of abnormally high permeability have been
found in arteries of rabbits, dogs, pigs, and rats (17-19). Some
may represent early forms of injury; however, in two studies a
structural basis for the different functional behavior was not
found, and local hemodynamic differences were sought as a possible
explanation (18, 19). It has even been reported that capillary
permeability (and ultrastructure) may vary at different depths of
ventricular myocardium in the rat (20). Thus, in the micro- as
well as in the macrocirculation, the endothelium is a very heterogeneous membrane.

Despite this variety, it is possible to classify all endothelia (and capillaries), as presently understood, into a few groups
(Fig. 1); we can still follow, with some retouches, the classification used in the previous review (1) which considered three
groups, based on the continuity of the endothelial barrier: (A)
continuous: this category can be retained, but new data on the
junctions suggest two sub-groups: with pleomorphic junctions
(characterized by a multiplicity of junctional arrangements, ranging from the focally tight "gap junctions" to open junctions;
example: blood vessels of muscle) and with tight junctions only
(example: brain); (B) fenestrated: this category can be retained
as previously described (with open or closed fenestrae); (C) discontinuous: two corrections are required: first, the discontinuities are not only intercellular but also trans-cellular (sect.
4a); second, the category as a whole cannot be equated with sinusoids, because the lining of the sinusoids in the bone marrow is
continuous (sect. 4a).

Although useful, this classification is not entirely satisfactory. it emphasizes the barrier properties of the endothelium
and neglects others, such as metabolic activities and phagocytosis.
Tight and non-tight junctions can occur side by side in the same
capillary loop and on opposite sides of the same endothelial cell.

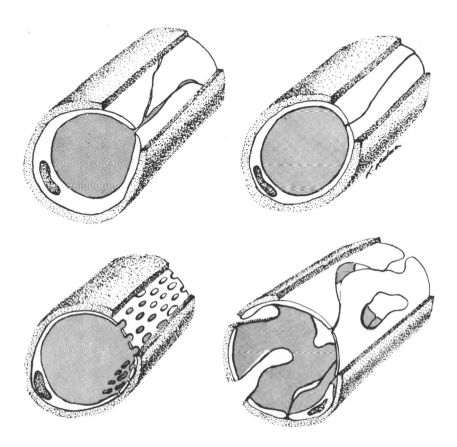

Figure 1. Main types of endothelium. Top: continuous, which includes two main varieties: with pleomorphic junctions, i.e., varying from tight to open (left) or with purely tight junctions
(right). Below: fenestrated (left) and discontinuous (right).
The latter has intercellular as well as trans-cellular openings.
(Modified from Forssmann, 22).

Occasional fenestrae can be found also in endothelia that are (on
the whole) continuous: in normal adult rat muscle, for instance,
it has been reported that one of about 60 cross sections of capillaries contains fenestrae (21); this agrees with our own experience.

Furthermore, the scheme of Figure 1 could be expanded to include more sub-groups: e.g., continuous endothelia include micro-
villous variants (sect. 3b) as well as the "high endothelium" of
the post-capillary venules of the lymph nodes (sect. 4b).

2.   TECHNIQUES

In the field of permeability studies, many new tracers have
been defined and used. To the group of particulate tracers, such
as ferritin (110 Å), were added graded dextrans (120-200 Å) and
glycogens (250-300 Å) (23). Yet finer crevices were probed with
"mass tracers" (10): horseradish peroxidase (50 Å) (24); myoglobin (34 Å) (25); cytochrome C (33 Å) (26); and hemepeptides obtained by enzymatic hydrolysis of cytochrome C: heme-undecapeptide (HIIP, "microperoxidase," 27) and heme-octapeptide (H8P)
both about 20 Å 928); heme-nonapeptide, recently reported as being
comparable to other heme-tracers and non toxic even in high concentrations (29); and polyethyleneimine, a synthetic polymer which
yields colloidal solutions of cationic particles; depending on
the process used for imparting contrast to the particles, their
size ranges from 100 to 300 Å (30). All permeability studies
based on tracers remain subject to the possible criticism of
changes caused by the tracer itself; in the guinea pig, for instance, horseradish peroxidase causes vascular reactions possibly
mediated by prostaglandins (31).

Freeze-cleaving has helped to clarify the structure of junctions (sect. 3d) and the advent of scanning electron microscopy
has led to scores of papers on endothelial surfaces: the latter
technique, however, is especially prone to artefacts, and a number of published results are misleading; a word of caution has
been published recently (32). With regard to the study of large
blood vessels, especially arteries, it is being realized that many
artifacts can develop in the endothelium if the blood vessels are
not fixed at physiological pressure (33, 34). For human material,
of course, this is not possible; thus human and experimental material cannot always be directly compared, a consideration that is
often forgotten. New methods have appeared for the study of the
endothelium en face (35) and for metabolic studies in vitro (36).
Tissue culture has made great contributions (sect. 8). Promising
new fields are the study of isolated capillaries (8, 37) and of
endothelial cells obtained from the microvasculature (38).

3. MORPHOLOGY

a) Light Microscopy

The only significant novelty that we could find is the identification of sex chromatin in endothelial cells (39, 530, 531):
perhaps not a surprising fact, but a useful tool in the field of
grafts (sect. 10). With suitable techniques, sex chromatin can be
recognized also in capillaries, using paraffin sections; the frequency of Barr bodies in female endothelium was 54% (human), 43%
(dog), 46% (rabbit), and 28% (rat, which was difficult to analyze).
In guinea pigs the method was not applicable (531).

b) The Endothelial Surface

At this level, one previously uncertain structure is here to
stay: the so-called endo-endothelial layer. This was first demonstrated by Luft using ruthenium red, an old technique (40). It
appeared as a fuzzy layer, and as such encountered at first some
skepticism. At present we must conclude that, although fuzzy, it
is real; further studies will have to establish its nature, extent,
and significance in various parts of the vascular system.

A criticism of the ruthenium red method has been that it only
demonstrates negative charges without providing information as to
the type of molecule that bears them. This objection does not
apply to the new technique based on concanavalin A, a plant agglu-
tinin (lectin) extracted from the jack bean. This molecule has
two active sites, both of which can react with sugars of glycoproteins that contain an appropriate branch terminal. When the sugar
is in an insoluble form, as in a cell coat (or in the endo-endothelial layer), concanavalin A attaches to it with only one of its
two active sites; the other is then free to operate as an acceptor
for any sugar secondarily added to the system: horseradish peroxidase can be bound in this manner because it is a glycoprotein
containing 18% of carbohydrates. All one has to do at this point
is to demonstrate the peroxidase histochemically. Weber et al.
used this method to demonstrate the endo-endothelial layer on the
surface of the aorta in laboratory rodents, normal as well as
hypercholesterolemic (41, 42). Another well-documented study has
been published by Stein et al., who used rat heart perfused with
a solution of concanavalin A (either native or radioactively
labeled) (43). It is possible that the glycoproteins demonstrated
by the concanavalin method serve in part as a barrier, in part as
specific receptors for molecules which, once captured, will be
transported across the endothelium. A similar conclusion was

reached by others (44, 45). Loudon et al. (46) studied the rate
of labeling of endothelial vesicles in mesenteric capillaries of
the frog, using ferritin, and concluded that there was a diffusion
barrier at the level of the neck of the caveolae. This constric-
tion could depend on the presence of an endo-endothelial layer,
or on the diaphragms described by Palade and Bruns (47).

Heparin-related mucopolysaccharides have been detected on the
surface of the endothelium (sect. 5); it has also been shown that
heparin injected intravenously, intraperitoneally or subcutaneously
becomes attached to the surface of the endothelium (48, 49):   one
hour after intravenous injection, the concentration of heparin
connected with the endothelium was 30-500 times greater than the
concentration in the blood. In the renal glomerulus, Latta et al.
studied the glycoprotein coat of the endothelium and other cell
types, using ruthenium red (50, 51); the endothelial surface was
covered with a fuzzy layer of width varying from negligible to
about 120 Å (rarely 600 Å).

In the lung, a composite layer (plasma protein and polysaccharide) has been described (52, 53). Several specific proteins
have been demonstrated or assumed to be bound on the endothelial
surface: a proteinase inhibitor, alpha-2-macroglobulin, lipoprotein lipase (sect. 5b) and fibrinogen (which was found also on the
surface of the erythrocytes) (54). The notion of a fibrin layer
on the surface of the endothelium (55) is not supported by current
evidence.

The surface characteristics of the endothelium should be
related to the sticking or "margination" of circulating white
blood cells; this premise has led to several studies of the adhesion of lymphocytes and granulocytes to endothelial cells culti-
vated in vitro (56, 57). Especially interesting, along these lines,
are the studies of MacGregor et al., who found that granulocyte
stickiness to nylon fiber columns (58) as well as to cultured

---

Figure 2. Demonstrating the importance of particle charge for
endothelial permeability. Four sections of glomerular capillary
wall 6-8 min. after perfusion with 4 different kinds of ferritin
(mouse; capillary lumen downward). From top to bottom: native
ferritin, isoelectric point (pI) 4.6; cationized ferritin, pI 7.4-
8.4; ferritin C, pI 8-9; ferritin D, pI 8.8 and higher. Positively
charged ferritins penetrate far more easily, suggesting that the
barrier function of the capillary wall depends in part on its
electrophysical properties (intrinsic negative charges). 50,000 x
(Rennke et al., 61).

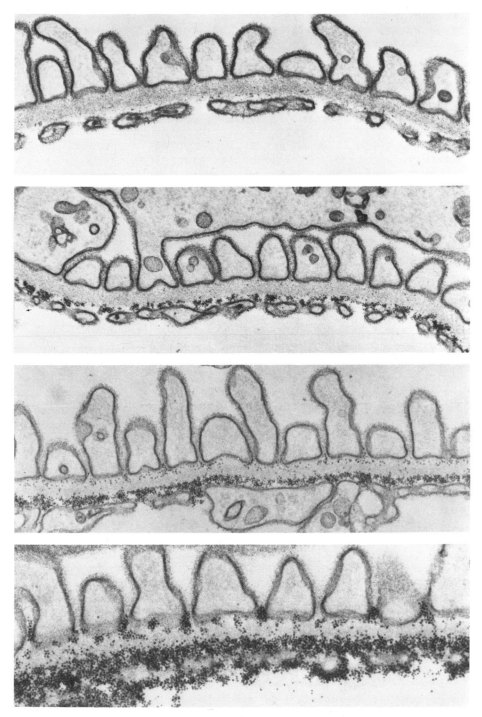

Figure 2

human endothelium (59) is increased by a factor present in inflammatory exudate; it is inhibited by anti-inflammatory agents (60)
and by trypsinization of the endothelial surface (59).

An important new concept, in relation to the endothelial surface, is the role of molecular charge in relation to permeability.
This was beautifully demonstrated by Rennke et al. in a study of
the permeability of the renal glomerulus using native ferritin and
various cationized derivatives (61): it is now clear that the
passage of a given molecule across the endothelium depends not only
on its shape and size, but also on its electrical charge (Fig. 2).
The role of surface charges was also studied by Danon et al. on
the aorta and vena cava of the guinea pig, by means of cationized
ferritin (62-64). The subendothelial surface charge was at least
as great; about half the negative charges on the surface of the
endothelium, but not of the subendothelium, were removed by incubation with neuraminidase.

The electrical properties of the endothelial surface have
been discussed in a series of papers by Sawyer et al. (65). These
studies could prove to be very interesting, especially in relation
to endothelial injury and thrombosis; unfortunately, they are
highly technical and very difficult to interpret for the average
biologist. This may explain why they are rarely quoted in the
context of vascular physiology and pathology. However, there is
at least one physiologic study in which the negative charge of the
normal luminal capillary surface is taken into consideration, and
assumed to play a significant role in the elimination of CO_2 from
capillary blood in the lung (66).

An occasional feature of the endothelial surface are cylindrical microvilli about 1 μ in length. A three-dimensional recon-
struction based on TEM of capillaries of the rat Gasserian ganglion
and testis suggested a truly villous endothelium (67). Microvilli
have also been described in countless SEM studies of large vessels
(68). A second look at the first published documents of this kind
(69) suggests that some of the early microvilli were artifacts;
however, their existence is unquestionable. Their function and
their peculiar abundance in certain vessels (67) remain a baffling
problem.

c) Intracellular Organelles

The mystery of the Weibel-Palade bodies is still well guarded.
but a few new data have been gathered. Since they lack acid phosphatase activity, a close link with lysosomes is ruled out (70);
their origin has been traced to the Golgi apparatus (71). In the
frog, their distribution in the vascular tree has been carefully

mapped; it forms a biphasic curve, with the lowest numbers in the endocardium and in the capillaries (72, 73): the message that lies behind this very specific topography has not yet been deciphered. Santolaya and Bertini studied their distribution in the arteries and veins of 17 species (74): they were present in the rat, cat and oppossum, but not in a fourth mammal, the armadillo; they were absent in chickens and pigeons, but present in the dove; they were present in four reptiles, four amphibians and one fish. In the latter three classes they were more abundant than in mammals or birds, and not quite the same, being spherical or oval; in the fish they occupied as much as 70% of the cell volume. The same authors succeeded in preparing a cell fraction of the granules from the toad aorta (75); when sonicated and injected into the rat, this material produced a rise in blood pressure: perhaps a hint as to the biologic function of the granules. Another hint comes from Burri and Weibel (76), who list several theoretical and experimental arguments suggesting a pro-coagulative action of the granules. Epinephrine caused pro-coagulative material to be liberated by rabbit aorta; and rabbit aortas incubated with epinephrine lost a significant number of granules, which were possibly secreted into the lumen.

Despite all their mysteries, the Weibel-Palade bodies have acquired an important function as markers of endothelial cells: in this capacity they have helped unravel the histogenesis of Kaposi's sarcoma (sect. 93); and in tissue culture their presence is the safest morphologic indication that the cells being cultured are truly endothelial. In this regard, cultures of capillary endothelium should be at a disadvantage, since Weibel-Palade bodies are practically absent in this milieu; indeed, in the first cultures of this type none could be found (37). There is a single report of Weibel-Palade bodies in human capillaries (77). The published electron micrographs suggest that the vessels are actually venules; however, this report is significant in that the rod-shaped bodies were present also in pericytes: so far the best (but unconfirmed) evidence that endothelium and pericytes are closely related cells.

Much new information is available on the vesicles through further studies from Palade's laboratory (the term caveolae is sometimes used for vesicles open at the cell surface; stoma refers to the opening of a caveola). A three-dimensional model was reconstructed from a segment of endothelium (78). Especially significant are structural modulations such as the presence of a diaphragm across the stoma, and flask-shape deformations, features presumably related to the "ferrying" function (47). Morphometric data are now available on vesicles in several endothelia (79-81). In their studies of pulmonary capillaries (82, 83), Smith et al. described caveolae with knobs on either side of the opening, interpreted as possible cross sections of a ring-like structure;

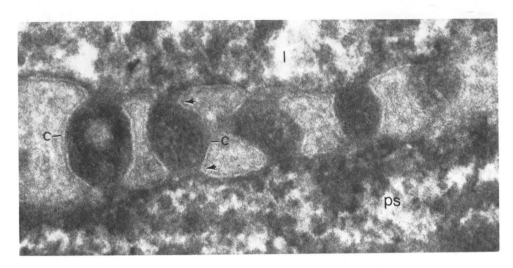

Figure 3. Capillary endothelium of rat cremaster, 5 min. after
local interstitial injection of heme-undecapeptide. Dark reaction
product marks the lumen (1), pericapillary space (ps), and transendothelial channels (c) formed by single vesicles. Note continuity between plasmalemma and vesicle membrane (arrows). 180,000 x
(Simionescu et al., 28).

the inner, concave surface showed regularly spaced globules, possibly enzyme clusters or binding sites (82).

    An important new finding has derived from studies with heme-
peptides as markers (28). In a thin portion of the endothelial
cell, a single vesicle can fuse with the luminal and abluminal
cell membrane and give rise to a short channel. Collision of two
or more vesicles with each other (and fusion with both cell membranes) can give rise to longer transendothelial channels (Fig. 3);
ring-shaped strictures persist at the points of fusion. These
channels are conceived as transient; their frequency still remains
to be established. Diaphragms can sometimes be seen across their
openings, similar to those found at the stoma of plasmalemmal vesicles or across the openings of fenestrated endothelium. Thus it
becomes apparent that single vesicles, fused vesicles, channels
and fenestrae can now be conceived as dynamic parts of a single
system for transcellular exchange of water-soluble molecules (10).

    Coated vesicles have been described in the capillary endothe-
lium of rodents (47) as well as in the aorta of the dog (84); in
the latter they fell into two groups: large (700 Å) located near
the cell surface, and small (400 Å) located near the Golgi appara-

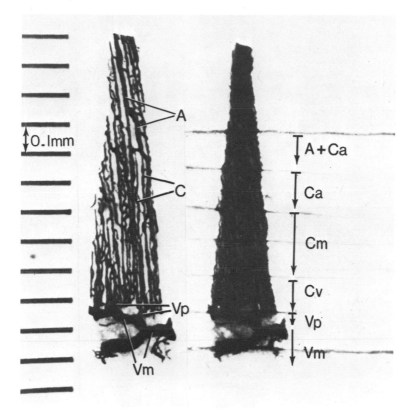

Figure 4. Example of the bipolar microvascular field of mouse diaphragm that allowed precise ultrastructural identification of microvascular segments. Left: fixed and reacted for microperoxidase; A = arteriole, C = capillaries, Vp and Vm = pericytic and muscular venules. Right: same specimen embedded in epon, and ready to be cut into 6 blocks of known topography. Even capillaries can be subdivided into arterial, middle and venous segment (Ca, Cm, Cv). 90 x (Simionescu et al., 87).

tus (with which they may be related, 85). The "coat" or corona (47) consisted of radiating projections 200 Å in length spaced by 200-250 Å. In the sinusoids of the rat bone marrow, large coated vesicles formed rapidly upon the intravenous injection of colloidal carbon black, and took up the particles (86). The endocytic function of the coated vesicles is well established (for ref., see

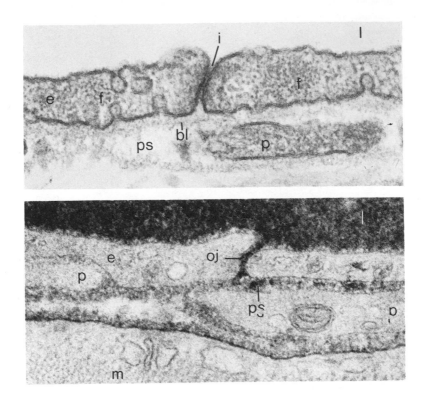

Figure 5. Top: endothelial junction (i) with gap of about 60 Å, in a pericytic venule of mouse diaphragm; e = endothelial cell, f = filaments, bl = basal lamina, ps = pericapillary space, p = pericyte, l = lumen. 72,000 x. Below: similar venule, 25 sec. after i.v. injection of heme-undecapeptide; the junction is "open" (oj), as shown by the dark reaction product (Simionescu et al., 88).

86). In human fibroblasts, coated vesicles have been shown to arise from specialized coated regions of the plasma membrane equipped with receptors for LDL (533).

d) Intercellular Junctions

A major advance in this area is reported by N. Simionescu, M. Simionescu and G. Palade (87, 88). It promises to settle a vexed question: the permeability of the "capillary" junctions, a topic beset with contradictions and uncertain results (e.g., 89). The answer is that the word "capillary" is not precise enough. In the mouse diaphragm, these authors were able to identify micro-circulatory fields in which the sequence arteriole-capillary-venule is bipolar, i.e., arranged in a straight line, so that sequential cross sections will show vessels precisely identifiable as to their topography (Fig. 4) (87). The main results are the following (88): in the arterioles, and along the entire length of the capillaries, the junctions are tight, i.e., closed to the probe molecule, heme-undecapeptide (20 Å). In the pericytic venules 25 to 30% of the junctions are normally open (Fig. 5): the gap measures 30-60 Å and is rapidly permeated by the H11P. The size limit for the mole-cules that may negotiate this gap is not yet certain, but preliminary experiments suggest that it lies between 50 and 70 Å (90). As a re-sult of this key study many previous data become obsolete; it is no longer possible to discuss junctional permeability without reference to the precise location of that junction along the microcirculatory loop. In the usual tissue samples, this is practically impossible, hence the confusion that had prevailed to this time.

A previous study by the same group, on vascular fields of the rat omentum and mesentery (91), had shown that junctions differ considerably in arterioles, capillaries and venules as seen by the freeze-cleaving technique. The principle of this method cannot be dealt with here (92); suffice it to mention that it cracks apart the two leaflets of the cell membrane and allows them to be seen from the inside, in small areas. Thus, it can provide certain data on the topographic arrangement of the junctions (93, 94) (but not directly) on their overall permeability. It does show that the junctions, which appear by TEM as buttons often appear as strands; but it does not indicate whether these strands ever form continuous belts around the cell. A correlation of these images with TEM is difficult (91). Despite these limitations, the study mentioned above (91) certainly suggests that the junctions are tighter and more complex in arterioles, where they include gap junctions or maculae communicantes; whereas they are simpler, as well as loosely organized in the venules.

e)   Basement Membrane

The mechanism whereby endothelial cells remain attached to their basement membrane is not fully understood. Stehbens de-scribed focal attachments which resemble the half-desmosomes of the dermal-epidermal junction (95); these structures certainly represent points of firm attachment, because when the endothelium is arti-fically injured, it tends to become lifted from its base but remains attached at these points (96). A curious observation is

that vinblastine causes the endothelium to become detached at certain sites in the glomerular capillaries (97).

        If the basement membrane is exposed to the blood stream,
platelets do adhere to it; but despite the fact that the basement
membrane contains collagen (sect. 5), the platelet reaction that
ensues is different from that observed with interstitial collagen:
the platelets do not aggregate, but simply spread and form a
"pseudoendothelium" (98). Similar observations were made in vitro
(99).

        The functions of basement membranes in general have been
reviewed by Vracko (100). Much attention is currently given to
the reduplication of the basement membrane in the microcirculation,
perhaps because it is one of the few morphologically recognizable
"capillary diseases." This topic will be discussed in sect. 9a,
b. A survey of normal skin biopsies showed that the reduplication
is so constant on the venous side of the microcirculation that
its very presence helps to identify the vessel (101). In other
words, it can be a normal phenomenon. The thickness of the basement membrane is better evaluated after fixation in osmium tetroxide only rather than after fixation in glutaraldehyde (sect. 9b).
The chemical nature and origin of the basement membrane are discussed in section 5.

4.   SPECIALIZED ENDOTHELIA

a) Sinusoids

        The vessels grouped under this name are now known to be so
heterogeneous that their main common characteristic is that of
being unlike common capillaries. There have been many TEM and SEM
studies on the sinusoids of the liver, spleen, and bone marrow,

---

Figure 6. Top: SEM of liver sinusoid (rat); note sieve plates.
3,800 x. Middle: SEM of bone marrow sinusoid (rat): continuous
endothelium. 3,800 x. (Courtesy of R.P. Becker, P.P.H. De Bruyn
and S. Michelson). Bottom: left to right: (1) SEM of bone marrow sinusoid, showing marrow cell emerging through a hole in the
endothelial cell; interendothelial junctions are clearly visible
nearby. 8,800 x (Becker and De Bruyn, 119). (2) SEM of an endothelial bulge, presumably formed by a marrow cell about to emerge;
note fenestrae forming over the bulge. 36,000 x (De Bruyn et al.,
122). (3) TEM showing fenestrae forming under similar conditions,
in rat leukemia. 22,500 x (De Bruyn et al., 122).

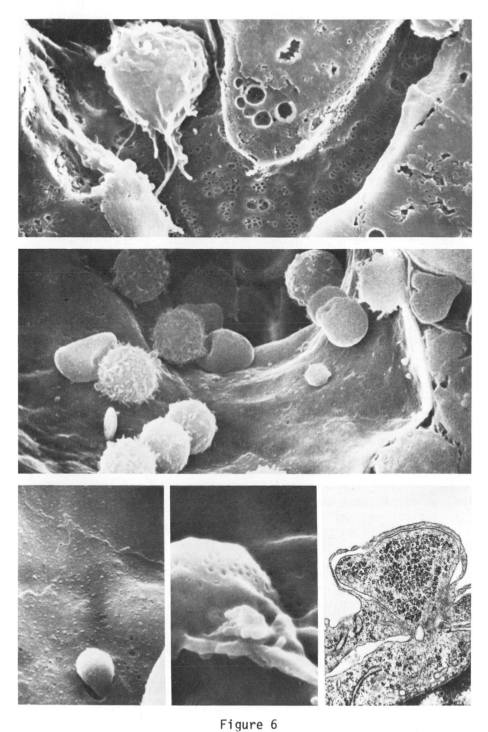

Figure 6

concerning their morphology (102-108) as well as the mechanism of
uptake of colloidal particles injected into the blood stream (109-
111). The difference between liver endothelial cells and Kupffer
cells has been studied by histochemical means (112-114); it has
also been possible to isolate these two cell types in preparations
suitable for biochemical assay (115).

Scanning electron microscopy has been of great help in the
study of sinusoids. It has shown that those of the liver (116)
show patches of trans-cellular perforations or "sieve plates."
(Fig. 6, top) If the venous outflow from the liver is obstructed,
these sieve plates are replaced by large fenestrations (117). By
contrast, in the bone marrow, the margins of the endothelial cells
are apposed throughout (Fig. 6, middle), an unexpected fact in
view of the heavy cellular traffic that flows through it. Here,
too, SEM has provided new data: this cellular traffic occurs
through the endothelial cells, rather than through the junctions
(118-120); the published electron micrographs would be difficult
to refute. This view is adopted in a recent textbook (121). A
similar sequence of events was described in rats with myelogenous
leukemia (122): the emerging myelocyte begins by impinging on the
endothelium, and causes it to bulge into the lumen; the bulge then
becomes covered with fenestrae, and eventually the myelocyte pops
out (Fig. 6, bottom). It should be mentioned here that scattered
fenestrae are present also in normal marrow sinusoids (110); they
are never as frequent as in typical fenestrated endothelia (e.g.,
in the renal glomerulus), thus the marrow sinusoids are best considered as a special variety of continuous endothelium.

b) The "High Endothelial" Venules of Lymphatic Tissue

Despite much new work by TEM and SEM, the best three-dimensional model of these peculiar, gland-like vessels, critical to the
life-cycle of lymphocytes, is an artist's view (Fig. 7). A debate
has raged concerning the pathway followed by the lymphocytes in
traversing the "high endothelium," on the way from the blood to the
lymph. On the basis of sequential (but not fully serial) sections,
supplemented by statistical analysis, Schoefl concluded that, contrary to previous belief, lymphocytes followed an intercellular
pathway (123). Subsequent investigators tended to agree with her
point of view (124-128). However, the problem has been restudied
recently by a method that would appear to be unimpeachable: multiple batches of complete serial sections (about 100 for every
single lymphocyte). The results indicate that the lymphocytes
first penetrate into the endothelial cells, then move laterally
toward the intercellular junction, through which they complete their
emigration (129). The thoroughness of this study strongly suggests
that the problem may be settled.

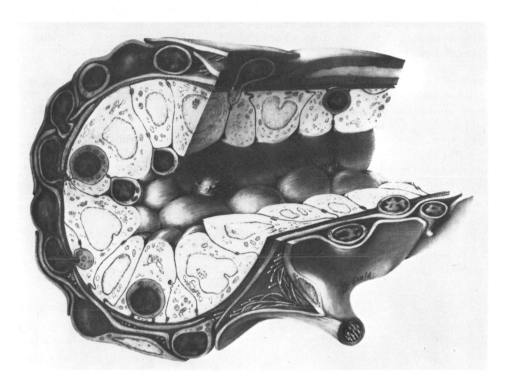

Figure 7. An artist's concept of a high-endothelial venule from a lymph node, showing lymphocytes at various stages of their trans-mural migration (Anderson et al., 125).

An interesting side product of Schoefl's work has been the finding that lymphocytes are perhaps the only cells which perform diapedesis in such a manner that the direction of their movement can be recognized even on electron micrographs: their "tail" or uropod is a welcome dynamic detail on electron micrographs, in which directional information is generally difficult to obtain.

Why is this endothelium so high? Schoefl has speculated that this feature may protect it from becoming excessively permeable as a result of the intense cellular traffic - assumed by her to be intercellular. If indeed the traffic were intercellular, the idea would have some support in known facts: first, this high endo-thelium is indeed very permeable to peroxidase; second, it does not have continuous tight junctions (130); and third, particles

of colloidal carbon did pass from the blood to the spaces between
high endothelial cells, but crossed the basement membrane only
where lymphocytes were also crossing it (124). However, in view
of recent evidence that the lymphocyte passage is first trans-,
then intercellular, Schoefl's suggestion becomes less cogent.
Transcellular traffic is obviously well tolerated by the very low
endothelium of the bone marrow sinusoids. Pertinent evidence from
other sources is meager; in the human thymus, the thickened endothelium found in patients with myasthenia gravis and other conditions has been interpreted as an indication of lymphocyte recircu-
lation (131). It is often said that, in chronic inflammation,
continued diapedesis causes the endothelium to become thicker, but
the single paper always quoted in this context (132) shows very
little evidence to support the notion.

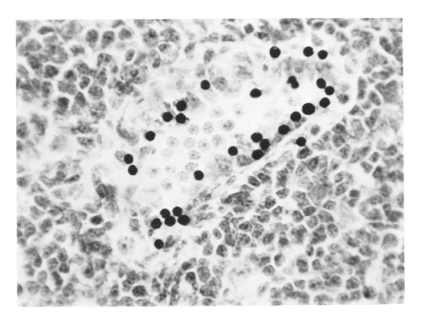

Figure 8. Demonstrating the selective affinity of lymphocytes for
high-endothelial venules. This is a cryostat section of a rat
lymph node, which was overlaid for 30 min. with a suspension of
thoracic duct lymphocytes (TDL), then stained with methyl-green-
thyonin, which stains the TDL very dark. Note that the TDL have
become adherent to a high-endothelial venule. 180 x (Stamper and
Woodruff, 137).

Histochemical studies have shown that the high endothelium has characteristics of its own (133). There is also structural and histochemical evidence that it appears "activated" in lymph nodes that drain skin allografts (134) or an injection of Freund's adjuvant (135).

The mechanism whereby circulating lymphocytes "home" in the high-endothelial venules of the lymph nodes has been studied recently (136-139); a specific attachment of lymphocytes on these vessels can be demonstrated also _in vitro_, on tissue sections (137-139) (Fig. 8).

c) Fenestrated Endothelia

Two findings are especially noteworthy. First, experiments with tracer particles show that the diaphragms stretched across the fenestrae, although morphologically similar, appear to behave in a different manner: some are capable of retaining probe molecules as small as ferritin, others allow them to pass (140). It is especially surprising to see particles as large as carbon black working their way through a diaphragm in the rat bone marrow (sect. 4a). The proportion of permeable fenestrae, when tested with glycogens and dextrans, varied from 20 to 70% (141). Whether this dual behavior reflects two different types of diaphragms, or different functional states of the same structure, is not known. When the diaphragm is absent (as in the renal glomerulus) the primary filtration barrier is the basement membrane (142).

The other finding of interest is the occasional presence of fenestrae in capillaries with continuous endothelium, as mentioned above in relation to marrow sinusoids. Electron microscopists are familiar with this fact, which is usually brushed off as a freak finding, but it has now been quantitated: in rats, in samples of various striated muscles, about 1 in 60 cross sections of capillaries contained one or more fenestrations (up to clusters of 20). The permeability of these fenestrae has never been tested; thus their significance in physiologic studies cannot yet be established.

In the jejunal villi of mice, fenestrae are about 12 times more frequent at the venous end (143). Not too surprisingly, biochemical analysis showed that the fenestrated capillaries of the intestinal mucosa are more permeable to albumin than to colloidal HgS (144).

There is evidence that fenestrae are rather labile structures, that can form and disappear under a variety of circumstances (see sect. 9e).

d)   Other Specialized Endothelia

The special properties of brain endothelium will be discussed in sect. 6e; a review of pulmonary endothelium was recently published (15).

5.   SYNTHETIC AND METABOLIC ACTIVITIES

It had long been an intriguing fact that certain endothelia, especially in large vessels, are endowed with abundant endoplasmic reticulum and a prominent Golgi apparatus, the hallmarks of synthetic activities. It has now become abundantly clear that the endothelium, besides functioning as a filter, is also an active factory, capable of synthesizing a number of substances and of modifying (activating or inactivating) circulating molecules (8). In the following summary we will separate, somewhat artificaly, synthetic and metabolic activities.

a)   Synthetic Activities

Most of the information is obtained from cultures of endothelium of large vessels; the potential of capillary endothelium remains to be explored. That endothelium could synthesize its own basement membrane had been suspected even before the advent of tissue culture (1), and on the basis of experiments with collagenase it was suggested that the principal component was an unusual form of collagen (145). Both points were confirmed using tissue cultures (146-148); the collagen was identified as belonging mainly to Type IV, which is characteristic of other basement membranes. Electron microscopy of cultured human endothelial cells also showed material recognized as elastin, associated with the typical microfibrils (146), and sulfated mucopolysaccharides could be identified biochemically (149). Predictably, endothelial cells are able to incorporate acetate into lipids (150) and to synthesize sterols (151). The synthesis of prostaglandins (152, 153) has been considered elsewhere in this volume.

"Factor VIII" is a term applied to a glycoprotein important as an initiator of blood coagulation and for platelet function. Although its composition is not yet fully established, it seems to consist of proteins with three functionally distinct components: an antigen, a clot-promoting factor, and von Willebrand factor (154). Two of these are known to be synthetized by endothelium: the antigen (155-158) and von Willebrand factor (159, 160).

Using an antibody to Factor V, the presence of this factor was demonstrated in the liver, as anticipated, and also on all

Table 1.   Handling of Biologically Active Materials in the Pul-
           monary Capillary Bed (From Fishman & Pietra, 165)

Metabolized at Endothelial Surface Without Uptake from Plasma

> Bradykinin - inactivated
> Adenine Nucleotides - inactivated
> Angiotensin I - activated

Metabolized Intracellularly After Uptake from Plasma

> Serotonin
> Norepinephrine
> Prostaglandins E & F

Unaffected by Traversing Lungs

> Epinephrine
> Prostaglandin A
> Angiotensin II
> Dopamine
> Vasopressin

Synthesized Within Lungs and Released Into Blood

> Prostaglandins E & F

Discharged from Intrapulmonary Stores Into Blood

> Histamine
> Prostaglandins
> Slow-reacting substance of anaphylaxis
> Kallikreins
> Eosinophil leukocyte chemotactic factor of anaphylaxis

endothelia; whether this represents synthesis, or absorption, is not yet known (161). Also with the use of immunohistochemical methods, tissue factor (thromboplastic) activity was found in endothelial cells of the rabbit (162) and later also in cultured human endothelial cells (163). The list of endothelial products is certain to continue (164, 168).

b) Metabolic Activities

A number of biologically active materials are metabolized either at the endothelial surface or within the endothelial cell itself, particularly in the lung (15, 165, 166) (see Table 1). Substance P, a vasoactive peptide, is also inactivated by human endothelial cells in culture (167).

The uptake of serotonin by pulmonary endothelial cells (166, 168-170) has been clearly demonstrated also by radioautography (170). In rats breathing pure oxygen, and therefore subject to lung damage, serotonin clearance was depressed by 35% after 48 hours; this is all the more interesting, in that it may correlate with changes in systemic circulatory hemodynamics and peripheral vasculature reported as manifestations of oxygen poisoning (171).

Studies of the type just mentioned are usually restricted to the lungs (15). However, recent findings by Shepro et al. have shown that pulmonary endothelium is not alone in being able to take up serotonin. Endothelial cells isolated from bovine aorta took up labeled serotonin, and several drugs could sharply reduce this uptake (172).

All these activities of the endothelium imply the existence of surface receptors, and indeed a number of papers discuss such receptors (173-176) (some of the evidence is still tenuous). A series of papers by Ryan et al. has dealt with the cellular and subcellular localization of the angiotensin-converting enzyme in the lung (177-181). Converting enzyme activity has also been found outside of the lung, in endothelial cells isolated from the aorta of the pig (182). Another vasoactive substance that can be inactivated by the lung is AMP. This may be important in crush injury followed by shock, which may be due, in part, to the release into the circulation of vasoactive substances, including adenine nucleotides (183).

An enzyme that contributes to the surface activities of the endothelium is lipoprotein lipase. This is an intriguing enzyme. Its very origin is unclear (184); perhaps it is secreted by fat cells and secondarily adsorbed onto the endothelial surface (185). It was identified in the intima scraped off bovine aorta (186).

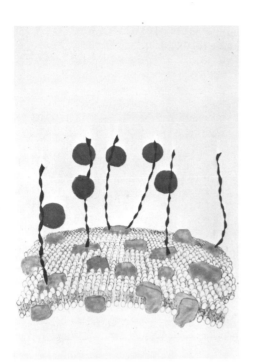 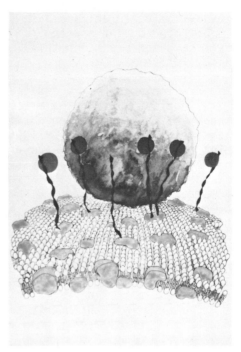

Figure 9. Hypothetical model of the mechanism of action of lipoprotein lipase at the surface of the endothelium, according to
Olivecrona et al. (187). Left: the enzyme (dark spheres) is bound
by electrostatic interaction to polysaccharide chains (spiral
threads) inserted onto proteins embedded in the bimolecular leaflet of the cell membrane. Right: a particle of VLDL is attached
to the cell membrane; lipase molecules have moved toward their
substrate by lateral diffusion - within the cell membrane - of
the proteins carrying the polysaccharide chains.

A very attractive hypothesis is illustrated by Olivecrona et al.
(185, 187): circulating molecules of lipoprotein lipase could be
captured by polysaccharide molecules attached to the endothelial
surface and waving in the blood stream (Fig. 9). The high affinity of this enzyme for negatively charged polysaccharides would
explain this trapping phenomenon (188, 189); it would also explain
the removal of the enzyme (by competition) by heparin injected
intravenously. Carbohydrates are certainly present on the endothelial surface (sect. 3b).

Proteolytic activity has been demonstrated by biochemical means on the surface of bovine aortic endothelial cells (190). Paradoxically, an antiprotease (alpha-2-macroglobulin) was also demonstrated on the endothelium of human blood vessels and lymphatics; other plasma proteins, including fibrinogen, were not found (191).

Fibrinolysis by the endothelium has received considerable attention (192-196; 8); material having the properties of a plasminogen activator has been obtained from the endothelium of large blood vessels of cattle (192); it may be responsible for the loosening of thrombi on the vascular surface (194). In human arteries and veins, fibrinolytic activity was found to be low in the intima and media, strong in the adventitia (197). Human veins obtained by surgery also contained much more plasminogen activator in the adventitia then in the intima (198). This supports our current interpretation of the adventitial "veil cells," extremely thin cells which we visualize as active phagocytes, and representing an outer barrier and disposal system for materials seeping out of the arterial wall (199). As regards histochemical studies, some have already been mentioned; histochemical reactions of the endothelium have been studied especially in the large vessels (200, 201). The useful, but poorly explained "silver staining" of the endothelial junctions has been reviewed by Gottlob and Hoff (202).

6. PHYSIOLOGY

a) Endothelial Responses

If the endothelial cells are so richly endowed with receptors, and thereby the target of so many vasoactive agents, one may wonder whether they may also be able to respond with some functional change. There is strong evidence for a contractile response to histamine-type mediators, largely limited to endothelial cells in the venules (203) (sect. 6f). The intimate contact of endothelium with pericytes (204) and especially with smooth muscle (205) have suggested that the endothelium may transmit messages to the underlying cells (206). It may be mentioned here that certain capillaries of cat brain have been said to receive an innervation (207). Endothelial cultures respond to serotonin, platelet components and other agents by enhanced proliferation (208, 209) and ornithine decarboxylase activity (535); serotonin can increase multiplication by as much as 150-1,000% (208). Phagocytosis is another activity that endothelial cells undertake when "pushed" to do so (210). Using multiple biopsies of skin and internal organs in twenty-six patients, iron could be found histochemically 1 hour after infusion of saccharated iron oxide; macrophages showed a diffuse reaction, whereas the endothelial cells contained only granules; it was therefore concluded that they represented "an overflow iron store" (211).

All these examples indicate that appropriate stimuli may turn endothelial cells into an "activated" state, as was mentioned earlier in relation to high-endothelial venules of lymph nodes. The basic question here is whether their transport activities may also be accelerated, as is often suggested. This question will be addressed below.

b) Vesicular Transport

This mechanism is now an accepted reality (212, 213). The morphologic documents are overwhelming. Suffice it to mention that in muscle capillaries a particulate tracer, such as ferritin, never passes through junctions; yet it is soon found in vesicles, and 10 minutes later in the extravascular spaces (214). A vast number of experiments with particulate as well as with mass tracers have confirmed this mechanism, which can be separated into the predictable phases: uptake, transfer, discharge (11). Reverse transport has also been demonstrated (215; 11). Thus, at this point, the data are so clearcut and consistent that the "theory of vesicle transport" can safely be referred to as the "mechanism of vesicular transport." Skeptics would have to bear the burden of providing another interpretation of the data, i.e., a new, secret pathway across the endothelium -- not a likely item for the next review.

The transport across the cell is probably accomplished, in part at least, by Brownian motion; attachment and detachment between vesicle and cell membrane are conceived as energy-requiring processes (10). The time required for surface-to-surface transport was calculated (216-221) with results varying from 1 second to 15 minutes. When measured on electron micrographs, it increased as expected with the size of the probe: 25 seconds for H11P, 45-60 seconds for myoglobin, 5-8 minutes for horseradish peroxidase, and 10 minutes for ferritin (28).

Modulations of vesicular transport may well occur, but convincing proof is difficult to obtain. A current tendency is to equate activity of transport with numbers of vesicles. In extreme cases this may be admissible (no vesicles/no transport). Thus, since vesicles are exceedingly scarce in the fetal capillaries of the human placenta, it may well be that transport in this endothelium is controlled mainly by the cytoplasm (222). And, if it is true that the retinal capillaries of day-active geckos have more vesicles than those of night-active geckos, this may imply that vesicles take part in active transport of metabolites (223). However, it should be self-evident that an increased number of vesicles on an electron micrograph does not necessarily imply more active transport: it could also indicate a traffic jam. A comparable condition could be that of passive congestion, which implies more blood in the vessels, but less flow.

We found 8 studies primarily focused on a change in the number of vesicles, or altered transport, as a result of some experimental treatment (ischemia, X-rays, edema, lanthanum poisoning, thyroid hormones, serotonin, cAMP, and kidney extract). Ligature of the iliac artery or vein in the rat for 20-40 minutes did not appear to cause an absolute change in the number of the vesicles in capillary endothelium of thigh muscles (224). Irradiation of the cerebral cortex of the rat caused, within an hour, a transient increase in the number of vesicles filled with horseradish peroxidase. It should be recalled here that, in the normal brain, the vesicles are usually not seen discharging their content on the abluminal side (225). A study of normal dog lungs, isolated and perfused under "normal" or "edematous" conditions due to increased outflow pressure showed that vesicular volume was increased twofold in edematous lungs; unfortunately, the size of the vesicles was not mentioned (226). An interesting approach is being attempted by Weihe et al. (227) who perfused the testis of the rat and studied the penetration of peroxidase into the endothelium. When lanthanum is introduced into the system, micropinocytic transport in both directions appears to be reversibly inhibited. This could be a promising avenue. Less dramatic is a freeze-etching study of endothelial cells in the thyroid of normal mice, compared with mice treated with hormones causing hyper- and hypo-function (228). The authors counted the number of vesicles in the freeze-etched preparations, and found 29.1 + 3.68 per square micron in the normal mice, 33 + 4.39 in animals treated with TSH for six days, and 25.3 + 2.68 in mice treated with thyradine. The situation described by Westergaard as enhanced vesicular transport deserves to be restudied (229). The author had previously found that, in the mouse brain, the endothelium of some small vessels breaks the rule (and the blood-brain barrier) by transporting some peroxidase toward the basement membrane. In the present study, serotonin was perfused for 30 minutes through the cerebral ventricles; a definite increase in peroxidase transport was seen in arterioles, less in the venules. Cell damage was never observed. The effect was somewhat erratic and not dose-dependent; sham-operated animals were unfortunately not studied. The author speculates that serotonin may stimulate the adenylcyclase in the endothelial membrane, and thus raise the intracellular level of cyclic AMP. (See Addendum.)

Worthy of confirmation is also a recent study from Japan, concerning nephrectomized rats made hypertensive with a kidney extract; the authors examined the capillaries of the intestinal muscularis, and found an increased outward passage of ferritin (230); they also described a significant increase in the number of vesicles labeled with ferritin (12.0 + 5.8 versus 4.9 + 4.4 in controls, P < 0.005; measurements 65 min. after injection of ferritin). It was concluded that "kidney extract contains substance(s) which increase capillary permeability for plasma proteins...via increased vesicular transport, resulting in tissue edema." Angiotensin did not have this effect. Although interesting, this study remains open to question, because it is now known that the rate of vesicular transport can vary from the arterial to the venous end of the capillary (88); this factor may have influenced the counts, since only 7 capillaries were examined for each group.

It may become possible to study the acceleration of endothelial uptake, but not transport, with preparations of isolated capillaries. One such method has been published by Wagner et al. (231) who conjugated ferritin with rhodamine, and thereby obtained a tracer molecule that is visible by electron microscopy as well as fluorescent by light microscopy. Using a suspension of capillaries isolated from the epididimal fat body, these authors found that they could obtain a quantitation of micropinocytosis by gauging the fluorescence of the endothelium.

Oddly enough, no electron microscopist, the authors included, has seen fit to perform a very obvious experiment whereby vesicle transport should truly be accelerated and decelerated: warming and cooling the tissue. Since vesicles are thought to move, at least in part, by Brownian motion, this experiment could be critical. Pappenheimer et al. performed such experiments a quarter of a century ago on perfused limbs (232) and Renkin pursued the lead (233, 234); Chinard et al. are now tackling the problem with the dog lung (235) and we have started to examine it by electron microscopy.

c) Lipid Transport

Since human LDL and HDL are about 200 and 100 Å in diameter (236) one might expect them to be taken up by plasmalemmal vesicles. According to Stein et al. this did occur, at least in their model (237). Human lipoproteins were labeled in the protein moiety and perfused through an isolated rat heart-aorta preparation. Radioautography detected the label in the wall with all lipoproteins; by TEM the endothelium was intact (an essential control). Biochemical evidence of passage of lipoproteins into the aortic wall was found by others (238). Y. and O. Stein have calculated that vesicle transport alone could amply account for the amount of lipoprotein cholesterol accumulating in the human aortic intima with age (236). In the perfused rat lung (239) results were somewhat different: rat or human LDL were not taken up, whereas VLDL were selectively taken up and the corresponding protein moiety was catabolized. With cultured endothelium results are interesting but fragmentary; human cells take up human LDL, and HDL reduce the uptake, possibly by competing for binding sites

(240). Calf cells take up human VLDL, but do not hydrolyze its
triglyceride moiety, as if they lacked the necessary lipoprotein
lipase (241). This would be consistent with the theory, mentioned
earlier, that endothelium picks up lipoprotein lipase from its
normal environment.

    Chylomicrons are too large for vesicle transport (0.05-0.5 μ),
(242); the current concept is that they are trapped at the surface
of certain endothelia, and reduced in size by lipoprotein lipase
located on the cell membrane (Fig. 9). Histochemical studies by
TEM show that further hydrolysis to fatty acids is accomplished
within the endothelium and possibly also by pericytes (243). The
complex literature on the role of capillary endothelium in the
clearance of chylomicrons has been reviewed recently (242) and will
only be mentioned here in relation to Scow's new concept of lipid
transport by lateral diffusion in cell membranes (242) (Fig. 10).
Lipoproteins are water-soluble, although their surface monolayer
contains a number of fat-soluble molecules. A special situation
may arise when chylomicrons or lipoproteins are hydrolyzed on the
surface of the endothelium, giving rise to a shower of fat-soluble
products: diglycerides, monoglycerides, free fatty acids. In
theory, these molecules could be carried across the endothelium by
carrier proteins, but a number of reasons make this very unlikely
(including the fact that these lipids would have to move in and
out of two lipid layers, a slow and inefficient process). Studies
with artificial membranes suggested a different process: the products of lipolysis could dissolve into the outer leaflet of the
cell membrane and diffuse rapidly along it. They could then reach
a cell junction and glide toward the outer surface of the cell;
conceivably they could also glide into caveolae and thus be caught
in vesicle transport, or move outward along a temporary channel
formed by coalescing vesicles. Thereafter they could reach other
cells by points of membrane contact (in Fig. 10 we have only indicated contact with a pericyte). This transport process would be
not only fast, but also economical: loss by diffusion into the
extracellular spaces would be minimal, the molecules being deliv-
ered directly to the surface of the "customer" cell. Further
studies will have to verify the possible role of this mechanism.
It certainly fits well with Olivecrona's model of lipoprotein
lipase function (Fig. 9).

                d) Endothelial Permeability

    We have previously touched upon this topic and will now attempt
to review it. The endothelium is more permeable to water and solutes than most epithelia; furthermore, it is permeable to large
water-soluble molecules (11). How is this permeability achieved?

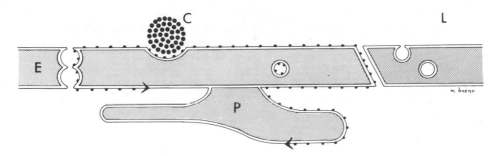

Figure 10. Hypothetical model for movement of lipid from a chylomicron to extravascular cells by lateral diffusion within the outer
leaflet of cell membranes (modified from Scow et al., 242). L =
lumen, E = endothelial cell. A chylomicron (C) is hydrolyzed in
contact with the endothelial membrane, and lipid-soluble products
of hydrolysis (small dots) dissolve into the cell membrane; transport across the endothelium can occur along clefts and channels or
by vesicle transport; extravascular cells can be reached by direct
contact (only a pericyte, P, is shown here).

This question has been tackled by physiologists and morphologists
by means so radically different that the result has been, rather
than a collaboration, a confrontation that is now in its third
decade. The background of this historic and constructive debate
has been recounted many times (1, 10-12, 212, 213) and will not be
repeated here except in briefest outline. Most of the discussion
to follow will refer to the microcirculation; much less is known
about the endothelium of large blood vessels.

     The first comprehensive theory of capillary permeability was
proposed by a group of physiologists (Pappenheimer et al. (232))
several years before the dawn of electron microscopy. At that time
the capillary wall could only be studied "as an abstract membrane"
(212), and its permeability was seen as the result of two passive
processes, diffusion and convection. Thus arose the original pore
theory of capillary permeability, based on the perfusion of cat
hind limbs; it postulated the existence of a single pathway, consisting of a system of pores with a radius of 30 A, or of slits
40 A wide, occupying less than 1% of the capillary surface. Later

work showed that a single pathway model could not account for the
size of molecules appearing in the lymph; it became necessary to
assume the existence of a set of "large pores" occupying a much
smaller cross-sectional area. The diameter of the small pores was
subsequently revised, and other models were proposed, based on
different classes of pores (see 212). Today the most widely
accepted concept is that of two pore sizes, small (about 90 Å) and
large (500-700 Å) (10-12).

Electron microscopy advanced independently of physiology, and
the number of possible outward pathways, for blood-borne molecules,
is today at least eight. These are summarized in Figure 11, in
which:

(1) represents the trans-cellular pathway, limited to water,
lipid-soluble solutes and very small molecules (diameter of the
pores = 8 to perhaps as much as 20 Å) (213). This pathway is
thought to be important for the rapid diffusion of respiratory and
anesthetic gases (213). (2) represents the lateral diffusion pathway for fat-soluble molecules, discussed earlier. Although presently based only on theoretical considerations, this pathway is
beginning to gain recognition (212, 185). (3 and 4) represent
extreme conditions of interendothelial junctions, either open or
closed; (5) shows vesicular transport, and (6) the related transendothelial channels, presumably temporary structures; (7) represents fenestrae, either open or closed by a diaphragm; the latter
should be visualized as having different degrees of permeability
(sect. 4c).

In attempting a synthesis of physiologic requirements and
structural findings, it is immediately apparent that ultrastructure offers an excess of pathways, none of which fits precisely
the dimensions and frequency postulated by calculation. A partial
reconciliation is currently outlined as follows (10, 11):

- continuous endothelium, large pores: plasmalemmal
  vesicles are considered as the only candidates,
  being the only structure capable of accepting molecules 100-300 Å in diameter. (This pathway is
  firmly established by TEM, but we believe that in
  physiologic experiments on perfused limbs its contribution is most likely contaminated by other
  pathways, as will be discussed below.)

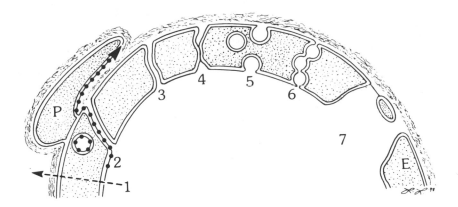

Figure 11. Scheme of possible pathways across the endothelial barrier: (1) direct trans-cellular pathway: (2) lipid transport by
lateral diffusion; (3 and 4) non-tight and tight junctions; (5)
vesicle transport; (6) transendothelial channels; (7) closed and
open fenestrae.

- continuous endothelium, small pores: this category could
  include: (a) the venular junctions, open to molecules
  smaller than 60 Å (this pathway would represent a pore size
  smaller than predicted); (b) the transendothelial channels
  derived from vesicles, assuming that they would offer
  restrictions by means of their diaphragms, or by annular
  strictures remaining where the vesicles fused (80-100 Å);
  (c) possibly a contribution from small molecules going
  through the "large pore system" (vesicular transport).

- fenestrated endothelium, large pores: obvious candidates
  are those fenestrae that are "compliant," i.e., permeated
  by the 100-300 Å probes; oddly enough, the number of observed fenestrae is in excess of calculations (141). A
  secondary contribution could derive from plasmalemmal vesicles, where present.

- fenestrated endothelium, small pores: these could correspond to the non-compliant fenestrae, and possibly to venular
  junctions.

If the calculated and the observed pathways are compared, several discrepancies are observed, not only with regard to the diameter and frequency of the pores, but also at the conceptual level. In continuous endothelia, for instance, the large pore system is based largely on a mechanism which is, to some extent, a form of active transport (the ferrying activity of plasmalemmal vesicles) which was not anticipated. Furthermore, the vesicles appear to represent only one aspect of a dynamic, unstable system consisting of vesicles, fused vesicles, channels, and fenestrae, all related and constantly interchanging.

It would be presumptuous to hazard a guess as to future correlations: but if we may offer the biased opinion of two electron microscopists, it is the following. There is, at present, too wide a gap between the detailed observations based on electron microscopy with molecular probes, and physiologic experiments based on perfusion of whole organs or of whole limbs. By perfusing whole limbs it has been possible to establish the basic limits of microvascular permeability; today, such preparations may have outlived their usefulness. They have led to the expression "dog paw capillaries" (213). This is a dangerous abstraction. We have never read, in the context of physiologic experiments, a discussion of the variety of capillaries included in a dog paw. The skin includes a rich population of fenestrated capillaries around glands and hair follices (244). If dog skin is similar to rabbit skin, fenestrated venous capillaries occur also in the subcutaneous fascia (245), while the muscle itself may include a sparse population of fenestrae, as shown in the rat (21). Worse yet, the paw contains bones and thus bone marrow, where endothelial fenestrae are incapable of retaining carbon particles as large as 200-380 A, while other particles are taken up by coated vesicles (109). It is difficult to see how such a heterogeneous system could be of any further help in clarifying matters.

We also believe that some of the large pore contribution may represent vascular damage, pre-existing or experimentally induced (144). Electron microscopic evidence of injury is not rare in electron microscopic samples, although they are collected with extreme care; yet this is never considered in the interpretation of physiologic data. The simple device of labeling potential leaks with an intravenous injection of a small dose of carbon black (246) is essential for checking the non-leaky condition of the chosen vascular field, before or after the experiment (247). Perhaps this method is too simple to qualify as scientific; in any event, it is never used, and a necessary control is thereby lost.

Thus, as matters now stand, we think that perfusion experiments need to be refined and brought closer to the range of microscopic structures; ideally, to the range of single capillaries. In such

preparations, the approach would be reversed: rather than searching for structures to fit postulates, one could measure the functional significance of demonstrated structures.

The problem mentioned above of the prevailing disregard for
pathologic changes in supposedly physiologic experiments deserves
further comment, because it is still causing, in our opinion,
pathologic results. In an oft-quoted series of studies of the uptake of albumin by the "endothelial surface" of the isolated carotid artery of the dog (248) the delay between excision and commence-
ment of incubation ranged from 30 to 90 minutes. Not surprisingly,
"there was no evidence that the length of this period, within these
limits, affected the results," and the study finds that the "uptake
process was primarily passive." There could not have been much
functional endothelium left; and had any been left, the artery in
some of the experiments was filled with the animal's own serum, a
highly abnormal fluid containing a host of vasoactive agents, and
therefore often used in experimental pathology for producing vascular leakage (249). None of this, however, may have mattered,
because oxygen was not bubbled into the surrounding incubating
medium. The same procedure was used in other studies, including
one on "pinocytic vesicle function" as affected by vibration (250).
Precise quantitative data based on such preparations can only lead
one astray.

e) Vascular Permeability in Specific Organs

In the lungs, vascular permeability and ultrastructure (251-
255, 15) have been studied especially in relation to blood volume
and pressure: myoglobin did not penetrate junctions under normal
conditions, but did so when pulmonary pressure was raised three-
fold above normal (254). In mice, horseradish peroxidase did not
penetrate the junctions unless blood volume was increased by a
large volume of intravenously injected fluid (255). The different
reactivity of the two pulmonary circulations, as regards histamine-type mediators, is noteworthy: only the bronchial venules
respond (254).

The many aspects of the blood-brain barrier cannot be reviewed
here (256-262), but we must at least recall that the cerebral endothelium, besides constituting a barrier restricting the exchange
of ions, proteins, and lipid-insoluble non-electrolytes, also has
a unique property: it possesses mechanisms for the rapid transfer
of specific molecules (260). To date, no less than 8 independent
transport systems have been described; they concern hexoses, mono-
carboxylic acids, neutral amino acids, basic amino acids, choline,
purines, nucleosides, and acidic amino acids (262). The operation

of these eight bidirectional active transport systems must impose
a considerable energy demand on the endothelium of the cerebral
capillaries; this may explain why these cells have 5 times more
mitochondria than comparable cells in muscle capillaries (262).

The blood-brain barrier itself is not absolute: if 24-48
hours are allowed, intravenously injected protein does appear in
extracellular fluids. One bypass may correspond to the choroid
plexus; another appears to be vesicular transport in certain arte-
riolar segments (263).

f) Endothelial Contractility

The notion of endothelial contractility in mammals had long
been discarded when electron microscopic studies gave it a new role
(264, 265, 203). A more detailed review of this topic will be published elsewhere (266). Briefly, we proposed in 1966 that the
histamine-type mediators of inflammation induce vascular leakage
by causing endothelial cells to contract, primarily in the venules.
Thus it became possible to reconcile the two apparently separate
effects of these mediators, contraction of smooth muscle and increased microvascular permeability. Our original evidence for
contraction was ultrastructural; the criteria we used for suggesting, on an electron micrograph, that an endothelial cell was contracted were the following: (1) change in shape of the nucleus,
which becomes more rounded; (2) formation of nuclear folds, especially tight, "pinched" folds; (3) shifting of cytoplasm and organelles towards the center of the cell; (4) annular profiles of
endoplasmic reticulum, suggestive of cytoplasmic flow; (5) folds
and protrusions of the cell membrane in the zone beneath the
nucleus; (6) presence in the cytoplasm of bundles of fibrils sometimes with evidence of cross-banding. We pointed out the difficulty
of interperting these features when the vessels are collapsed (i.e.,
not fixed under physiologic pressure). Corresponding observations
were also made in vivo: endothelial cells were observed to bulge
next to leaks in the wall of venules (267). Meanwhile, new findings on endothelial filamentous structures were published (268,
269), and other workers provided data supporting the notion of
endothelial contractility by demonstrating the presence of contractile and relaxing proteins in endothelial cells (270, 271).
Myosin was later extracted from cultured human endothelium and
demonstrated by immunofluorescence (Fig. 12) (272); the thin filaments of lymphatic endothelial cells were "decorated" with heavy
meromyosin, and could therefore be definitely identified as actin
(273). Thus all the basic components of the intracellular contractile apparatus have been identified biochemically. (See
addendum.)

The variety and significance of the cytoplasmic fibrils has
received much attention. Especially intriguing are the bundles of
cross-striated fibrils, with a period of 0.6-0.7 µ (269, 274),
first described in normal myometrial arterioles of the rat by Rohlich
and Olah (269), who pointed out the analogy between these dense,
periodic striations and the Z-lines of striated muscle. It has
been proposed that structures such as these are the contractile
units responsible, at least in part, for the contraction of the
splenic sinusoids (275). The periodic banding was found to be
enhanced in contracted vessels, suggesting that their function is
vasoconstriction (205). Similar striated bundles were found in
the endothelium of hypertensive rats: in cerebral arteries and
arterioles (276) as well as in the aorta (277). Striated bundles
were found also in lymphatic endothelial cells, in association with
centrioles (278).

It is now clear that not all intracellular filaments are contractile. At least 3 types of filaments have been described in
the endothelium as well as in other cells: thin (40-70 Å) identified as actin; thick (about 150 Å) identified as myosin; intermediate (100 Å) of uncertain function but not contractile (279-281).
Pollard has suggested that the contractile proteins (especially
actin, which is often present in excess) could also function as a
cytosekelton (282).

It should be noted that the endothelial contraction described
by us, as a result of histamine-type mediators, was observed predominantly in endothelial cells of the venules, much less in other
segments of the microcirculation. A similar effect on arterial
endothelium (283) could not be confirmed in our laboratory.

Twelve years since it was proposed, the notion of endothelial
contraction appears to be generally accepted; the arguments submitted against it (284) are either obsolete or not relevant. On
the other hand, excessive enthusiasm has led to some uncritical
applications. Published electron micrographs (285) certainly do
not support endothelial contraction as a basic mechanism of atherogenesis. Yet the presence of banded fibrils in cells of the
aortic endothelium needs to be explained. Could these cells be
contractile in the same sense as those in the venules? Or are
their fibrils just an adaptation to shear stress? This is certainly
possible: the endothelium of hypertensive animals contains more
fibrils (276, 277) and it resists better than normal endothelium
a sudden pressure increase (286).

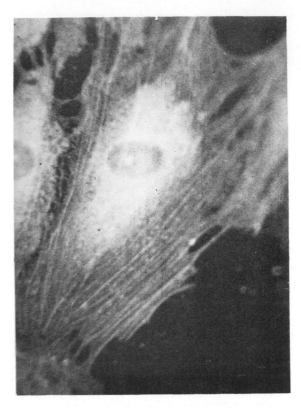

Figure 12. Demonstration of myosin in endothelium. Human endothelial cell in culture; fibrillar pattern obtained by immunofluorescence, with rabbit antiserum to platelet myosin followed by
fluoresceinated goat antiserum to rabbit IgG. (Moore et al., 272).

7. INTERACTION WITH PLATELETS

The relationship between platelets and endothelium (287, 288)
was first understood to mean that the platelets, somehow, support
the endothelium. There is now evidence of a two-way interaction:
the endothelium is partly responsible for the normal function of
the platelets.

a) Effects of Endothelium on Platelets

Endothelium produces two of the components of Factor VIII;
50% of this becomes attached to the surface of the platelets, and

is required for their normal function (289). Endothelium also
produces prostacycline, a potent inhibitor of platelet aggregation
(153).

b) Effects of Platelets on Endothelium

There is no doubt that platelets exert a beneficial effect on
the endothelial cells; obvious evidence is thrombocytopenic bleeding. The first electron microscopic studies of this phenomenon
(on irradiated guinea pigs) reported that the erythrocytes escaped
by holes through individual endothelial cells (290, 291). This
was not confirmed in the recent work of Dale and Hurley, who used
rats and guinea pigs made thrombocytopenic by antiplatelet serum
or by irradiation; the red blood cells escaped through loosened
endothelial junctions (292); changes in the structure of the endothelial cells were not reported. The latter statement conflicts
with two recent papers by Kitchens and Weiss, who used rabbits
made thrombocytopenic with antiplatelet serum or busulfan, studied
punch biopsies of the tongue, and reported that the endothelium
became rapidly thinner, to the point of developing fenestrae,
within less than 24 hours (293) (Fig. 13). These changes could
be prevented or reversed with prednisone (294). More work is
needed to explain this contradiction; perhaps we are dealing with
a species difference. In any event, in view of the many regional
differences in the biology of the endothelium, future experiments
on thrombocytopenic animals should sample several types of endothelium. Yet another approach to this problem is the work of
Gimbrone et al., who perfused isolated dog thyroids with plasma
(295, 296): if the plasma was platelet-poor, by 5 hours vascular
resistance increased rapidly, fluid accumulated within the thyroid,
and electron microscopy showed extensive endothelial damage; if
platelets were added to the perfusing medium, the vessels were
better preserved, and if the thyroid was subsequently perfused with
whole blood, "reflow purpura" did not occur. This study certainly
lends weight to the notion that the platelets exert a "maintenance"
effect toward the endothelium. Confirming evidence comes also
from recent studies on cultures of human endothelial cells (534):
when intact platelets were added, the cells became dispersed more
evenly; and a defect produced by making a scratch across the confluent primary culture healed more rapidly. If the cultures were
maintained as long as 4 days, an increase in cell growth was noted;
and by TEM some endothelial cells were found to contain platelets
within their cytoplasm. The stimulation of growth produced by
platelets on cultures of endothelium may be due to serotonin and
ADP (sect. 6a). Another effect produced on cultured endothelial
cells by serotonin (as well as by serum and by thrombin) is an increase in ornithine decarboxylase activity: this is the rate-limiting step in the synthesis of polyamines, 535).

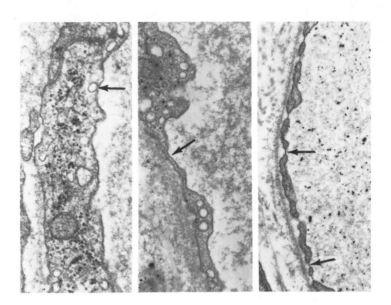

Figure 13. Effect of thrombocytopenia on the endothelium of capillaries (rabbit tongue). Left: normal control. Center and right:
a "thin spot" and fenestrations, after 3 days of maximal thrombocytopenia (average endothelial thickness about 1/2 normal).
20,000 x (Kitchens, 294).

        Whether the serotonin content of platelets is important to
the endothelium in vivo is not clear. It is often implied in the
current literature that vasoactive amines liberated by platelets
cause leakage; this could certainly be true for the microcirculation, but the evidence regarding large vessels is controversial
(see sect. 6f). This is but a part of the broader problem - whether platelets may cause damage to the endothelium. Large platelet
thrombi may certainly damage the endothelial surface by interfering
with its nutrition; a more subtle type of injury could be inflicted
on the endothelial surface by platelet lysis, since it was reported
that platelets contain an enzyme capable of degrading heparin sulfate (297). A thorough discussion of the possible roles of platelets as injurious agents can be found in a paper by Mustard and
Packham (298).

c) Similarities Between Platelets and Endothelium

An antigenic relationship between endothelium and platelets
has been suggested (532), but on the basis of experiments whereby
dogs were sensitized with endothelium obtained from washed aortas
of other dogs, the possibility of platelet contamination cannot be
excluded. Rafelson et al. have studied the platelet-endothelium
interaction in vitro by comparing the behavior of platelets and of
cultured endothelial cells after brief exposure to thrombin (299).
Within 1 to 12 seconds both cell types rapidly extruded parts of
their cytogel, which then contracted. The authors believe that
this phenomenon may help understand the interaction between injured
endothelium and platelets.

8. ENDOTHELIAL GROWTH AND REGENERATION

In large vessels, the turnover of endothelial cells is fairly
slow (300-308, 9) and depends on their location: for guinea pigs,
a rough estimate of the life span in areas around the mouths of
branches was 60-120 days, as compared with 100-180 days in control
areas (301); in pigs, the rate was higher in areas stained by intravenous Evans blue (308). In the aorta of 3-month old rats 0.3
to 1.5% of the total population entered DNA synthesis each day
(305). In capillaries of adult mice the same approach gave a figure of 0.01 percent for the retina; in the myocardium the rate
was at least 14 times greater (309). The turnover time for retinal capillaries was estimated to be 3 years of more; there was also
evidence that some endothelial cells could become polyploid (309).

A vast literature has accumulated on endothelial culture (8,
310-317; see also sect. 8). The growth of aortic and portal vein
endothelia have been compared in vitro; results suggest that arterial endothelium is more sensitive and less adaptable to the conditions of tissue culture (316). Long-term cultures of endothelium have given rise to two cell types, one mononucleated, the
other multinucleated (307). Large human and non-human vessels
can be maintained in vitro under conditions of organ culture (318,
319) so that endothelial regeneration can be studied en face (319).
Endothelial cells have also been grown from capillaries isolated
from rat epididyimal fat (37).

As to the stimuli that bring about endothelial proliferation
(8), ocular trauma was shown to cause mitoses in retinal vessels
(320). The expansion of endothelial surface during the growth of
collateral arteries in the coronary tree is accompanied by the
adherence and penetration of many monocytes, possibly attracted to
the intima by a MIF-type factor produced by the proliferating
endothelial cells (321). Cholesterol feeding for three days is

enough to induce a burst of endothelial proliferation in the aorta of swine (322, sect. 9a). A single injection of estrogen in adult female rats causes a multiplication of endothelial cells in the liver; the peak effect occurs on the third day (323). The hair growth cycle in rat skin (324) and the delayed hypersensitivity reaction in the guinea pig (325) are also accompanied by endothelial proliferation.

A major step forward was accomplished by Folkman and collaborators, who studied the phenomenon of angiogenesis induced by tumors and identified a tumor angiogenesis factor (TAF) (9, 326-328). It was somewhat surprising to find that confluent cultures of endothelial cells, which regenerate promptly if a culture is "wounded," (315) did not respond to TAF (312) nor to factors known to stimulate fibroblasts in vitro (329). However, this may reflect a "stringent control" of cell growth, necessary for the function of these cells in vivo (9). Others have reported success in stimulating cultures with tumor cell homogenates (330) as well as with tumor-conditioned medium obtained from rat and human tumors or the central nervous system (331). Simultaneous growth culture of Sarcoma 180 and pig aortic endothelium also indicated that the tumor produced a diffusible growth-stimulating factor (332). Another endothelial growth-stimulating factor has been isolated from bovine salivary glands (333). Endothelial cultures are also stimulated by platelet components (208) and by at least one potent fibroblast growth factor extracted from bovine brain or pituitary glands, which appears to be essential for the survival of bovine vascular endothelium (334). Conversely, it was found that human endothelial cells are capable of stimulating granulopoiesis in agar cultures of human bone marrow cells (335).

Inhibition of endothelial growth has been obtained with cartilage extracts (336-338); this may be related to the antiproteolytic activity of such extracts (336) and may explain the relative resistance of cartilage to invasion by tumor. Artificial seeding of endothelium has been attempted experimentally to accelerate the cellular covering of artificial vascular surfaces (339, 340, 8).

Finally, we should mention a bizarre and potentially harmful effect of regenerated endothelium (341). In rabbit aortas, deendothelialized with a balloon catheter, the endothelium regenerated in focal areas corresponding to the ostia of branches; if hyperlipidemia was induced, the largest amount of deposited lipid was present in areas covered by regenerated endothelium. This paradoxical effect of regenerated endothelium is still unexplained; it may imply that the circulating lipid is not passively infiltrating the exposed surface, but actively taken up and transported toward the media by the endothelium. However, this hypothesis is not supported by studies of cholesterol accumulation in the rabbit

aorta: the penetration was greater in areas of defective endothelium (342).

9. PATHOLOGY

a) Varieties of Experimental Injury

The following selection from hundreds of papers can only serve
as a guide to the variety of approaches in this field.

In large vessels, total removal of the endothelium by means
of a balloon catheter has become a popular procedure (343-346);
it does not provide information on endothelial injury per se, but
has been useful for studying endothelial regeneration and the
adaptation of the arterial wall to the lack of an endothelial cover. A similar effect was produced in the rat by drying the intima with a stream of air, in a blood vessel temporarily isolated
from the circulation (347). These denudation experiments have
proven beyond doubt that smooth muscle cells can provide a temporary, non-thrombogenic surface (pseudoendothelium): an important
evolutionary adaptation. A comparable denudation method for the
microcirculation is lacking.

Shear stress is a particularly important mechanism of injury,
because it occurs naturally. Fry studied acute effects in the
dog, by introducing into the aorta a cylindrical plug; a channel
gauged along one side of the plug forced the blood into a narrow
stream, where the endothelium was exposed to increased shearing
forces (348). Within one hour severe endothelial injury ensued, as
evaluated by light microscopic methods. Further studies along
these lines are needed. Acute shear stress was also studied in
the dog renal artery after anastomosis with the inferior vena cava
("high flow shunt") (349). The reported first change (10 minutes)
was an aberration in the ruthenium red staining; after 30 min.
evidence of injury appeared in most endothelial cells, some of
which sloughed off. At two hours, thrombosis and leukocytic infiltration were noticed. (However, some of the changes reported
in this paper, such as reduplication of the basement membrane
at 15 minutes, cannot be attributed to the experimental procedure.)
Chronic hemodynamic effects were studied by Stehbens, who anastomosed the external jugular vein in sheep to the common carotid
artery, then studied the jugular vein by light (350) and electron
microscopy (351). The changes observed between 4 and 56 months
included severe endothelial injury. In the microcirculation,
shear stress may explain the endothelial damage observed experimentally in dog kidneys perfused with pulsatile flow, an accepted
mode of kidney preservation prior to grafting (352).

The effect of freezing and thawing was studied under visual control in the hamster cheek pouch (353) and in the hind paw of the mouse (354); both studies describe TEM changes. In the second study there was evidence of no-reflow upon thawing. Local freezing was also applied to the rat aorta (355). Whole body chilling (5-7°C for 22 hours) seems to affect the permeability of venular endothelium of the nasal mucosa in the rat: the localization of colloidal gold was significantly higher in this area as compared with that of control rats (356). This interesting study should be correlated with TEM changes.

Mild heat applied to the skin of rats (54°C for 20 seconds) induced discrete changes in the endothelium of small vessels (357): an irregular dilatation of interendothelial clefts, with partial damage of the endothelial cell membrane. Passage of ferritin through these areas was not seen until 30-60 minutes later. These junctional changes, presumably due to direct injury, may help understand the pathogenesis of the so-called "delayed leakage" after certain forms of injury.

The inflammatory reaction after thermal injury was accompanied by endothelial proliferation (358). The number of replicating endothelial cells was gauged by ^{3}H-thymidine labeling. It was concluded that electron microscopic images previously ascribed to activation, recovery or regenerative transformation of endothelium "represent, in the main, endothelial proliferation." We are sure that this is a correct interpretation, but still feel on general grounds that it should be possible to induce, with appropriate stimuli, some form of "endothelial activation" (see sect. 6a).

It is often stated that chronic inflammation per se, because of the constant emigration of white blood cells, can modify non-lymphoid venules and cause them to resemble the "high-endothelial venules" of lymph nodes. As mentioned earlier, the paper quoted in this context (359) only shows a blood capillary with thick endothelial cells in a granuloma produced by the injection of adjuvant. The point would deserve to be investigated further. Acute, massive diapedesis certainly caused endothelial damage in large veins (360).

The effect of long-wave ultraviolet rays and of sunlight was studied by biopsy in two patients with erythropoietic protoporphyria (361). The damage was confined to the superficial vessels, whereas the epidermis showed no abnormalities. It was concluded that the endothelial cells are the primary cellular targets for the photodynamic reaction in this disease (the striking multilayered basement membranes observed in this condition will be discussed in sect. 9b, Fig. 14). The effect of X-rays on endothelial growth was studied in rats (362, 363) and on cultured endothelial

cells (364, 365) without TEM investigations. Ultrasound was found
to have highly destructive effects on the central artery of the
rabbit ear (366); whereas a laser beam produced, in the bat wing,
platelet aggregation without visible endothelial damage (367).

In large vessels, the effect of anoxia was studied in vivo
(368-370) as well as in vitro, with preparations of rabbit aorta
incubated in Krebs-bicarbonate buffer containing 6% albumin and
glucose (371). Aerobic incubation for 1 hour produced no electron
microscopic changes: 2.5 minutes of anoxia caused widespread
endothelial swelling, and 10 minutes of anoxia caused marked and
wide-spread endothelial changes, including gaps seen by transmission as well as by scanning electron microscopy. Chronic hypoxia
in vivo was studied in the large vessels of cattle (368) and rabbits (369); the severest changes were found in rabbits exposed
for 14 days to 15.3 and 11.7% oxygen; intimal edema was noticed,
as well as the formation of large subendothelial "vacuoles" (the
mechanism of intimal edema is here attributed to endothelial contraction, but the evidence is again not convincing). Large vessels
submitted to acute ischemia have been studied by TEM as well as
by SEM (372-374). Among the earliest changes observed is a deposition of platelets on the endothelium (in the absence of flow),
which could possibly be explained by a change in the charge of the
endothelial surface from negative to positive (374).

In the microcirculation, the injurious effects of ischemia
were often described (375-384). The changes reported vary a great
deal from one organ to another, also because the surrounding
structures vary in their response: at one extreme, in the brain,
the glial cells have been reported to swell within a few minutes,
enough to nearly occlude the capillaries (378). At the other
extreme, in the skin, ischemia for as long as 6 hours does not
cause necrosis upon reflow (380), suggesting that endothelium, at
least in the skin, is rather resistant to ischemia. In most
studies endothelial swelling is the basic finding; however, in
striated muscle of the rat hind limb, after 2 1/2 hours of ischemia
the average thickness of the endothelium had decreased (379).

An important ramification of the ischemic effect is the concept of no-reflow or impaired reflow; if endothelial injury in
the microcirculation is severe, it may impair the return of blood
flow once the obstacle is removed (376, 377). Mesangial and endothelial swelling were found to be severe 60 minutes after clamping
of the renal artery, and sufficient to explain the failure of
reflow (384). The extensive literature on the no-reflow phenomenon
can be found by consulting the latest contributions (382, 384, 385).
In spite of all the controversy, it seems impossible to argue
against the notion that endothelial swelling must be an obstacle
to flow and reflow. There is at least one condition in which

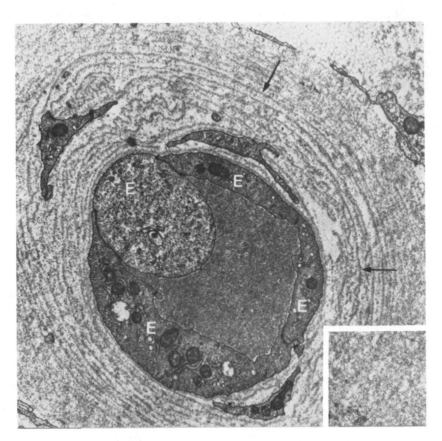

Figure 14. Multilayered basement membrane (arrows) around a small
vessel of the superficial dermis in pathologic human skin. This
condition closely mimics diabetes, but it is actually erythropoietic protoprophyria (EPP), in which the primary target of the
photodynamic lesion by long-wave UV appears to be the endothelium
(the biopsy was taken from the back of the hand, an exposed region). This finding clearly supports the notion that repeated
injury leads to multilayered basement membranes. E = endothelium.
Inset: flocculent material typical of EPP lesions. 10,800 x;
inset 20,000 x (From Gschnait et al., 361).

endothelial swelling seems to be the key factor and almost path-
ognomonic: eclampsia (386). This change, known also as endothe-
liosis, has also been observed in a primigravid chimpanzee (387).

     The microcirculation of the gastrointestinal tract in puppies
was severely affected by anoxia (breathing 7% oxygen for 2 hours)
and by severe reduction of blood volume (388). The reported

changes were similar to those observed in necrotizing enterocolitis of the newborn. Hemorrhagic shock is known to produce "shock lung," which is characterized by an abnormal leakiness of capillary endothelium; a freeze fracture study of the intercellular junctions in shock lung (in the dog) showed changes in the endothelial zonulae occludentes (389).

The effects of venous stasis have received very little attention. In the rabbit, changes found in the endothelium of the vena cava after complete ligation were reported as signs of increased metabolic activity after 3 days; vacuolation and "vesiculation" after 5 to 7 days; large vacuoles and advanced injury by 14 and 20 days (390). Greatly needed are TEM studies correlated with physiologic experiments on increased venous pressure (391).

Studies using endothelial regeneration as a marker showed that the target of oxygen toxicity is the endothelium of capillaries and larger thin-walled adjacent vessels; no effect was observed in the larger pulmonary veins and arteries, nor in the systemic vasculature (392, 393).

A number of physical and chemical agents were tested in rats (changes in pH, osmolarity, anoxia, temperature, vasoactive amines, various enzymes and surfactants). The illustrations show drastic non-specific cellular injury; none of these changes, however, may be accepted as suggesting "contraction of the endothelial cells in response to the stimuli" (394).

Among inorganic toxic agents, cadmium chloride was shown to produce discrete changes in the interendothelial junctions of small vessels in certain target organs (testes, gasserian ganglion) (395). These changes do not result in visible leakage until a few hours later. The mechanism is unknown; other physical or chemical agents are known to have a selective effect on the junctions. We must conclude that the interendothelial junction is an especially sensitive portion of the endothelial lining.

Pellets of lead acetate implanted into the brain of adult rats produced a number of changes, including the appearance of fenestrated blood vessels (396), probably a non-specific response. Certainly the "striking increase in pinocytic vesicles" is not supported by published pictures. Contrast media used in angiography were shown to produce severe vascular damage (397, 398).

Treatment with rifamycin was shown to produce renal failure; in one case a biopsy suggested that the basic lesion was a swelling of the glomerular endothelial cells, similar to that of toxemia of pregnancy (399). Rifamycin probably becomes antigenic in vivo by binding to plasma protein. Even the mild penicillin has been

shown to produce severe endothelial damage experimentally. The
toxic action of penicillin derivatives on the endothelium appears
to be related to their capacity to bind proteins, and to solubilize
cholesterol (400). The pulmonary toxicity of bleomycin was also
linked to endothelial lesions (401).

The effects of endotoxin on vascular endothelium have been
studied in the lung (402) and other organs (403) and its relation
to endothelial cells turnover was measured by H-thymidine incorporation (404). In normal rabbits nuclear labeling was greater
in certain areas, such as the aortic arch, presumably as a result
of a "spontaneous hemodynamic condition." In treated animals
these differences were intensified, possibly reflecting a greater
susceptibility to endotoxin-induced injury in areas that were
already "minimally injured." The endothelial injury induced by
endotoxin is not mediated by complement, as shown in complement-
depleted rats (405). The pulmonary effects of endotoxin shock were
compared with those of hypovolemic shock (406). Intravenous colloidal carbon was used as a marker of increased vascular permeability. During the first hour, leakage was detected only from
venules of the bronchial circulation; hypovolemic shock produced
no such leakage. Thus the pattern of leakage was similar to that
obtained in the lung after the administration of histamine or bradykinin. The effect of endotoxin shock was also studied on the
aortic endothelium of the rat, by a variety of methods (407).

In a light microscopic study, chronic alcoholism was said to
produce small vessel disease in the myocardium (408); the evidence,
however, is not very convincing. The effects of smoking were also
studied by comparing the ultrastructure of human umbilical arteries
in the offspring of smoking and non-smoking mothers (409): if the
drastic differences demonstrated could be confirmed, this paper
could become a flag for an anti-smoking campaign.

The bite of crotalid and viperid snakes produces, among other
effects, hemorrhage; this was studied both in vivo and by TEM using
the venom of Trimeresurus flavoviridis (410). The mechanism of
erythrocyte diapedesis, however, was not established.

An interesting poison is dehydromonocrotaline which, when
injected intravenously into the rat, produces endothelial damage
with a latency of 6-8 hours. This injury is primarily capillary,
and reversible; the result is very similar to the delayed-prolonged
vascular leakage observed after thermal injury (411).

Hypercholesterolemia, in the rabbit, produced discontinuities
of the endothelial lining and other more subtle changes (412).
Light microscopic endothelial changes were also observed by others
(413). The mechanism whereby hypercholesterolemia affects the

endothelium is not clear; equally intriguing is the fact that it
stimulates the mitotic activity of the endothelium (414-416).

Low density lipoproteins, added to a culture of human endothelial cells, caused injurious effects: the cells underwent extensive morphologic changes, and became detached from the bottom
of the culture dish (417).

A surface active agent, triton WR1339, produces a hyperlipemia in the rat, and extensive uptake of lipid particles by the
arterial endothelium (418). The endothelial reaction was different from that of dietary-induced hyperlipemia, because some of
the lipid particles (100-1200 Å) were transported intact to the
sub-endothelial space. The intimal changes were severe and accompanied by diapedesis of mononuclear cells. The changes, however
complex, appear extremely interesting and might yield further data
on active transport of lipids by the endothelium.

Acute lipid mobilization by ACTH produces even more severe
endothelial injury (419). In 11 of 12 rabbits, the aortic endothelium showed changes varying from vacuolation to detachment of
the endothelial lining.

Two other hormones have been implicated with endothelial
changes: oestradiol, which induces escape of plasma in the myo-
metrium of immature female rats; electron microscopy showed the
mechanism of this edema to be partially similar to that of acute
inflammation (transient gaps in the endothelium) (420). However,
the predominant pattern of leakage was capillary, and it was of
long duration, quite unlike the short-lived venular leakage typical of the histamine effect. Evidence of endothelial contraction
was not sought in this model. It was also reported that estrogen
injected into female rats (0.25 mg of ethinylestradiol every 4th
day for 16 days) increases the susceptibility of the endothelium
to injury by several test-substances washed over the aortic intima
for 5 minutes immediately after death (421); the evidence, however,
is highly indirect. The role of platelets in endothelial injury
was discussed in sect. 7. Thrombin, in the rabbit, was said to
produce endothelial injury, but the experimental conditions were
highly artificial: thrombin and other test substances were maintained in an isolated segment of the aorta (without circulation)
for 15 mintues (422).

The endothelial injury of homocystinemia was brought to attention as a model for the production of arteriosclerosis (423).

Vitamin E deficiency in the rat causes brown pigment granules
to appear in the endothelium of splenic sinusoids (424) and if
a vitamin E diet is combined with a diet high in unsaturated fats,

an acute necrotizing encephalophaty develops in the chick; ceroid-
like dense bodies accumulate in the endothelial cells, which later
swell and break down. The pathogenesis is interpreted in the
light of lipid peroxidation as a result of excess uptake of unsaturated fatty acid in the absence of vitamin E (425). The endothelial changes illustrated are striking.

Lipofuscin was found in cerebral capillary endothelium in
the monkey, especially in young animals; it was suggested that in
young animals there is a normal removal of lipofuscin from nerve
cells to capillary endothelium (426).

Lipofuscin can apparently be decreased, by mechanisms yet
unknown, with certain drugs used in the treatment of presenile
and senile confusion states (426). One such drug, dimethylamino-
ethyl-p-chlorofenoxy-acetate (Helfergin) allegedly dissolved and
removed lipofuscin from neurons and capillaries in guinea pigs.
Vacuoles in the endothelium apparently represented dissolved lipofuscin granules (unfortunately, the effect of severe weight loss
in the treated animals was not studied) (427).

In scorbutic guinea pigs, regenerating capillaries (in wounds
in the cremaster muscle) showed structural abnormalities (428).

The effect of hypertension on the endothelium is not yet
clear (429-433). An essential requirement is to separate the
mechanical effect of increased intraluminal pressure from the
possible biological effect of the circulating agents which are
responsible for the hypertension and may also, conceivably, alter
the endothelium. A careful study by Huttner et al. did separate
these two effects, but the results are somewhat puzzling (432):
by mechanical coarctation both peroxidase and to a lesser extent
ferritin showed increased passage; peroxidase was seen passing
through the junctions, but ferritin was never found in that location. The possibility of accelerated vesicle transport comes to
mind. The authors suggest that the junctions may be dynamic
structures capable of stretching as a result of increased pressure, without a permanent change in the permeability of the endothelium. If this is true, we believe that such dynamic changes
would disappear during fixation at physiologic pressure. In a
study of retinal capillaries in DOCA hypertension (433), the rats
were perfused with a mixture of fixative and lanthanum (pressure
not stated). The tracer permeated the junctions in the hypertensive animals only, but there was no detectable endothelial injury.
The authors conclude that an increase in permeability may occur
without evidence of injury to the junctions. In future studies
along these lines, fixation at hypertensive pressure may help
unravel some of the present difficulties. An interesting recent

finding is that the microcirculation of spontaneously hypertensive rats are better able to sustain an acute increase of blood pressure (286).

Are there any diseases of the endothelium? Today the most definite candidate is probably von Willebrand disease (sect. 5a), but it has no known ultrastructural equivalent, hence we do not know whether all endothelia are affected. Diabetes is next in line, with its intriguing replication of the basement membrane; this change has often been described and reviewed (434-438); it has been demonstrated also in prediabetic patients (434, 438) and the controversy over its validity seems to be settled, since it is now apparent that fixation in osmium tetroxide (and not in glutaraldehyde) is required to fully appreciate it (438). The mechanism whereby the basement membrane acquires its multiple layers recalling onion skin is not yet clear; the only satisfying explanation is that of Vracko and Benditt, who found that the basement membrane becomes multilayered as a result of repeated cell death and replacement (439); a similar sequence could take place in diabetes (440). It will now be necessary to find out whether endothelial cells, pericytes, or both actually have a shorter life span in diabetics and prediabetics. It has also been stated that diabetes implies a decrease in thickness of the capillary endothelial cell membranes: but this study was based on a single human eye, and a single rat treated with streptozotocin (441). Endothelial changes have been noticed in giant axonal neuropathy, a congenital disease of cytoplasmic microfilaments (442) and in dermatomyositis of childhood; regarding the latter disease, Banker believes that the fundamental lesion is in the wall of the intramuscular blood vessels (443).

b) Effects of Endothelial Injury

The variety of endothelial catastrophies just listed corresponds to a variety of effects, from which a few generalizations may be drawn. An increase in permeability is among the commonest results; it is necessary to distinguish between leakiness due to cell damage (direct injury) and to an active cellular response (contraction) (249). Whether the cytoplasm itself can become permeable to large molecules (444; see also 249) without irreversible cellular injury is not settled. There is some evidence that the peripheral part of the cell is more sensitive to direct injury. Whenever the increase in permeability occurs in an organ equipped with a "blood barrier," it is somewhat surprising to observe that no drastic perivascular damage seems to occur (445, 446). Cellular swelling, a common effect of injury of endothelium as of other cell types, can itself become the source of further injury by reducing blood flow: hence the concept of the "no-reflow phenomenon"

and its therapeutic implications. Thinning of endothelial cells
may correspond to a state of paralysis; it is commonly observed
in ischemic injury, and its reversibility is not yet known. The
new findings on activation and inactivation of hormones by the
endothelium, especially in the lung, now raise the possibility of
syndromes of endothelial deficiency after extensive injury, e.g.,
by oxygen poisoning of the lung: a mechanism that will need to
be explored further. Thrombosis remains a typical effect of endothelial injury; its pathogenesis has become increasingly complex
(447-449). Chronic, repeated injury was shown to leave its mark
in a reduplication of the basement membrane, due to the fact that
each regenerating endothelial cell and pericyte provides its
own new layer (450, 451). This concept, which was introduced by
Vracko and Benditt and is still the only likely explanation of
diabetic microangiopathy, is beautifully illustrated and confirmed
by the multilayered basement membranes of skin capillaries in
protoporphyria: a condition in which endothelial cells are being
constantly destroyed by UV rays and replaced. The published electron micrographs illustrating this condition can match any that
have been shown in diabetics (Fig. 14). Thus, capillaries share
with bone tissue a rare characteristic: that of maintaining, in
their structural makeup, a trace of their past history.

c) Infection

By TEM, several intra-endothelial pathogens have been identified: Meningococci in the skin of patients with acute meningococcemia and maculo purpuric lesions (452), Corynebacteria in a jejunal biopsy obtained from a patient with untreated Whipple's disease
(453), Rickettsiae in guinea pigs (454, 455), crystalline virus
arrays in human Coxsackie myocarditis (456). In laboratory animals,
careful study has allowed Margolis et al. to obtain striking pictures of virus-infected endothelial cells even by light microscopy
(457-460).

d) Tubulo-Reticular Aggregates (TRA)

These puzzling structures are mentioned here not because they
are necessarily related to infection, but because they recall the
structure of viruses. Dozens of papers have reported them in
human and experimental tissues. Typical TRA have definite ultrastructural features: they consist of several convoluted, branched,
and interwoven components, usually tubular in cross sections, and
with an outside diameter of 180-260 Å. They are usually enclosed
within dilated cisternae of endoplasmic reitculum, but may also
be free within the cytoplasm (461). In some cases they appear to
arise as dimplings of the membrane of the endoplasmic reticulum

(462). The association with measles (463) and with herpes (464-466) would appear to suggest a viral nature, but structural details weigh against this interpretation. Their frequent appearance in lupus (467-471) is so striking (89% in one series of renal biopsies, 471) that their presence has been considered as a diagnostic aid in this condition. They have been seen in scleroderma (472), dermatomyositis (473, 474) and other skin diseases (475), in human wounds (476), in synovial vascular endothelium in lupus, and in a case of undiagnosed transient arthritis (477), in endothelial cells of the human liver from a case of malignant melanoma (478), in retinoblastoma (479), in certain pituitary adenomas (480, 481), and a host of other locations and conditions ranging from congenital infantile nephrosis (482) to the cerebral arteries of the normal rat (483). It has been suggested that they are related to immunoglobulin synthesis (484). It is quite likely that not all the structures described under this heading correspond to the same entity; some of the reported crystalline or pseudocrystalline inclusions (485, 486) are neither compatible with any known virus nor fitting with the definition of typical TRA. Such are the inclusions that we found incidentally in the arterial endothelium of a dog (Fig. 15).

The nature of the TRA and the little that is known of their chemical constituents have been repeatedly reviewed (461, 462). The current trend is to interpret them as non-viral structures of unknown significance. Because of their broad but irregular distribution, we believe they represent a response to mild injury.

e) Neoplasia

Several interesting endothelial neoplastic growths have been studied by light or by electron microscopy (487-489). One case of Kaposi's sarcoma was studied at autopsy; Weibel-Palade bodies were found in the cytoplasm of the tumor cells, thus establishing their nature as endothelium (490). Cultured vascular endothelium has been transformed in vitro with SV40 DNA (491). Blood vessels of tumors have been studied in many organs, including brain (492). Lack of space does not allow us to adequately cover this topic, which would require a review of angiomas.

f) Metaplasia

Metaplasia of endothelium has never been studied as such. We will include under this heading the many published instances of continuous endothelium becoming fenestrated, and vice versa. That this type of metaplasia should occur is consistent with the notion, already mentioned, that the fenestrae are labile, dynamic structures. Fenestrated endothelium was seen to appear in the alveolar

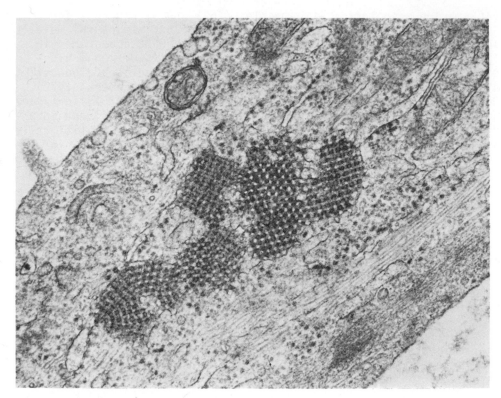

Figure 15. Tubulo-reticular aggregates with unusual crystalline arrangement, lying within dilated cisternae of endoplasmic reticulum (dog, arterial endothelium). 60,000 x.

capillaries during experimental pulmonary fibrosis (493). In the guinea pig, transplants of vas deferens and ureter into the anterior chamber of the eye developed capillary fenestrations only in relation to epithelium, suggesting that this tissue may have been responsible in inducing that specific change (494). Metaplasia of continuous to fenestrated endothelium was reported in experimental thrombocytopenia (293); focally, in the endothelium of the bone marrow over the bulge produced by a marrow cell pushing its way toward the lumen (Fig. 6); in experimental allergic encephalomyelitis (495); in certain naevi and in many tumors (496) and in a variety of other conditions (497).

One report claims that material from the intermediate lobe of
the hypophysis causes metaplasia of renal glomerular endothelium
into cells of erythroid line (498).

10. IMMUNOLOGY

The immunologic properties of the endothelium have come to
the forefront because "the vascular interface is an important
battleground in graft rejection" (499). In the field of grafting,
however, seniority undoubtedly belongs to the fetus and placenta.
Szulman has studied the distribution of ABH-major transplantation
antigens in the human placenta, with fascinating results (500, 501).
Trophoblast was negative to all three antigens, presumably because
it must maintain absolute antigenic neutrality. Placental capillaries contained only the H antigen, which is characteristic of
group O and consists chemically of a truncated form of the AB
antigens. In the vessels of the umbilical cord there was a progressive transition to the full AB endowment, with a corresponding
reduction of the strength of the H antigen within a few centimeters
of the body wall. This modulation of the endothelium along a single vessel has no known precedent in the literature. The antigens
of the HL-A group have also been identified in cultured human
endothelial cells (502, 8).

There is now evidence that endothelial cells contain their
own specific (E) antigens (503-505), a potentially very important
development. In kidney transplantation, donor and recipient are
usually matched with regard to HL-A antigens; the matching is performed with the use of lymphocytes, by the MLC method ("mixed lymphocyte culture," see below). Yet some recipients of transplants
thus matched reject the grafts, even though they do not develop
lymphocytotoxic antibodies. On the other hand, kidney transplant
recipients develop antibodies that react with cultured endothelium from umbilical cord vein, but are not cytotoxic for lymphocytes from the same donor. Curiously, these E antigens are
expressed also in blood monocytes (504, 505); a tantalizing
observation for those who feel that monocytes are able to take the
place of endothelial cells.

Another important development in this field is the discovery
of an anti-endothelium antibody that may be present in the blood
of normal individuals, and appears to be of great help in predict-
ing the outcome of renal grafts (506-508). The test can be performed by immunofluorescence, using frozen sections of arteries
obtained at the time of transplantation, or suspensions of endothelial cells obtained from umbilical cords (508). The antigenic
properties of the endothelium have also been explored using mixed
cultures of lymphocyte and endothelial cells. Mixtures of lymphocytes from two genetically dissimilar individuals result in

blast transformation of some of the participating cells (the "MLC"
phenomenon); cells other than lymphocytes are mostly unresponsive
in this test. However, endothelial cells of dog and man can stimulate allogeneic lymphocytes (509, 510).

The normal interaction between endothelium and lymphocytes
has also been studied in vitro, using cultured endothelium from
the aorta of the pig, and autologous lymphocytes (511): aortic
endothelium in situ has less binding capacity than cultured endothelium; the lymphocyte binding component was stable to trypsin,
but labile to neuraminidase and papain. Curiously, endothelium
from umbilical veins never showed the capacity to bind lymphocytes
(perhaps another indication of immaturity of umbilical cord endothelium).

An important problem is the fate of donor endothelium in a
graft. Is it ever replaced by recipient endothelium? This question was tackled with the use of sex chromatin (499, 512-514, 531).
The results are ambiguous. All investigators find some evidence
of host endothelial cells in the graft; Williams et al. (514), working on experimental animals, believe that this repopulation is
significant; de Bono (513), working with human renal grafts, is
inclined to believe the contrary. Sinclair studied 45 human kidney allografts; definite endothelial chimerism was present in 3,
but these were the most severely damaged kidneys, hence the conclusion that host repopulation cannot explain graft adaptation
(531). However, while studying the problem of host-repopulation,
Williams et al. made an important contribution. Using rats, they
grafted aortic segments from male donors to female recipients;
some of the Lewis recipient rats were made into chimeras by infusion of bone marrow cells. Then, using the sex chromatin marker,
they found not only that some endothelial repopulation occurs in
large vessel allografts; but also that cells derived from the bone
marrow can lodge among normal endothelial cells and become morphologically identical to them. There was considerable individual
variation, but as many as 1/25 to 1/10 of the cells could be of
bone marrow origin. This is, to our knowledge, the best evidence
that monocytes can take the place of endothelial cells. (These
results will need to be confirmed, and some control will be
needed in order to exclude that some of the "bone marrow cells"
may be, in fact, bone marrow endothelium.)

Antibody- and cell-mediated damage to the endothelium has
been studied in various systems (515-517). A cross reaction has
been described between Streptococcus pyogenes and human endothelial cells as well as fibroblasts and astrocytes (518). Antibodies
against endothelial basement membrane were found in the blood of
patients with a variety of gastrointestinal diseases (519).

Finally, a unique TEM observation made by Wiener et al. on skin allografts in mice: areas of fusion were noticed between the surface membranes of emigrating polymorphonuclear leukocytes and the endothelium of these vessels. Some of the leukocytic granules were found to be spilled into the endothelial cytoplasm. At least one of the published electron micrographs (Fig. 2) seems unquestionable; the significance of this observation with regard to immune damage will need further study (520).

11. CELLS RELATED TO ENDOTHELIUM

Included here will be endothelial cells in the wrong place, non-endothelial cells taking the place of endothelium, and cells similar to endothelium. Endothelial cells can be found in the circulating blood after endotoxin injection and in the generalized Shwartzman reaction (521, 522), in anaphylactic shock (523), in caisson disease, in anoxia and after the administration of certain drugs (304). Conversely, it has been said that circulating white blood cells (presumably monocytes) can assume the role of endothelium. The evidence was summarized recently (524); in our opinion many of the experiments are open to criticism, but the transformation of monocytes to endothelium remains a tempting possibility, as mentioned in sect. 10.

The very thin cells of the perineurium are strikingly similar to vascular endothelium, including the presence of plasmalemmal vesicles. Thus, they have been called "perineurial endothelium" (525). The pericytes, cells very similar to the endothelium, have been the object of very few studies (526). Intimate contact (interdigitation) with endothelial cells in the human choroid and retina suggested exchange of "information concerning the blood circulation" (204).

It is now abundantly clear that when the endothelium is artifically removed, a temporary non-thrombogenic covering, a pseudo-endothelium, can be formed by other cell types. Clearly competent in this respect are the smooth muscle cells. Less clear is the role of the monocytes. They can certainly form a pseudoendothelium after experimental aortic injury (527). Whether they can become permanently settled, as suggested by the experiments of Williams et al. (sect. 10) is not clear, and remains an important question in endothelial biology. A pseudoendothelium can also be fleetingly formed by platelets (528).

Trophoblast functions as "de facto endothelium," and is indeed continuous with the endothelium of maternal vessels (500); its immunologic adaptation to this function is most interesting (sect. 10).

The mesothelium is occasionally used as a model to be compared with endothelium (529, 16); attempts have also been made to
use it surgically as a vascular lining (for ref., see 8).

CONCLUSION

By comparing the chapter headings of this review with those
of the previous one (1) progress on many fronts is obvious. The
"endothelial family" has become even more varied than anticipated;
tissue culture has singled out differences between arterial and
venous endothelium, and differences have been found even between
the two ends of the umbilical vessels. The permeability properties
of the endothelium are far better understood; vesicular transport
has become firmly established; the variable anatomy of the junc-
tiosn has been recognized. A partial correlation with the pore
theory has been accomplished, but a closer synthesis with physiologic measurements may have to wait until physiologists find means
of working with smaller units. At present, the size of the samples
used by physiologists (whole paws) and by electron microscopists
are about 14 orders of magnitude apart.

It is now recognized that endothelial cells, under given circumstances, are able to respond to stimuli. Observed responses
include metabolic changes, contraction, and proliferation. The
immunologic properties of endothelium have come to the forefront
due to practical circumstances - organ transplantation; and many
synthetic properties have been recognized. Thus a true endothelial
deficiency disease has been identified (von Willebrand disease)
and it is possible that extensive endothelial damage, as in shock
lung, may bring about other deficiency syndromes. In some respects,
we are no longer dealing with an endothelial membrane but with an
endothelial organ weighing about 200 grams, which produces clotting
factors, inactivates hormones, and resembles, in both respects,
the liver. Endothelium has become, in this sense, the ultimate
endocrine organ.

ADDENDUM

Modulations of vesicular transport (sect. 6b). A paper that
was not retrieved by our MEDLARS search came to our attention at
the last minute (536). The purpose of this work was to study
whether the blood-brain barrier may break down by an increase in
vesicular transport. Mice were injected intraperitoneally with
a lipid-substituted derivative of cyclic AMP (dibutyryl cAMP) and
killed 5 and 20 minutes later; the number of vesicles per square
micron of endothelial cytoplasm was counted in capillaries of the
parietal cortex and cerebellar vermis. At 5 minutes there was a

significant increase in the number of free vesicles (from 7.09
+ 0.10 to 14.85 + 0.18) and of basal caveolae (from 0.41 + 0.02
to 4.88 + 0.1); there was a comparable increase at 20 minutes;
coated vesicles behaved in similar fashion. The figures appear
interesting, but of course they cannot be taken to represent
"facilitation of pinocytosis" as proposed.

Histamine-induced vascular leakage (p. 34). Joyner et al.
(537) studied the effect of histamine on blood-lymph "transport"
(i.e., passage) of plasma protein in dog paws. Their calculations
led them to conclude that the increased "transport" of both small
and large molecules occurred "through a barrier of unchanged
porosity." They did not test the permeability of the barrier by
an injection of colloidal carbon black, which would have labeled
endothelial leaks; thus it is difficult to reconstruct their
observations. In any event, they state that the phenomenon of
histamine-induced endothelial gaps has been demonstrated "largely
on rodents and lagomorphs," and imply that it is not significant
for dogs. The facts are otherwise: histamine increases vascular
permeability by the same mechanism in rats, in cats, dogs (246),
and humans (538).

ACKNOWLEDGMENTS

The compilation of this review was supported in part by grants
HL 16952 and HL 21843 from the National Institutes of Health.

We are indebted to Mrs. Karen E. Melia, Deborah E. Gossel,
Allyson J. Soell, and Miss Jane M. Manzi for the preparation of
the manuscript, and to Mr. Peter W. Healey for the photographic
work.

ATHEROSCLEROSIS AND INFLAMMATION

Isabelle Joris and Guido Majno

Department of Pathology
University of Massachusetts Medical School
Worcester, Massachusetts

It is probably safe to state that atherosclerosis is the sum of several different processes. Each one of the past and current theories of atherosclerosis emphasizes one of these processes. Thus, if we open a contemporary textbook of pathology (1), we find at least four theories: (1) lipid insudation, (b) structural or metabolic alteration of the arterial wall, (c) intimal stress or injury, (d) thrombogenesis or encrustation. To these we should add the two newer theories that emphasize a further aspect of the process, cell proliferation: the theory of Ross et al. (2, 3) which gives platelets the stimulating role, and the theory of Benditt (4, 5) in which the proliferation is considered akin to neoplasia.

Whichever pathogenetic theory one may choose, it is always implied that the arterial wall is injured, to the point of suffering cell death and necrosis. Now, in most organs, tissue injury implies an inflammatory reaction. Does any reaction of this kind occur in the arterial wall? This question, to our knowledge, is not being asked; currently there is no "inflammatory theory" of atherosclerosis, presumably because it is assumed that the vascular wall, being devoid of a microcirculation, cannot develop an inflammatory response.

The purpose of this short paper is certainly not to propose a new theory of atherosclerosis, but to analyze the relationship between atherosclerosis and inflammation -- and thereby to offer a perspective that may have conceptual and practical implications.

We should hasten to add that the idea is over 100 years old. Virchow is credited with having proposed an inflammatory theory of

atherosclerosis (6). However, his concept of inflammation was so
far removed from today's that his statement cannot be taken literally, in the context of the inflammatory process as we now understand it.

The first step should be to define what is meant by inflammation. We will adopt a current definition, whereby inflammation
represents a response of living tissue to local injury, leading to
the local accumulation of fluid and blood cells (7). We must
therefore analyze four points: (1) Is there local injury? (the
term injury is used here in the passive sense of damage). (b) Can
the arterial wall "respond" in a manner comparable to that of other
tissues? (c) Is there a local accumulation of fluid? (d) Is there
a local accumulation of blood cells?

ATHEROSCLEROSIS AND ARTERIAL INJURY

Whether primary injury is required as a triggering event of
atherosclerosis depends on the pathogenetic theory: the neoplastic
theory does not imply any pre-existing endothelial damage; the
"platelet" theory of Ross et al. does presuppose some form of endothelial damage, so that the platelets may accumulate locally and
initiate the presumed chain reaction, beginning with smooth muscle
cell proliferation. Secondary injury obviously occurs, leading to
cellular death (8-11) of which atheroma is the ultimate expression.
Thus tissue injury is a definite component of atherosclerosis; certainly as a secondary event; probably also as a primary event.
Would it be severe enough to initiate an inflammatory response? We
have no means of measuring it, nor do we know precisely the extent
of cell death required for the purpose; however, we can empirically
evaluate (on histologic sections) the extent of cell death in atherosclerosis: it is prominent, and experience suggests that - in
other tissues - it should be adequate for triggering the inflammatory response.

As a matter of fact, the adventitia of atherosclerotic vessels
often shows chronic inflammatory infiltrates. Schwartz and Mitchell
(12) have summarized the pertinent literature, and concluded that
two mechanisms could account for these infiltrates: an autoimmune
reaction is a possibility; but the likeliest hypothesis is that
these foci represent a reaction to abnormal material arising from
atheromatous lesions.

ON THE CAPACITY OF THE ARTERIAL WALL TO RESPOND

In the typical inflammatory process, the response to injury
includes changes (i) in the microcirculatory blood vessels and (ii)
in the surrounding stroma.

(i) In an arterial wall, a microcirculatory network exists only in the adventitia (and at most in the outer media). However, the intima is another blood-tissue interface which, on theoretical grounds, should allow the outpouring of fluid and of cellular exudate. There is no reason to limit the notion of "inflammatory exudation" to the endothelium of the microcirculatory vessels. (ii) As to the stromal reaction, the cellular population of the media is highly specialized, being composed of smooth muscle cells only; but it is now known that in response to injury these cells can partially dedifferentiate and act as a multifunctional mesenchyme (13). Thus, although the arterial intima and media cannot respond to injury exactly in the same manner as vascularized connective tissues, they certainly have the potential to develop a response that can be defined as inflammatory.

INCREASED ENDOTHELIAL PERMEABILITY IN ATHEROSCLEROSIS

In advanced lesions the endothelial lining has disappeared altogether; hence an increase in permeability occurs a fortiori. More pertinent here is the possibility of an increased permeability in the early stages. It is well established that - in large animals - aortas that appear grossly normal show patches of increased permeability demonstrable by injecting Evans blue intravenously a few hours before sacrifice (14-18). This is precisely the technique used for the demonstration of increased permeability in inflammation (19). These "blued" patches occur in areas that are also known as atherosclerosis-prone in older animals; hence there is good reason to believe that these simple lesions are, or can be, precursors of typical atherosclerotic lesions. Correspondingly, in histologic sections, an interstitial (intimal) accumulation of fluid has been described - in fairly recent times - as characteristic of certain early lesions of human atherosclerosis (gelatinous lesions) (10, 11). The presence of fibrin in this edema testifies to the increased endothelial permeability; the edema itself is described as "serofibrinous insudate" (11), only a semantic step away from "serofibrinous exudate".

Thus, there can be no question as to the existence of an increased intimal permeability in atherosclerosis. However, when we compare this phenomenon with the vascular leakage of inflammation, we must remember that there are two basic mechanisms of increased permeability (20): (1) a histamine-type effect, which is an active cellular (endothelial) response to local chemical mediators, such as histamine, bradykinin, and the like; and (2) direct injury, a passive change, i.e., endothelial damage due to the noxious agent acting directly on the vessels (trauma, heat, etc.). This distinction has important implications, especially as regards therapy: the histamine-type response can be inhibited by pharmacologic means,

such as anti-histamine drugs; direct injury is far more difficult
and perhaps impossible to prevent with drugs.

In summary, then, atherosclerosis shares with inflammation
the phenomenon of increased endothelial permeability. To establish
its significance (and its susceptibility to anti-inflammatory drugs),
it will be essential to determine whether it is due to an active
cellular response, or - as appears more likely - to cellular injury.

EXUDATION OF WHITE BLOOD CELLS IN ATHEROSCLEROSIS
AND IN EXPERIMENTAL ARTERIAL LESIONS

The papers describing hematogenous cells in the intima of
large arteries can be counted by the dozen. In 1957, Duff, McMillan and Ritchie saw foci of "monocytoid" cells in the intima of normal rabbits, and assumed them to be hematogenous (21). A year later,
Poole and Florey published beautiful light microscopic illustrations
of macrophages performing diapedesis in the aorta of atherosclerotic rabbits (but could not decide whether the cells moved in or
out...) (22). Again in rabbits - on a high cholesterol diet - Still
and Marriott noticed significant numbers of lymphocytes and monocytes in superficial areas of the aortic lesions; sometimes these
cells could be caught in the act of "breaching the endothelium."
Similar observations were made in early atherosclerotic lesions of
human aortas (23). Studies from F.J. Mustard's laboratory have
shown patches of edematous intima stained with Evans blue in rabbits and pigs; similar patches were found in young human subjects;
the edema was correlated with the presence of leukocytes over and
beneath the endothelium (24, 25). One of the papers just mentioned
contains an electron micrograph of diapedesis in the aorta of the
pig (25). Clowes et al. have also illustrated diapedesis across
the endothelium of the carotid artery in hypercholesterolemic rats
(26, 27) and there is evidence that hypertension increases the
penetration of lymphocytes and monocytes (28, 29).

We have examined - by light and by electron microscopy -
early lesions of atherosclerosis in aortas obtained at autopsy
(i.e., both fibrous plaques and "gelatinous lesions"). The presence of inflammatory cells was obvious, especially at the periphery of the lesions; the cells included basophils (presumably the
same cells described by others (23, 30) as mast cells). These
studies will be reported elsewhere. At this time, the only point
we wish to make is that inflammation should be considered as one
of the major components of the atherosclerotic process, and that
work is needed along these lines, aimed at correlating the atherosclerotic process with the vast amount of information now available
on the inflammatory process.

Experimental studies directly pertinent to this approach are
almost nonexistent. The single exception - to our knowledge - is
a report published by Hollander et al. in 1974 (31). It does not
deal with either permeability or cellular infiltration, but with
local cell proliferation of smooth muscle cells. Reasoning that
cellular hyperplasia is a major component of the atheromatous fibrous plaque, these authors produced atherosclerosis in rabbits,
and studied the effect of treatment with a number of anti-proliferative and anti-inflammatory drugs. Some suppression of fibrous
plaque formation was obtained. Obviously the intent of this study
was not, strictly speaking, to inhibit inflammation: the purpose
was to suppress cellular proliferation, and it so happens that
some of the most effective anti-proliferative drugs are also anti-
inflammatory. However, the results are encouraging.

In conclusion, there are theoretical, experimental and even
therapeutic reasons for assigning inflammation a significant role
in the pathogenesis of atherosclerosis. Somehow this concept
appears self-evident - but we felt that it should be formally proposed, since it is not mentioned in any of the recent reviews on
atherosclerosis (32-35).

REFERENCES

1. Robbins, S.L. (1974) in Pathologic Basis of Disease, W.B.
    Saunders Co., Philadelphia, pp. 595-600.

2. Ross, R., and Glomset, J.A. (1976) N. Engl. J. Med. 295, 369-
    377; 420-425.

3. Ross, R., Glomset, J., and Harker, L. (1977) Am. J. Pathol.
    86, 675-684.

4. Benditt, E.P., and Benditt, J.M. (1973) Proc. Natl. Acad. Sci.
    USA 70, 1753-1756.

5. Benditt, E.P. (1974) Circulation 50, 650-652.

6. Haust, M.D., and More, R.H. (1972) in The Pathogenesis of Ath-
    erosclerosis (Wissler, R.W., and Geer, J.C., Eds.), Williams
    and Wilkins, Baltimore, pp. 8-9.

7. Ryan, G.B., and Majno, G. (1977) Am. J. Pathol. 86, 184-276.

8. Imai, H., and Thomas, W.A. (1968) Exp. Mol. Pathol. 8, 330-357.

9. Imai, H., Lee, S.K., Pastori, S.J., and Thomas, W.A. (1970)
    Virchows Arch. Abt. A. Path. Anat. 350, 183-204.

10. Haust, M.D. (1971) Human Path. 2, 1-29.

11. Haust, M.D. (1974) Adv. Exp. Med. Biol. 43, 35-37.

12. Schwartz, C.J., and Mitchell, J.R.A. (1962) Circulation 26, 73-78.

13. Wissler, R.W. (1968) J. Atheroscl. Res. 8, 201-213.

14. McGill, H.C., Jr., Geer, J.C., and Holman, R.L. (1957) Arch. Pathol. 64, 303-311.

15. Caplan, B.A., Gerrity, R.G., and Schwartz, C.J. (1974) Exp. Mol. Pathol. 21, 102-117.

16. Somer, J.B., Gerrity, R.G., and Schwartz, C.J. (1976) Exp. Mol. Pathol. 24, 129-141.

17. Katora, M.E., and Hollis, T.M. (1976) Exp. Mol. Pathol. 24, 23-34.

18. Adams, C.W.M., and Bayliss, O.B. (1977) Atherosclerosis 26, 419-426.

19. Payling Wright, G. (1958) in An Introduction to Pathology, Longmans, Green and Co., London, pp. 112-113.

20. Cotran, R.S., and Majno, G. (1964) Ann. N.Y. Acad. Sci. 116, 750-764.

21. Duff, G.L., McMillan, G.C., and Ritchie, A.C. (1957) Am. J. Pathol. 33, 845-873.

22. Poole, J.C.F., and Florey, H.W. (1958) J. Pathol. Bact. 75, 245-253.

23. Still, W.J.S., and Marriott, P.R. (1963) J. Atheroscl. Res. 4, 373-386.

24. Packham, M.A., Rowsell, H.C., Jørgensen, L., and Mustard, J. F. (1967) Exp. Mol. Pathol. 7, 214-232.

25. Jørgensen, L., Packham, M.A., Rowsell, H.C., and Mustard, J.F. (1972) Lab. Invest. 27, 341-350.

26. Clowes, A.W., Ryan, G.B., Breslow, J.L., and Karnovsky, M.J. (1976) Lab. Invest. 35, 6-17.

27. Clowes, A.W., Breslow, J.L., and Karnovsky, M.J. (1977) <u>Lab.</u>
     <u>Invest.</u> 36, 73-81.

28. Still, W.J.S. (1968) <u>Lab. Invest.</u> 19, 84-91.

29. Still, W.J.S., and Dennison, S. (1974) <u>Arch. Pathol.</u> 97, 337-
     342.

30. Geer, J.C., and Webster, W.S. (1974) <u>Adv. Exp. Med. Biol.</u> 43,
     9-33.

31. Hollander, W., Kramsch, D.M., Franzblau, C., Paddock, J., and
     Colombo, M.A. (1974) <u>Circ. Res.</u> 34-35 (Suppl. 1), 131-141.

32. Constantinides, P. (1976) <u>Triangle</u> 15, 53-61.

33. Gorlin, R. (1976) in <u>Coronary Artery Disease</u>, vol. 11 of Major
     Problems in Internal Medicine (Smith, L.H., Jr., Ed.), W.B.
     Saunders Co., Philadelphia, pp. 29-39.

34. Wissler, R.W., Vesselinovitch, D., and Getz, G.S. (1976) in
     <u>Progress in Cardiovascular Diseases</u>, vol. 18, (Sonnenblick,
     E.H., Ed.), Grune & Stratton, pp. 341-369.

35. Wissler, R.W. (1977) <u>Cardiovasc. Res. Ctr. Bull.</u> 15, 69-86.

ACKNOWLEDGMENTS

     This study was supported in part by grant HL 16952 from the
National Institutes of Health.

DISCUSSION FOLLOWING FIRST PLENARY SESSION:

CONCEPTUAL ASPECTS

D.B. Zilversmit: Dr. Gotto, as you have indicated, the cholesterol-rich chylomicron remnant may well be quite atherogenic.
Recent evidence in the rabbit indicates that a large proportion of
hypercholesterolemia, induced by cholesterol feeding, is the result
of chylomicron remnants that can be identified by their retinol
content after feeding a meal containing retinol. Do you not think
that in studies on human subjects, and in screening for susceptible individuals, greater emphasis should be placed on lipoprotein
concentrations and metabolism in the post-prandial state instead
of in the post-absorptive state?

A.M. Gotto, Jr.: Non-fasting measurements of lipids provide
useful information and I suppose that is why they have been so
determined at the Donner Laboratory. In population studies, and
in individual patients, it is difficult to standardize for dietary
differences. For this reason, fasting determinations have become
popularized, although they may not reflect the metabolic state during the course of the day.

D.B. Zilversmit: Dr. Gotto, do you think that it would be
worthwhile to measure rates of catabolism of chylomicron remnants
in man?

A.M. Gotto, Jr.: Yes, I think such measurements should be
done in normal and hyperlipidemic subjects and under varying dietary conditions.

Question: Dr. Gotto, is there available information about the
frequency of lipoprotein lipase deficiency in the population?

A.M. Gotto, Jr.: To the best of my knowledge epidemiologic
data are not available. Adipose tissue lipoprotein lipase is completely absent in familial lipoprotein lipase deficiency, an extremely rare disorder. The enzyme is probably depressed in type V
hyperlipoproteinemia. The frequency of type V may be estimated
from the Lipid Research Clinics Prevalence Study, when its results
are published.

T.N. Wight: On your last slide, I think you suggested that sulfated glycosaminoglycans bind to circulating lipoproteins and therefore constitute part of the surface receptor of the endothe- lial cell. Is this merely a suggestion or do you and/or others have data to indicate that sulfated glycosaminoglycans are indeed part of such receptors?

A.M. Gotto, Jr.: There is only indirect evidence from the studies of DiFerrante et al., who found a circulating glycosamino- glycan which is extremely potent in its ability to bind LDL. It is present in very small concentrations in plasma.

M.R. Malinow: With regard to Dr. Wissler's presentation, I would like to raise a point concerning semantics. "Regression" is the progressive decline in size or severity of a manifestation of disease. Regression, then, was used correctly by Dr. Wissler be- cause arterial lesions show a decline in size. However, it is a matter of interpretation whether the decrease in size and in lipids is associated with a decline in severity of the atherosclerotic process. When one compares normal arteries to "regressed" lesions in monkeys, the lesions show intimal thickening with increased mucopolysaccharides and collagen, as well as breaking and partial disappearance of the internal elastic lamina. These changes indi- cate an increase in the severity of the fibrotic process, although one would expect blood flow to be less compromised by arterial lesions that have decreased in size.

To avoid ambiguity, and thus a rise in false hopes, when de- scribing the reduction in size of the arterial lesions and the pro- bably hemodynamic consequences, should we not use a term without implications of severity? I wonder, then, if you would consider advocating use of "shrinkage" or a similar word in this context such as "metagression," where the prefix meta- means change or transformation in the progression of atherogenesis.

R.W. Wissler: I believe regression is a very good term and as I pointed out in the presentation, there are also elements of healing and of remodeling in the changes that occur following the sustained lowering of the serum cholesterol.

I think that there is little doubt that these regressed lesions are less severe functionally and less dangerous clinically not only because the lumen becomes larger but also because the intimal sur- face endothelium is less thrombogenic both physically and chemi- cally. While collagen may become more dense during regression there is evidence that it and other fiber proteins do decrease in absolute (per anatomical unit) terms if the regression regimen is sustained, i.e., 18 months or more in the rhesus monkey.

M.J. Karnovsky: Could Dr. Wissler clarify a conceptual point for me? Is the proliferation of smooth muscle basic and necessary for the accumulation of lipid, e.g., by positioning of target cells in the intima, or are these possibly two concommitant phenomena, not necessarily interrelated?

R.W. Wissler: Although I do not think it is possible to give a definitive response to this question, we do see in the butter fat-cholesterol-fed rhesus monkey model a rather remarkable build-up of lipid droplets in the smooth muscle cells of the intima and inner media without very much evidence of smooth muscle cell migration into the intima or of smooth muscle cell proliferation. On the other hand, some food fats such as peanut oil or coconut oil, fed with cholesterol, results in remarkable smooth muscle cell migration and proliferation relatively early in the process of plaque formation. The Albany group (Thomas, Lee, etc.) has published data indicating that excessive smooth muscle cell proliferation begins very soon after an animal is shifted to a high fat, high cholesterol diet. I don't know of any in vitro (cell culture) data as yet that would give a definitive answer to your question.

A.B. Chandler: Early studies of the thrombogenic theory of atherosclerosis emphasized that fibrin in thrombi may serve as a scaffold for the growth of connective tissue. F.B. Mallory compared the organization of fibrin-rich thrombi to that of organizing fibrinous exudates on serosal membranes. Some years ago, Woolf and others demonstrated the frequent presence of fibrin antigen in fatty streaks. Dr. Wissler now refers to the work of Dr. Elspeth Smith who has shown that fibrinogen/fibrin accumulates progressively in plaques and seems to accompany plasma lipoproteins. Would Dr. Wissler comment on the possibility that fibrinogen/fibrin might also be a stimulant for connective tissue growth.

R.W. Wissler: That is an interesting idea! While I agree that fibrinogen and/or fibrin is a macromolecule that becomes "trapped" or "bound" and accumulates along with low density lipoproteins in plaques of all ages,* I know of no convincing evidence for or against its role in stimulating connective tissue (collagen, elastins or glycosaminoglycans) synthesis by the arterial smooth muscle cells of the plaque.

K.T. Lee: Dr. Schwartz, you presented a slide showing the frequency of thrombotic occlusion in patients with myocardial infarction. In cases with sudden unexpected cardiac death the frequency of thrombotic occlusion was only approximately 30%, whereas

---

*Kao, V. and Wissler, R.W. A study of the immunohistochemical localization of serum lipoproteins and other plasma proteins in human atherosclerotic lesions. Exp. Mol. Pathol. 4, 465-479, 1965.

occlusive thrombi were found in over 90% of cases with myocardial infarction. Some years ago, a Russian pathologist visited us and told us that in Russia they believed thrombosis is a secondary phenomenon occurring after myocardial infarction, since the frequency of thrombi in patients who died soon after the onset of chest pain was very low, while the frequency increased with the length of time between the onset of symptoms and the death of the patient. How do you explain these phenomena?

C.J. Schwartz: Dr. K.T. Lee's question relates to one of the important controversies in this field. I have already indicated that a consensus has emerged, indicating that recent transmural myocardial infarction is associated with occlusive thrombi in over 90% of cases; moreover, the occlusions show a distinct spatial and temporal relationship to the infarctions. At present, much of the available data suggests that we should not equate sudden cardiac death and acute myocardial infarction. This is verified by Dr. Cobb's findings in Seattle, where only approximately 16% of patients successfully resuscitated after dying suddenly go on to develop pathological Q waves and enzymatic evidence of transmural myocardial infarction. In other words, not all cases of sudden death appear to be due to myocardial infarction and ischemia in the traditional sense; the data help to explain, in my opinion, the low frequency of occlusive coronary thrombi in sudden unexpected cardiac death. The problem is discussed in greater detail in the text.

S. Moore: Dr. Schwartz has emphasized the need for more experimental study in the area of coronary thrombosis and embolism. We have performed experiments in dogs examining the myocardial lesions which result from occlusive and non-occlusive (mural) thrombi. Occlusive thrombi were in all cases associated with transmural infarction. Mural thrombosis was associated with a variety of lesions including myofibrillar degeneration, focal round cell infiltration, focal fiber necrosis, and focal small infarcts. These lesions occurred primarily in the subendocardial region and in the inner third of the ventricular wall. Dogs that died did so in ventricular fibrillation, which was preceded by runs of premature ventricular contractions. We are now attempting to define the pathogenesis of these events by labeling platelets with ^{51}Cr to study the embolic process. So far, the results are consistent in showing more uptake of radioactivity in the area of myocardium served by the artery containing a mural thrombus.

A. Nordøy: Could I ask Dr. Moore a question in relation to his comment on the accumulation of platelets in the subendocardial areas during sudden death in experimental animals? Have you labeled the red cells also, and do they, as the platelets, accumulate?

S. Moore: No, we have not.

S. Wessler: Dr. Schwartz, you showed arteriographically a
coronary artery occluded presumably by atherosclerosis and thrombosis with the implication that when it recanalized it was "through
and through" recanalization from the proximal to the distal end.
Is it possible that the recanalizations are only partial and that
the blood flow is provided by overlying interarterial collaterals,
some of which could enter and leave portions of the recanalized
vessel or bypass it entirely? Is your suggestion only for the
specific case presented or is it meant to be a general phenomenon?

C.J. Schwartz: The illustration referred to by Dr. Wessler is
a microradiograph of a recanalizing coronary artery thrombus in the
left coronary artery of a young man who died after his second myocardial infarction. Specifically, this slide showed multiple channels of recanalization, which traverse the whole length of the occlusion, restoring continuity to the circulation at this point.
These channels occur within the thrombus, as confirmed histologi-
cally; their physiological significance in restoring significant
blood flow to the myocardium is speculative.

Dr. Wessler is correct, however, in pointing out that some so-
called collaterals may occur in the adventitia, bypassing the occlusive site completely. Additionally, not all new vessels within
the thrombus restore continuity to the circulation; these non-com-
municating vessels are part of the process of revascularization, as
distinct from recanalization.

G.C. McMillan: This question concerns a slide shown by Dr.
Schwartz on the incidence of pulmonary embolism. As you know, there
have been remarkable decreases in the death rates from coronary
heart disease and stroke in the U.S.A. SInce 1970, these decreases
(all ages) have amounted to about 15% for CHD and about 19% for
stroke up to 1976. When the data are displayed by decade of age at
death, the decreases between 1963 and 1976 are roughly about 25%
in CHD death rates at ages under 65 years and roughly about 30%
for stroke death rates in each age decade under 75 years.

Are there equivalent data relating to pulmonary embolism or
other thrombotic phenomena?

S. Wessler: Unlike the recently observed decrease in cardiac
and cerebral deaths in the U.S. to which you referred, there has
been no evidence of any decrease in the incidence of pulmonary embolism at autopsy over this same time span.

R.W. Wissler: Dr. Mustard, I am interested in the models
which you have called attention to in which lipid-containing plaques
with some features of atherosclerosis have been produced by sustained severe intimal injury, either by indwelling catheters or
immunological mechanisms. But I think we have to be very cautious

in assuming this is a common mechanism in human atherogenesis --
it may be in patients with lupus erythematosus or hemocytonemia,
but epidemiologically at least we know that there are many human
populations with chronic or repeated endothelial damage from
cigarette smoking or from hypertension that show virtually no
clinical or pathological evidence or progressive atherosclerosis.
The big question (which may be very difficult to answer) is how
much of the atherosclerosis we see in people has a significant
endothelial injury component.

J.F. Mustard: Dr. Wissler may have misunderstood my point
and what I see as the relationship among serum LDL levels, endothelial injury, and atherosclerosis. Epidemiological studies are
heavily influenced by genetic as well as environmental factors.
Therefore, there may well be people upon whom cigarette smoking
does not have a major effect on endothelial injury. We know that
not all smokers get lung cancer and recent evidence suggests that
genetic factors may influence susceptibility.

Hypertension may only damage the endothelium when there are
sharp changes in blood pressure.

The evidence indicates, in my opinion, that injury to the
endothelium is a major factor in causing atherosclerotic lesions.
Since elevated serum lipids can damage the endothelium, it is impossible to dissociate the serum lipid and endothelial injury aspects of atherosclerosis. There seems little point in promoting
separate hypotheses for atherosclerosis at this state.

R.W. Wissler: I agree that these two fields of endeavor and
investigation are getting closer together as Dr. McMillan indicated
in his introductory presentation. I simply wanted to inject a word
of caution as to how we interpret the "chronic intimal injury -
hypocholesterolemic" atherogenesis. I thought you were too enthu-
siastic in your emphasis on these exceptions to the hypercholesterolemic association with atherogenesis. I find them very helpful
to explain the paradoxical or exceptional cases as I said in my
opening talk.

D.N. Fass: Dr. Mustard, is there evidence, in your balloon
denuded vessels, that there is platelet:platelet interaction on
the surface and that there is thrombin generation and fibrin deposition on the denuded vessel?

Does the increase in platelet adhesion seen in the indomethacin
treated vessel, result from platelet:wall or platelet:platelet
interaction? Are the 20,000/mm platelets a saturation density?
Then, the indomethacin may be interpreted as increasing the rate
of adhesion, is that not so?

J.F. Mustard: There is no morphological evidence in our rabbit experiments for fibrin disposition. This suggests that there
is not much fibrin information.

The increased platelet adherence seen when the vessel wall is
trapped with non-steroidal anti-inflammatory drugs like aspirin and
indomethacin is due to increased surface area coverage because the
tests are carried out before the surface is saturated. Therefore,
it could be increasing this rate of adhesion.

J.C. Lewis: Dr. Mustard, a report has recently been published
by Dr. Mason's group which suggests that plasma lipoproteins are
one of the factors responsible for modulation of platelet adhesion
to artificial surfaces. Although Dr. Mason's experiments were done
under in vitro conditions, the demonstration that lipoproteins may
be involved in regulation of platelet to surface interaction is
important. Could you comment on the implications these in vitro
studies have with respect to the response of platelets to subendothelial elements.

J.F. Mustard: Your question about the effect of lipoproteins
on platelet adherence to surfaces is important. One could broaden
the question to include all plasma proteins. We do know that albumin decreases platelet adhesion to the subendothelium. It could be
that lipoproteins will modify the adherence of platelets to the
subendothelium but I do not think anyone has tested it.

H.C. McGill, Jr.: Dr. Woolf, is it possible to examine large
numbers of human arteries from persons 20 to 40 years for fibrin
and platelets? We would like to know how often thrombotic material
is involved in the genesis of lesions in this age range, which is
the period of most active progression of fibrous plaques.

N. Woolf: It is, of course, theoretically quite possible to
do this. However, in the autopsy population available to me for
study, the number of patients in this age group has been too small
to allow adequate data to be collected.

A. Nordøy: Dr. Woolf, could you say something more about the
specificity of your platelet antibodies? You have stated that
they do not react with human fibrin/fibrinogen. How about the
reactivity to lipoproteins or smooth muscle cells?

N. Woolf: The anti-platelet sera, which are absorbed with red
cells and human kidney homogenates before use, do not cross react
with either lipoproteins or smooth muscle cells.

R.W. Wissler: Dr. Schwartz, I wonder if you can explain for
me the difference, if any, between the plaques that result from

experimental thrombotic emboli that organize and the usual plaque
that results from atherogenic stimuli, whatever they are, in human
subjects. I seem to remember some rather large differences being
reported between the lipid chemistry of the organized emboli and
regular plaques.

C.J. Schwartz: There is little doubt that the organization
of experimental thrombi may result in complex fibro-fatty plaques
with many of the histological characteristics of human lesions.
Dr. Craig and I studied the detailed lipid composition of such
lesions in the pulmonary arteries of the pig and found that although there was a significant increase in cholesterol esters with
time, the overall lipid profile did not evolve towards that characteristic of the human lesion, a difference that may be species
dependent. In other words, this model does not completely repro-
duce all the features of human atheroma; nevertheless, it does
establish that the organization of thrombotic material can
result in lesions morphologically similar to the lesions of man.

J.P. Strong: Dr. Woolf and Dr. Schwartz, how often do you
find large masses of fibrin and platelets in the intima of young
persons under age 40 using the most modern techniques? In the
International Atherosclerosis Project material, Geer, Robertson,
McGill and I examined over 500 coronaries of individuals 10-39
years of age using standard histologic techniques and found such
changes in only a few cases.

N. Woolf: While it is clear from a variety of experimental
studies that mural thrombi can cause lesions morphologically
resembling atherosclerotic plaques, the data which I presented
today cannot be evaluated from this standpoint. They do, however, indicate that incorporation of mural thrombi occurs frequently in relation to aortic atherosclerotic plaques (approximately 45% of such plaques) and that this process represents a
significant contribution to the latter stages of the natural
history of atherosclerosis.

C.J. Schwartz: I have the distinct impression that histological evidence of the constituents of residual thrombus in
atheromatous plaques is most prominent in older subjects. Thrombosis contributes to plaque growth, but this contribution appears
to occur later rather than earlier in plaque pathogenesis. Dr.
Woolf has already demonstrated both platelet and fibrin material
in a wide range of lesions, and has commented on the capricious
nature of fibrin-staining. I would appreciate hearing from Dr.
Chandler who also has studied the frequency of thrombi in the
arteries of young people; perhaps he would care to comment.

A.B. Chandler: In response to Dr. Strong, thrombi undergoing organization have not been frequently observed in younger age groups. However, the question is, in fact, quite unanswered because so few studies directed at this problem in this age group have been undertaken. In a recent survey of the reported frequency of incorporated thrombi found in atherosclerotic lesions, most studies were of cases 40 years of age or older.* In one autopsy study of serial sections at a specified site in the left coronary artery from subjects 12-30 years of age, incorporated microthrombi were found in a few instances, all in subjects 25 years or older and all on established plaques. Considerably more work is needed to determine at what age and at what stage in plaque formation, thrombi begin to contribute to plaque growth, and if variances in the population exist.

---

*Chandler, A.B., and Pope, J.T. (1975) In Blood and Arterial Wall in Atherogenesis and Arterial Thrombosis (Hautvast, J.G.A.J., Hermus, R.J.J. and VanDerHaar, F. Eds.), E.J. Brill, Leiden, Netherlands, pp. 110-118.

FIRST WORKSHOP SESSION
INTERACTION OF PLATELETS AND
COAGULATION WITH THE ARTERIAL WALL

Harvey Wolinsky, *Session Chairman*
Departments of Medicine and Pathology
Albert Einstein College of Medicine
Bronx, New York

WORKSHOP 1a: ENDOTHELIUM

Ralph L. Nachman, Moderator
Participants: M.A. Gimbrone, Jr., E.A. Jaffe,
C.R. Minick, F.A. Pitlick, B.B. Weksler

WORKSHOP 1b: SMOOTH MUSCLE

Wilbur A. Thomas, Moderator
Participants: T.P. Bersot, M.J. Karnovsky,
S. Moore, J.F. Mustard

SUMMARY OF WORKSHOP a: ENDOTHELIUM

R.L. Nachman

Department of Medicine
Division of Hematology-Oncology
The New York Hospital-Cornell Medical Center
New York, New York

The endothelial cell activity modulates the response of the
blood vessel wall to physiologic and pathophysiologic stimuli.
The biosynthetic properties of endothelial cells are important
determinants of normal vessel physiology. Recent advances in the
study of cultured endothelial cells have shed new light on the
active role of endothelial cells in normal hemostasis. It is
probable that alterations in endothelial cell function significantly contribute to atherosclerotic processes.

ENDOTHELIAL CELLS AND HEMOSTASIS

E.A. Jaffe

Cultured human endothelial cells synthesize and secrete a pro-
tein(s) which has Factor VIII antigen, but which lacks Factor VIII
clot-promoting activity (1). The Factor VIII antigen synthesized
by cultured endothelial cells was found to contain the same polypeptide subunit (molecular weight, 200,000) present in plasma
Factor VIII antigen (2). Von Willebrand factor activity has been
identified in medium from cultured human endothelial cells. This
activity was demonstrated by the ability to correct the defect in
platelet adhesiveness of blood obtained from patients with von
Willebrand's disease. This activity also supported ristocetin-
induced aggregation of washed normal human platelets. The von
Willebrand factor activity from cultured endothelial cells has phy-
sicochemical and immunologic properties like those of the von
Willebrand factor activity and the Factor VIII antigen present in
human plasma and the Factor VIII antigen synthesized by human endothelial cells _in vitro._ Rabbit antibody to chromatographic frac-

tions containing endothelial cell von Willebrand factor inhibits
the platelet retention of normal blood in glass bead columns (3).

Subcellular membrane and granule fractions derived from human
platelets also contain Factor VIII antigen and von Willebrand factor
activity but not Factor VIII procoagulant activity. Circulating
platelets constitute a significant reservoir of plasma Factor VIII
antigen, containing approximately 15% of the amount of Factor VIII
antigen present in platelet poor plasma. Thus, normal platelets contain surface bound as well as internally stored von Willebrand factor, a protein synthesized by endothelial cells which is necessary
for normal platelet function in vivo. These studies suggest that
endothelial cells play an important role in the surface-oriented
modulation of hemostatic events.

Further studies were performed to determine if cultured human
endothelial cells synthesized basement membrane collagen. In culture, endothelial cells were attached to grossly visible membranous
structures which on light microscopy were composed of ribbons of
dense, amorphous material. On transmission electron microscopy,
these membranous structures consisted of amorphous basement membrane
and material morphologically similar to microfibrils and elastic
fibers. By immunofluorescence microscopy, these membranous structures stained brightly with antisera to human glomerular basement
membrane. Cultured endothelial cells incorporated [^{3}H] proline into
protein; 18% of the incorporated [^{3}H] proline was solubilized by
purified collagenase. When endothelial cells were cultured with
[^{14}C] proline, 7.1% of the incorporated counts were present as [^{14}C]
hydroxyproline. Cultured endothelial cells were labeled with [^{3}H]
glycine and [^{3}H] proline and digested with pepsin. The resulting
fractions on analysis by SDS-polyacrylamide gel electrophoresis contained two radioactive protein peaks of molecular weights 94,200 and
120,500. Both these peaks disappeared after digestion with purified
collagenase. Thus, cultured human endothelial cells synthesize material which is morphologically and immunologically like amorphous
basement membrane and biochemically like basement membrane collagen
(4). In addition, it has been recently demonstrated that endothelial
cells also synthesize fibronectin (cold insoluble globulin) which is
also a component of the subendothelium.

ENDOTHELIAL CELL MODULATION OF PLATELET FUNCTION

B.B. Weksler

Cultured endothelial cells derived from human umbilical veins
or bovine aorta produce a potent inhibitor of platelet aggregation.
The inhibitor, which is ether-extractable, is synthesized from sodium arachidonate or prostaglandin (PG) endoperoxides by a micro-

somal enzyme system. Tranylcypromine, a specific antagonist of prostacyclin synthetase, suppressed production of the inhibitor by endothelial cells. The inhibitor has been identified using a two step thin-layer radiochromatographic procedure and a synthetic PGI_2 standard. With this procedure, it has been shown that human and bovine endothelial cells convert $[^3H]$ sodium arachidonate to radio-labeled PGI_2 and 6-keto-PGI_{1_α}, as well as PGE_2 (5).

The ability of endothelial cells to synthesize PGI_2 suggests that PGI_2 may be the agent which normally prevents platelets from adhering to intact endothelium. Thus, a balance may exist between the effects of endoperoxide-thromboxane A_2 (produced by platelets in response to vascular damage) and PGI_2. The prostaglandin endo-peroxides may therefore serve as pivotal substrates since they can be converted by platelets or by endothelial cells into products with opposing actions. Damage to or loss of endothelial cells in a local area promotes thrombosis both by exposing subendothelium and by abating PGI_2 production. In turn, the adhesion of platelets to the subendothelium leads to their degranulation and subsequent release of smooth muscle cell growth stimulating factors and per-meability enhancing factors. This process, repeated over time, might result in atherosclerosis. It is likely that the prevention of these phenomena is dependent upon the normal synthesis and released of PGI_2 by endothelial cells.

ENDOTHELIUM AND TISSUE FACTOR

F.A. Pitlick

Effective hemostasis represents a delicate balance between blood coagulation, platelet aggregation and blood flow; if this balance is upset, thrombosis will result. A cell culture model of the various types of cells found in the vessel wall allows in vitro comparative studies of the possible contributions of each cell type to effective hemostasis. Studies of the initiation of coagulation by tissue factor (thromboplastin), have revealed that the amount of coagulant activity in cultured cells is regulated by four para-meters; cell integrity, cell age, cell type and response to phar-macologic agents (6, 7).

In all cell types studied, the undisturbed monolayer or cell suspension has minimal tissue factor activity. Trypsin digestion first releases the cell surface coat, then tissue factor, leaving the cell intact and ready for subculture.

The expressed activity of disrupted cells is also related to cell type hours after subculture. In endothelial cells, activity increases and reaches a peak at 5 hours after transfer (400 units/

10^5 cells), then returns to basal level. Fibroblast tissue factor activity starts at a higher basal level after subculture, increases 5 to 10 fold 12 hours after transfer (3000 to 1200 units/10^5 cells), then declines. Smooth muscle cells show a lag in reaching peak activity (30 hours or more), but may remain at a sustained high level (2000 to 30,000 units/10^5 cells). Thus, each cell type can be distinguished by the kinetics of tissue factor production after subculture and by the amount of activity each cell type generates.

Tissue factor production in each cell type exhibits distinctive responses to a variety of pharmacologic reagents. Butyrate inhibits while chloroquine enhances generation of activity in endothelial cells; in fibroblasts, both butyrate and chloroquine were stimulatory. Colchicine has little effect on endothelial cells, but depresses production in fibroblasts and smooth muscle cells.

Each cell type was also studied as a monolayer culture for interaction with ^{14}C-serotonin labeled platelet rich plasma and for hydrolysis of exogenous ADP. Endothelial cells did not provoke the platelet release reaction and had the highest rate of ADP hydrolysis at low ADP concentrations; the obverse was found for smooth muscle cells. It is possible that endothelium may be nonthrombogenic in part due to an active mechanism which removes ADP. With injury to the vessel wall, endothelial cells have low, but real, hemostatic potential. Smooth muscle cells, due to their intrinsic activities and greater numbers, are an important site for thrombosis and hemostasis.

ENDOTHELIAL CELL METABOLISM OF VASOACTIVE SUBSTANCES

M.A. Gimbrone, Jr.

In addition to functioning as a selective permeability barrier and nonthrombogenic lining for the vascular system, there is increasing evidence that endothelium actively participates in the metabolism of vasoactive substances. Endothelial cultures have proved especially useful for identifying metabolic products and characterizing the enzymatic activities involved. Cultured human endothelial cells contain an indomethacin-sensitive prostaglandin synthetase system capable of generating E-type prostaglandins, which are known to influence vascular tone and permeability, as well as the function of leukocytes and platelets (8, 9, 10). PGE production is stimulated by polypeptide hormones such as angiotensin II, perhaps through a receptor-coupled mechanism. Cultured human endothelial cells also contain a carboxyterminal dipeptidase which generates biologically active angiotensin II (octapeptide) from angiotensin I (decapeptide), and inactivates bradykinin. In

its molecular weight, cofactor requirements and inhibitor sensitivity, this enzyme resembles human and plasma angiotensin I converting enzymes. Further study of these metabolic capabilities may
help unravel the interrelationships of complex disease processes,
such as hypertension and atherosclerosis, and the role of vascular
endothelium in their pathogeneses.

ENDOTHELIAL CELL REGENERATION, INTIMAL
THICKENING AND LIPID ACCUMULATION

C.R. Minick

Experiments were performed to test the hypothesis that absence
of endothelium favors intimal thickening, lipid accumulation and
atherosclerosis. Rabbit aortas were de-endothelialized with a balloon catheter at day 0. Initially, all rabbits were fed a diet low
in lipid. Some rabbits, group I, were continued on a diet low in
lipid for 8-40 weeks after de-endothelialization. Beginning 4-16
weeks after de-endothelialization, other rabbits were fed cholesterol supplemented diets, group II, or semisynthetic lipid-rich
diets, group III, for from 4-16 weeks. In aortas of groups I, II,
and III the degree of intimal thickening was always significantly
greater in re-endothelialized areas. Intimal thickness was enhanced
in re-endothelialized areas of hypercholesterolemic rabbits of
group II but not in areas lacking endothelium. Fatty change in all
groups was significantly greater in thickened intima covered by
regenerated endothelium than in adjacent intima lacking an endothelial lining (11). There was also histochemical evidence of increased quantities of proteoglycan in re-endothelialized areas as
compared to adjacent areas lacking endothelium. Thus, results of
these experiments do not support the hypothesis that the absence
of endothelium particularly favors intimal thickening and intimal
lipid accumulation. Results indicate that intima covered by regenerated endothelium is significantly thicker and more likely to
accumulate lipid. Increased lipid accumulation in re-endothelialized areas may result from increased quantities of proteoglycan,
since low density lipoproteins have been shown to bind to proteoglycans.

REFERENCES

1. Jaffe, E.A., Hoyer, L.W., and Nachman, R.L. (1973)
   J. Clin. Invest. 51, 2757-2764.

2. Jaffe, E.A., and Nachman, R.L. (1975) J. Clin. Invest. 56,
   698-702.

3. Jaffe, E.A., Hoyer, L.W., and Nachman, R.L. (1974) Proc.
   Natl. Acad. Sci. USA 71, 1906-1909.

4. Jaffe, E.A., Minick, C.R., Adelman, B., Becker, C.G., and
   Nachman, R. (1976) J. Exp. Med. 144, 209-225.

5. Weksler, B.B., Marcus, A.J., and Jaffe, E.A. (1977) Proc.
   Natl. Acad. Sci. USA 74, 3922-3926.

6. Maynard, J.R., Dreyer, B.C., Stemerman, M.B., and Pitlick,
   F.A. (1977) Blood 50, 387-396.

7. Glasgow, J.E., and Pitlick, F.A. (1977) Fed. Proc. 36,
   1082. Abstract.

8. Gimbrone, M.A., Jr. (1976) In Progress in Hemostasis and
   Thrombosis. Vol. 3. (Spaet, T., Ed.) Grune & Stratton,
   New York, pp. 1-28.

9. Gimbrone, M.A., Jr., and Alexander, R.W. (1977) In Proc. of
   the International Symposium on Prostaglandins in Hematology.
   (Silver, M.J., Ed.), Spectron Publications, New York, pp.
   121-134.

10. Gimbrone, M.A., Jr. (1977) In International Cell Biology
    1976-77. (Brinkley, B.R. and Porter, K.R., Eds.), The
    Rockefeller University Press, New York, pp. 649-658.

11. Minick, C.R., Stemerman, M.B., and Insull, W., Jr. (1977)
    Proc. Natl. Acad. Sci. USA 74, 1724-1728.

DISCUSSION FOLLOWING WORKSHOP 1a: ENDOTHELIUM

K.M. Brinkhous: My comments relate to the impressive data
presented by Dr. Weksler in which she provides definitive evidence
that the previously known endothelial platelet inhibitor is indeed
prostacyclin. All of us are impressed with the rapidity with
which the nature of this inhibitor has been elucidated. My comments are twofold: 1) The first relates to the continuing work
of R.A. Johnson and his colleagues who originally described the
structure of prostacyclin (Prostaglandins 12, 915, 1976). This
group now has dozens of analogues of this compound, so that a
series of probes are potentially available for further study of
this specific inhibitor of platelet function. 2) Historically,
in 1974, a platelet inhibitor of endothelial origin was reported
by Saba and Mason (Thromb. Res. 5, 747) and partially characterized. This work was well known and the lack of reference to
it in Vane's 1976 articles led many people to assume that prostacyclin was possibly of some cellular origin other than endothelium,
since they used whole vessel wall as the source of tissue. Dr.
Weksler's paper nicely puts this development of knowledge in perspective and removes any doubts about the important role of endothelium in this regard.

G. Hornstra: Dr. Weksler, although PGI_2 is known to be extremely potent as an inhibitor of primary ADP-induced aggregation,
you showed the ADP (and collagen) induced aggregation to be rather
resistant to the aggregation inhibiting effect of endothelium.
Have you any idea as to the explanation of this apparent discre-
pancy?

In general, we were surprised to find that rat smooth muscle
cells in culture are perfectly capable of converting PGH_2 into
prostacyclin. On the basis of the amount of protein incubated,
they are at least as effective as rat (and human) endothelial cells.
Maybe there is a species specific effect. Did anybody perform
comparable experiments with human smooth muscle cells?

B.B. Weksler: Yes, there is a straightforward explanation
for the apparent differences in inhibition of platelet function.

I showed inhibition of platelet aggregation and serotonin release responses to threshold doses of aggregating agents, following platelet exposure to a concentration of endothelial cells which completely inhibited platelet response to arachidonate. Since arachidonate acts as a substrate for PGI_2 production by endothelial cells as well as a platelet aggregant, more PGI_2 was synthesized in the arachidonate stimulated system than in incubations in which other aggregating agents were used. In addition, the threshold concentration of each aggregating agent was that which produced full, irreversible aggregation. In the case of ADP and collagen-induced aggregation, the amount of PGI_2 produced in the presence of endothelial cells sufficed to inhibit secondary phase ADP aggregation and to diminish markedly collagen aggregation. If we were to use a weaker ADP or collagen stimulus, for example, a concentration producing only reversible primary aggregation, the same exposure to endothelial cells would completely inhibit the platelet response. As with other agents which raise platelet cyclic AMP levels, PGI_2 shows a dose-related inhibition of platelet function partly dependent on the strength of the opposing aggregatory stimulus.

We have found recently that human smooth muscle cells and fibroblasts (as monolayers or gently detached from tissue culture dishes with collagenase of low concentrations of trypsin) do produce prostacyclin when stimulated with arachidonic acid. Baenziger, Dillender and Majerus (Biochem. & Biophys. Res. Com. 78(1), 294, 1977) have recently published their findings that human fibroblasts and human arterial cells produce prostacyclin when injured, and Moncada has also suggested that arterial media is capable of prostacyclin production. Therefore, different layers of the vessel wall do seem capable of synthesizing PGI_2.

J.F. Mustard: I would like to briefly review some indirect evidence that supports Dr. Weksler's comments that unstimulated endothelial cells produce very little, if any, PGI_2. We have found, in an in vitro test system for studying platelet adherence to the vessel wall, that treatment of a normal vessel wall with aspirin or Indomethacin does not cause platelet adherence to the normal endothelium. Treatment of platelets, and treatment of the platelets and the vessel wall with these drugs, also does not cause adherence to normal endothelium. These drug treatments would be expected to inhibit PGI_2 production by the vessel wall. Thus, if PGI_2 is the factor which prevents platelet adherence to the normal endothelium lining, one would expect platelets to adhere to the endothelium when there is no PGI_2 available. This indirect evidence suggests that PGI_2 formation by the endothelium is not necessary to prevent normal platelets from adhering to normal endothelium.

B.B. Weksler: Our examination of the medium overlying resting monolayers of endothelial cells, or suspensions of endothelial cells following removal from tissue culture dishes strongly suggests that PGI_2 is not present in the medium in the absence of stimulation of the endothelial cells and thus supports your results in a platelet-vessel wall adherence system. Since injury results in PGI_2 synthesis, handling of the cells may initiate PGI_2 production and make a continuous synthesis appear to occur. However, since we are measuring PGI_2 by bioassays which do not measure the concentration of biologically inactive 6-keto PGF_{1a}, the main product of PGI_2, the possibility of a very low level production of the latter with rapid conversion in warm aqueous medium to the inactive derivative, cannot be excluded. This question will be directly resolved by radioimmunoassay or possibly by radiochromatography following labeling of endogenous substrate, such as arachidonic acid.

H.C. McGill, Jr.: We see different endothelial configurations in different organs -- for example, in the renal glomerulus, the liver, and so forth. Do we know whether the endothelium of the large muscular and elastic arteries has responses and functions similar to those of capillaries, veins, and arterioles? The answer would be important in determining the role of endothelium in the pathogenesis of atherosclerosis, which only affects these larger arteries.

M.A. Gimbrone, Jr.: This is an important area which deserves further study. Certain functional attributes of vascular endothelium, e.g., its blood compatability, are probably similar throughout the circulatory system. However, specialization and regional differences do appear to exist, in vivo, with respect to permeability to macromolecules, the response to inflammatory mediators, and the transit of blood cells. The in vitro study of biochemical functions thus far has been limited, for technical reasons (accessibility and ease of isolation), to large vessel endothelium. The next important task in the culture area will be the selective cultivation of specific endothelial cell populations for comparative functional studies.

G.C. McMillan: The question relates to the suggested role of proteoglycans in lipid accumulation in Dr. Minick's experiments. Is there coincidence in the location of stainable lipid and of stainable proteoglycans in the regenerated areas around the ostia of intercostal vessels?

C.R. Minick: Generally, there is a good correlation between the location of alcianophilic material in the arterial wall of both blue and non-blue areas, and the deposition of lipid.

M.J. Karnovsky: In support of Dr. Minick's findings we (A. Clowes and I) have found that exogenous tracers, such as peroxidase penetrate both the de-endothelialized and re-endothelialized areas, but the tracer persists in the latter, and diffuses away through the wall in the former case. This suggests possibly a binding of the tracer in the re-endothelialized areas.

K.T. Lee: Dr. Minick, have you studied ballooned rabbit aortas after regenerating endothelium has covered most of the denuded surface? If so, what happens to the lipid deposition which had been limited to the area near the vessel orifice, and what type of atherosclerotic lesions do you find? I still have a vague feeling that the lipid accumulation you observed in the area covered by the regenerating endothelial cells has something to do with the intimal cushions near the orifices of branches.

C.R. Minick: Following longer intervals after balloon injury, the accentuated intimal thickening and lipid accumulation occupies all of the re-endothelialized area. Moreover, similar findings are found at the junction between the normal and ballooned aorta and in the iliac arteries. These latter areas are at some distance from branch sites. Finally, the thickened re-endothelialized intima is often at some distance from branch sites and does not have the morphologic features of cushion areas.

A.L. Robertson, Jr: I would like to propose an explanation for Dr. Minick's very interesting observations on intimal thickening and lipid accumulation occurring under regenerating endothelium rather than beneath de-endothelialized areas.

In collaboration with Dr. Eugene L. Hirsch, we have been studying for the last two years a new model of endothelial injury and repair. Briefly, the method induces a predictable 2-3 mm wide longitudinal tract that, in contrast to balloon de-endothelialization, repairs very rapidly (approximately 96 hours) providing at the same time large areas of undisturbed endothelium in the same vascular segment.

In this model, ultrastructural evaluation shows that as repair takes place, proliferation and migration of endothelial cells results in an advancing line containing "plump" endothelial cells with considerable accumulation of extracellular material beneath the healing edge. I would like to suggest that in a similar fashion, regenerating endothelial cells following balloon injury allow extracellular entrapment of macromolecules, including lipoproteins, while areas still de-endothelized induce continuing removal and rapid turnover rates of blood components and cellular debris.

SUMMARY OF WORKSHOP 1b: SMOOTH MUSCLE

W.A. Thomas

Department of Pathology
Albany Medical College of Union University
Albany, New York

Atherogenesis is characterized in part by excessive proliferation of arterial intimal smooth muscle cells (SMC). Arterial SMC
proliferation can be produced by acute or chronic intimal trauma in
normo-lipidemic (NL) animals, especially if the endothelial cells
(EC) are denuded as with a balloon catheter. Also, intimal SMC
proliferation can be produced by making animals hyperlipidemic (HL)
by dietary manipulation without trauma to the EC.

The SMC proliferation feature could be a simple reaction to
injury with locally-produced mitogens involved only incidentally
in their physiologic role in the process or it could be caused
directly by mitogens from the blood stream (? platelets, ? lipoproteins, ? other) that enter the arterial wall through damage
points elsewhere and interact with the arterial SMC. It is also
quite possible that both of these mechanisms are involved.

Aspects of all of the above were discussed under five sections
in this workshop:

POPULATION DYNAMICS OF ARTERIAL SMC IN HL AND NL SWINE
WITH AND WITHOUT BALLOON CATHETER DENUDATION OF EC

W.A. Thomas

A modest increase (circa 50%) in mitotic (1) and tritiated
thymidine (^{3}HTdR) labeling indices of arterial SMC throughout the
arterial wall can be produced within 3 days after beginning an HL

diet. When overt intimal lesions appear 30-60 days later, the increase in ^{3}HTdR labeling induced in their SMC is 5-10-fold. Both
increases appear to be accompanied by increased deaths among arterial EC and SMC (2). Thus, the increased proliferative activity
could be a direct response to injury. It could also result at
least in part from interaction with a mitogen (LDL, platelet or
other) that enters the arterial wall at the sites of EC injury.
The initial modest response (3 days) occurs before there is any
demonstrable increase in lipids as determined by EM and biochemical
techniques. The greater response seen in overt lesions in HL
swine is virtually always accompanied by an increase in lipids in
the lesion tissue. Evidence derived from the "dilution of isotopic
label by division" technique was presented suggesting that the
overt atherosclerotic lesions in the HL swine arose from multiple
SMC; hence, these lesions are not monoclonal in origin (3).

When the aortas of NL swine are subjected to balloon-EC-denudation, SMC proliferative response occurs which is many-fold
greater than that seen in NL animals without trauma. This begins
shortly after the trauma and persists for about one month. After
that, it slowly disappears until activity has returned to normal
within a few months. If the ballooning procedure is accompanied
by an HL diet, increased proliferative activity persists for as
long as the HL diet is continued and the resulting lesions are
many times larger than with either procedure alone. Data from
studies of human populations (rural East Africans and Koreans)
with serum cholesterol levels below 150 mg/dl were also discussed,
suggesting that atherosclerotic lesions in such individuals almost
never reached a size that resulted in clinical complications such
as myocardial infarcts. Thomas concluded that though mitogens in
NL blood such as those associated with platelets may be factors in
atherogenesis, it is generally necessary to have hyperlipidemia
(with serum cholesterol levels at least in excess of 150 mg/dl) to
produce clinically significant lesions. An exception in regard
to experimental animals was presented later in this workshop by
Sean Moore indicating that chronic injury produced by an indwelling intra-aortic catheter could produce very large lesions in NL
rabbits.

Another question not resolved in this workshop was whether
or not NL blood could result in SMC proliferation in thrombocytopenic animals; in other words, is a substantial amount of platelet
mitogen required for proliferation. This question was at least
partly answered by Friedman in a later workshop. Rabbits made HL
and thrombocytopenic (less than 7000/mm^3) and then subjected to
balloon-EC-denudation had a marked SMC proliferative response,
whereas NL thrombocytopenic rabbits had essentially no SMC proliferative response after ballooning.

ROLE OF PLATELETS IN STIMULATING PROLIFERATION
AND MIGRATION OF ARTERIAL SMC

J.F. Mustard

There is good evidence from the in vitro studies of R. Ross
and co-workers (4) that for smooth muscle cells to grow in tissue
culture there is need for a factor released from platelets when
blood clots. This mitogen which has been partially purified has
a molecular weight of around 13,000 with another fragment present
of around 23,000. It causes both smooth muscle cell migration and
smooth muscle cell proliferation. The importance of platelets in
SMC proliferation in vivo following endothelial injury comes from
several lines of evidence.

First, if rabbits are made thrombocytopenic and an indwelling
cannula is left in the aorta, the animals will not develop significant atherosclerotic lesions, although they are readily produced
in animals with a normal platelet count.

Second, if rabbits are exposed to a single balloon catheter
injury to the aorta, they will develop arterial SMC proliferation
with intimal thickening within two weeks. If, however, the animals
are made thrombocytopenic before the balloon injury, the rabbits
do not develop proliferative lesions (5). Further, in the monkey,
Ross and Harker (6) have found that homocystine damages the endothelium, resulting in shortened platelet survival and the formation of smooth muscle cell intimal lesions containing lipid. If
the animals are treated with dipyridamole, the shortened platelet
survival is prevented and the proliferative lesions in the intima
are significantly inhibited. They have proposed that this drug
prevents platelet adherence to the damaged wall which, therefore,
minimizes the release of the platelet mitogen at the injury site.

Factors governing platelet adherence to the damaged vessel
wall and the release of the platelet mitogen are of some importance in understanding this reponse. The principal constituent in
the subendothelium with which platelets interact is collagen. The
platelets which adhere to the collagen release their constituents
including the mitogens. Therefore, factors which inhibit adherence
and release could be expected to inhibit the effect of the platelet
mitogen on the vessel wall. Anti-platelet-aggregators, such as
aspirin, do not inhibit platelet adhesion to the subendothelium
or to collagen. Furthermore, aspirin does not inhibit the release
reaction of platelets that are adherent to collagen. It is,
therefore, not surprising that aspirin fails to inhibit SMC proliferation following endothelial injury. Sulfinpyrazone also fails
to prevent platelet adherence to collagen and the release reaction
and does not prevent SMD proliferation following EC injury.

Following a single injury to endothelium in the rabbit, a
monolayer of platelets forms which disappears during the next 4 to
5 days. Few platelets interact with the wall once the initial
monolayer forms. Thus, there is not much turnover of rabbit
platelets in the damaged vessel wall. This means that the initial
platelet interaction is probably the most important as far as the
mitogenic effect is concerned. Furthermore, endothelial injury
in the rabbit does not shorten platelet survival. In contrast,
endothelial injury in the monkey does. This is probably due to
thrombus formation with fibrin trapping the platelets and causing
their loss from the circulation.

EFFECT OF CHRONIC INJURY TO THE ARTERIAL WALL
ON BEHAVIOR OF ARTERIAL SMC IN NL ANIMALS

S. Moore

Continual or repeated arterial wall injury in NL rabbits causes
raised lipid-containing lesions, fatty streaks and non-lipid containing fibromusculo-elastic plaques (7, 8). These lesions are
observed either with continued arterial injury caused by an indwelling polyethylene catheter or repeated immunological injury induced
by four injections at one-week intervals or human serum which is
cytotoxic to rabbit lymphocytes. During regression of raised,
lipid containing lesions after removal of the chronic injury stimulus, lesions typical of human fatty streaks occur and rapidly
disappear. Eventually only non-lipid containing streaks remain.

Repeated endothelial injury caused by balloon catheter denudation of the aortic endothelium of NL rabbits causes lesions resembling human fibrous plaques containing intracellular and peri-
fibrous lipid, with in some instances a central lipid pool. In
animals ballooned six times at two week intervals, lipid occurs
preferentially in areas that become covered by regenerating endothelium, and in animals examined six months and one year following
the last ballooning, lipid occurs exclusively in EC covered areas
around branch vessels.

Development of lesions can be inhibited by making the animals
thrombocytopenic either with anti-platelet serum or a combination
of anti-platelet drugs and anti-platelet serum.

The fact that lipid occurs in response to repeated endothelial injury in areas where endothelium has regenerated indicates
that the concept of the barrier function of the endothelium may
need modification. After a single ballooning, the raw surface is

covered by a monolayer of platelets. As shown by Stemerman, a later ballooning exposes the blood to collagen formed in the neo-intima and a thrombus including fibrin is laid down. Presumably, this process is repeated with subsequent removals of the endothelium with the balloon. The changes thus induced in the neo-intima apparently favor the deposition of lipid. Proteoglycans formed in this tissue may act to bind lipoproteins. That this does not happen in the areas where endothelial regeneration fails to occur is probably explained by recent experiments showing that such a surface rapidly becomes inert to further deposition of platelets and no thrombus forms.

FACTORS CAUSING INHIBITION OF ARTERIAL SMC PROLIFERATION FOLLOWING ACUTE INJURY IN NL RATS

M.J. Karnovsky

Following endothelial denudation in the carotid artery of rats, produced by air-drying, there is marked intimal SMC proliferation. As the elegant work of Ross and colleagues (4, 6) has invoked the release of a mitogen for smooth muscle from platelets adherent to the denuded surface, it was of interest to see whether drugs affecting platelet behavior had any effects on the degree of smooth muscle proliferation.

Aspirin, reserpine and flurbiprofen were given to rats in doses at which the platelets showed markedly diminished aggregation in response to ADP and thrombin (9). In denuded areas, platelet deposition was unaffected, nor was the degree of SMC proliferation influenced.

Continuous intravenous infusion of heparin, at doses which prolonged clotting times 3-fold or more, had a markedly suppressive effect on myo-intimal thickening. In vitro studies of SMC growth in culture also showed that heparin had a markedly suppressive effect (10). Whether this is due to anticoagulant or non-anticoagulant fractions of heparin is currently under investigation.

Lastly, the response of fawn-hooded rats was assessed. These rats have a form of platelet storage disease. In animals 6 months old, myo-intimal responses were normal, whereas at 10-13 months, SMC proliferation was suppressed. Studies carried out in vitro showed that extracts of platelets from normal rats could stimulate proliferation of normal and fawn-hooded smooth muscle, whereas extracts from fawn-nooded platelets could stimulate neither. However, the growth response of fawn-hooded smooth muscle was always less than that of normal muscle in response to normal serum or

platelet extract. It was concluded that in the old fawn-hooded
rat, the platelets apparently lack a mitogenic factor for smooth
muscle; but the situation is complicated by the age differential
responses, by the inherently weaker growth response of the smooth
muscle, and by the fact that these animals have a progressive
kidney lesion.

INTERACTION OF PLASMA LIPOPROTEINS WITH CULTURED
FIBROBLASTS AND OTHER CELLS

T.P. Bersot

Previous studies have shown that low density lipoprotein (LDL)
and HDL_c, a high density lipoprotein induced by cholesterol feeding to some experimental animals, bind to the high affinity receptor of fibroblasts in tissue culture (11-14). LDL has a single
major apoprotein constituent, apo B, while HDL_c contains the arginine-rich apoprotein (ARP) as its major apoprotein (11). Lipoproteins lacking apo B or ARP cannot bind to the high affinity receptor.

In addition to having this binding specificity, both HDL_c and
LDL inhibit cellular HMG CoA reductase activity and decrease cholesterol accumulation, when cells are incubated with these lipoproteins.

Our studies and those of others demonstrate that HDL_c and LDL
bind to the high affinity lipoprotein receptor of arterial smooth
muscle cells and fibroblasts in culture. This binding is mediated
by apo B in LDL and ARP in HDL_c. Similar primary structures or
charged regions of the apoproteins may account for the ability of
both to bind. Based on studies with cyclohexanedrone, arginine
residues are important in binding by both lipoproteins.

Relationships among the above properties and the ability of
certain lipoproteins to stimulate proliferation of arterial SMC
are not known at the present time.

REFERENCES

1. Florentin, R.A., Nam, S.C., Lee, K.T., Lee, K.J., and Thomas, W.A. (1969) Arch. Path. 88, 463-469.

2. Imai, H., Lee, K.J., Lee, S.K., Pastori, S., and Thomas, W.A. (1970) Virchows Arch. Abt. A. Path. Anat. 350, 183-204.

3. Thomas, W.A., Florentin, R.A., Reiner, J.M., Lee, W.M., and Lee, K.T. (1976) Exp. Molec. Path. 24, 244-260.

4. Ross, R., Glomset, J., Kariya, B., and Harker, L.A. (1974) Proc. Natl. Acad. Sci. USA 71, 1207-1210.

5. Moore, S., Friedman, R.J., Singal, D.P., Gauldie, J., Blajch-man, M.A., and Roberts, R.S. (1976) Thrombos. Haemostas. 35, 70-81.

6. Harker, L.A., Ross, R., Slichter, S.J., and Scott, C.R. (1976) J. Clin. Invest. 58(3), 731-741.

7. Moore, S. (1973) Lab. Invest. 29, 478-487.

8. Friedman, R.J., Moore, S., and Singal, D.P. (1975) Lab. Invest. 30, 404-415.

9. Clowes, A.W., and Karnovsky, M.J. (1977) Lab. Invest. 36, 452.

10. Clowes, A.W., and Karnovsky, M.J. (1977) Nature 265, 625.

11. Bersot, T.P., Mahley, R.W., and Brown, M.S. (1976) J. Biol. Chem. 251(8), 2395-2398.

12. Mahley, R.W., Weisgraber, K.H., and Innerarity, T. (1974) Circ. Res. 35(5), 722-733.

13. Patthy, L., and Smith, E.L. (1975) J. Biol. Chem. 250(2), 565-569.

14. Mahley, R.W., Innerarity, T.L., Weisgraber, K.H., and Fry, D.L. (1977) Am. J. Pathol. 87(1), 205-225.

SUMMARY COMMENTS

H. Wolinsky

Several studies described in these workshops and many others
presented at this conference elegantly demonstrate the rapid progress possible when vascular endothelial or smooth muscle cells
can be isolated purely and subjected to well-controlled stimuli.
The major contributions of the Albany group, the Boston group, the
Cornell group and the Seattle group to the development and estab-
lishment of this methodology as a major research tool in vascular
disease research deserve special mention. However, the first
blushes of success should not distract us completely from address-
ing certain questions. For example, in our zeal to get cells to
grow in these systems, we have largely ignored the vessel site of
origin. Perhaps it is time to see if we can answer the first
question put to this workshop on day 1 - "are there regional variations in cellular properties despite phenotypic similarities?" It
also would be helpful if information about the age and sex of the
animal source from which cultured cells are derived were consistently provided.

Perhaps even more fundamental from the standpoint of future
directions is the need to better define the relevance of results
obtained in tissue culture to in vivo circumstances in health and
disease (1). "In vivo" could include, of course, isolated flow
systems; what is important is that the complexity of the in vivo
state not be lost sight of completely. Do we take a risk of great
disappointment in too-rapid extrapolation from an isolated cellular system excruciatingly defined in vitro but missing many of
its touch points which are present in vivo? These missing factors
include among many others 1) the presence of a distending force,
2) close approximation to another mesenchymal cell type and 3)
exposure to plasma at high concentration for endothelial cells
which has never been frozen or supplemented with penicillin and
streptomycin. Will some of the mechanisms defined in vitro be
swamped by these factors?

Though none of these concerns may ultimately prove to be important, it seems reasonable to urge that attempts be made in
future work to allay them. At the same time, we anxiously wait
to hear reports of further stages of the stimulating advances
described in these workshops.

REFERENCE

1. Fowler, S., Shio, H., and Wolinsky, H. (1977) J. Cell Biol.
    75, 166-184.

DISCUSSION FOLLOWING WORKSHOP 1b: SMOOTH MUSCLE

J.F. Mustard: Dr. Thomas' concern about lipid in lesions produced by repeated endothelial injury is understandable. However,
in addition to the work which has been reported today, there are
some additional observations which suggest that the concept that
repeated injury is important. Bondjers and Bjorkerud have found
that repeated endothelial injury is more important than the level
of plasma cholesterol in determining lipid accumulation in the vessel wall in rabbits. The group working with Dr. Baumgartner showed
that following removal of endothelium in the rabbit, there is initially increased cholesterol accumulation in the wall due to permeability changes and possibly trapping. However, after about 2 weeks
there is no longer lipid accumulation in the wall even though the
endothelium has not regenerated. This may mean that for lipid to
accumulate in the wall, there has to be more than increased permeability and high plasma cholesterol levels. The concepts of Moore
and Minick, that proteoglycan is important for trapping cholesterol
is attractive. Thus, if repeated endothelial injury leads to increased proteoglycan accumulation, one would expect lipid-rich
lesions without the need for elevation of serum cholesterol.

H.J. Weiss: Dr. Mustard, you indicated that when ^{51}Cr platelets were given after balloon injury, fewer platelets adhered to
the subendothelium than if they were given before injury. Do you
think this is because the subendothelium becomes covered with a
layer of platelets that are now "unattractive" for other platelets,
or do the platelets that attach initially become totally removed,
leaving an altered subendothelial surface that is now "unattractive"
for platelets.

J.F. Mustard: In the experiments looking at platelet adhesion to the damaged wall in rabbits, three time periods were looked
at: 1) the percentage of the labeled platelets adhering when the
^{51}Cr labeled platelets are given before the endothelium is removed
with a balloon catheter; 2) the percentage of ^{51}Cr platelets adherent when the labeled platelets are given during the first 12

hours following injury; and 3) the percentage of labeled platelets
adhering when they are given 1 day or longer after balloon injury
to the aorta. About 0.1% of the platelets adhere when the labeled
platelets are in the circulation before removal of the endothelium.
However, in the second period, less than 1/10 of this number of
platelets adhere to the surface. This means that once the platelet monolayer has formed, it becomes a non-reactive surface.
During the third period when the platelets are lost from the surface, there is much less adherence than at the time of injury.
Thus the subendothelium rapidly becomes non-reactive to platelets.

R.J. Friedman: In support of Dr. Mustard, we have recent
evidence supporting the role of the platelet as an initiator of
the smooth muscle cell (SMC) proliferative response. Animals made
thrombocytopenic 1 hour, 3 hours and 1 day post-ballooning develop
SMC intimal thickening equal to that of controls. Animals thrombocytopenic prior to ballooning have marked inhibition of their SMC
proliferative lesions.

T.N. Wight: I would just like to add a comment concerning
the importance and relevance of glycosaminoglycans in atherogenesis
and to support perhaps some of the interpretive comments of Dr.
Moore and Dr. Minick regarding the trapping of lipid by these macromolecules in the arterial wall. We have been investigating the
ability of aortic cells cultured from atherosclerosis susceptible
White Carneau and atherosclerosis resistant Show Racer pigeons to
synthesize and secrete glycosaminoglycans. The data show that
the culture media from the susceptible breed contain 3 to 4 fold
greater amounts of glycosaminoglycans than comparable media from
cultures of the resistant breed. When the types of glycosaminoglycans are analyzed, no differences are found and the major type
is chondroitin sulfate A/C. These findings are interesting in
light of Dr. Kathleen Curwen's recent findings. She has found that
areas predestined and involved in the atherosclerotic process in
the White Carneau pigeon contain significantly more glycosaminoglycans than corresponding sites in the Show Racer and that the
major type present in vivo is chondroitin sulfate C. These studies
indicate the possible importance of glycosaminoglycan metabolism
in atherosclerotic susceptibility.

G.C. McMillan: Earlier today Dr. Karnovsky mentioned that
in balloon de-endothelialization experiments a tracer such as
peroxidase floods and is removed from the denuded area while it
accumulates under the endothelialized areas.

The analogous cholesterol feeding experiments have a continuously elevated lipid environment while I assume the tracer is a
short pulse and the tracer probably does not react with proteoglycans like lipoproteins do. Would Dr. Karnovsky comment further?

M.J. Karnovsky: I do not know the mechanism; the accumulation of tracer may be related to binding to proteoglycans and/or different solvent flux through the two areas.

M. Tiell: As Dr. Karnovsky has stated, our experience with older fawn-hooded rats, subjected to intra-arterial balloon catheterization, was quite different from his experience with these animals using the air dried endothelial cell injury model. In our hands, these animals developed fibromusculoelastic lesions comparable to those observed in Sprague-Dawley rats, which served as our controls, 2 weeks after injury. Our findings suggest these animals have platelets which do support the proliferation of their medial smooth muscle cells following intimal injury.

L.C. Smith: VLDL isolated from plasma of subjects with normal lipid values does not suppress $HMGC_oA$ reductase in normal cultured human fibroblasts; whereas VLDL from Types III, IV and V hyperlipoproteinemic plasma is effective in suppressing enzyme synthesis. The apoprotein compositions are qualitatively similar. In addition to the presence of apoB and apoE on the lipoprotein surface, other factors are necessary for the suppression of $HMGC_oA$ reductase. (Gianturco, et al., (1978) J. Clin. Invest. In press).

SECOND PLENARY SESSION
RISK FACTORS FOR
ATHEROSCLEROSIS AND THROMBOSIS

Henry C. McGill, Jr., *Session Chairman*

Department of Pathology
University of Texas
Health Science Center at San Antonio
San Antonio, Texas

RISK FACTORS FOR ATHEROSCLEROSIS

Henry C. McGill, Jr.

The University of Texas Health Science Center
San Antonio, Texas

Nearly three decades of intensive epidemiological investigation have identified a group of characteristics that predict an individual's probability of developing clinically manifest disease due to atherosclerosis -- myocardial infarction, sudden death, angina pectoris, stroke, or peripheral vascular disease. These characteristics are known as "risk factors," a descriptive but non-committal term which avoids the question of whether these characteristics are causative agents, intervening variables, early manifestations of disease, or secondary indicators of an underlying disturbance.

The major risk factors also are associated with more severe and more extensive atherosclerotic lesions as well as with more frequent clinical disease. We have various degrees of knowledge about the mechanisms of their effects on atherogenesis, but relatively little knowledge about whether they affect thrombosis as a terminal occlusive episode, and if so, how. The purpose of this section of the workshop is to focus attention on the potential thrombogenic effects of the established risk factors, effects which may contribute both to atherogenesis and to the terminal occlusive episode. The purpose of this presentation is to review briefly the status of knowledge of the risk factors for atherosclerotic disease. The purpose of succeeding presentations is to consider how they may affect thrombosis and how we may get better information on this issue.

THE RISK FACTORS

Age

As with so many chronic diseases, the incidence rates of all
atherosclerotic diseases increase with age. The simplest explanation of this association is an accumulation of responses to
injury as exposures to injury increase. This explanation may be
true in middle aged and older persons, but the early stages of
atherogenesis during adolescence show more specific age-dependent
changes. Aortic fatty streaks increase rapidly in extent between
8 to 18 years, and fibrous plaques begin to form from fatty
streaks in the coronary arteries at about 20 years (1). These age
trends suggest that the artery wall undergoes a systematic change
with maturation, that the artery wall is exposed to distinctive
atherogenic agents at those ages.

The concept of aging as a degenerative change after attain-
ing adult growth is not yet sufficiently refined to explain
progression of the advanced lesions of atherosclerosis in biochemical and physiological terms (2). The cumulative effect of repeated injuries and the associated scarring seem to account for
most of the age effects on lesions in adulthood, but a more
precise definition of aging of smooth muscle cells may change
this view.

Male Sex

Except for age, male sex is one of the best documented and
strongest risk factors for coronary heart disease, but not for the
other forms of atherosclerotic disease (3). Furthermore, the sex
differential in coronary heart disease is most marked in whites,
and is greatly attenuated or absent in nonwhites. The sex differential also is much attenuated in populations with low overall
incidence rates of atherosclerotic disease, and is reduced or
eliminated among diabetics. Despite the attractiveness of the
hypothesis that the estrogenic hormones of the female are responsible for her protection from coronary artherosclerosis, it
has become clear that exogenous estrogen administration does not
protect the male and may even be atherogenic or thrombogenic.
Neither does it appear that exogenous estrogens, as in oral contraceptives, add to the natural protection of the female. Females
have slightly lower levels of three major risk factors between the
menarche and the menopause (serum cholesterol, blood pressure,
cigarette smoking), but the lower levels of risk factors do not
seem sufficient to account for the differences in coronary heart
disease. Male sex in whites remains the most puzzling of all of
the risk factors, and the one for which we have the least coherent hypothesis regarding mechanism.

Hypercholesterolemia

Total serum cholesterol concentration has long been recognized as the strongest and most consistent risk factor for atherosclerotic disease other than age and sex, and reduction in serum cholesterol has received much attention as a means of preventing disease (4). Serum cholesterol concentration can be elevated in many animal species by feeding a human-like high fat, high cholesterol diet, and these animals develop intimal lipid deposits resembling human fatty streaks. Cholesterolemia maintained in the range of 200-400 mg/dl for several years leads to experimental lesions that are reasonable facsimiles of human fibrous plaques. However, in both humans and animals, there remains a high degree of individual variation in cholesterolemic response to an atherogenic diet; and at any level of serum cholesterol, there is wide variation in the response of the arterial wall in forming atherosclerotic lesions.

Knowledge about the cellular metabolism of low density lipoprotein (LDL), which carries most of the plasma cholesterol, provides an attractive hypothesis for the mechanism by which hypercholesterolemia initiates intimal lipid deposits and causes some of them to progress to fibrous plaques (5). Cells (including fibroblasts and smooth muscle cells) possess specific receptors which bind LDL and promote internalization. The uptake of LDL suppresses synthesis of cholesterol in the cell. Internalized LDL is degraded, and the cholesterol is hydrolyzed and re-esterified as cholesteryl oleate. The cell thus obtains cholesterol for membrane structures at lower energy cost than by synthesis. In the presence of excess LDL, lipoprotein is internalized by a nonspecific process which does not suppress cholesterol synthesis, and cholesteryl ester accumulates within the cell in excess. Prolonged accumulation leads to cell death, extravasation of cholesterol esters and other debris, and a consequent chronic inflammatory and reparative reaction which results in the fibrous plaque.

Since elevated serum cholesterol levels can be lowered by either diet modification or by drugs, a major question now is whether reduction in serum cholesterol slows progression or permits regression of advanced atherosclerosis. Clinical trials of lipid-lowering agents in postmyocardial infarction patients (secondary prevention) have shown no benefit, and early trials of lipid lowering regimens in relatively small numbers of apparently healthy middle-aged or elderly persons (primary prevention) have yielded suggestive but not conclusive results. Currently, large scale trails are underway (6). It may never be possible to conduct a controlled trial of maintaining low serum cholesterol levels from childhood, but much circumstantial evidence suggests that control in childhood is likely to be more effective than in adults.

The relationship of serum cholesterol concentration to atherosclerotic disease has been strengthened by the recent demonstration
of an inverse association with high density lipoprotein (HDL)
cholesterol (7). This epidemiologic observation is consistent with
current hypotheses that the metabolic function of HDL is to transport cholesterol from peripheral tissues to the liver for eventual
degradation and excretion.

Thus, knowledge of lipoprotein metabolism supports the link
between serum cholesterol concentration and atherogenesis by suggesting biochemical mechanisms for the relationship. Whether
elevation of serum cholesterol or a specific lipoprotein concentration contributes to risk of coronary heart disease by other
mechanisms, such as, for example, by predisposing to thrombosis,
remains a possibility that may provide additional links.

Hypertension

Like serum cholesterol concentration, increase in blood pressure
in all ranges is associated with increased risk of atherosclerotic
disease, and particularly cerebrovascular disease. Hypertension
selectively augments cerebral atherosclerosis (8). The most obvious
mechanisms of action of hypertension on atherogenesis are by increasing filtration of lipoprotein-rich plasma through the intima,
or by increasing the workload of smooth muscle cells of the artery
wall. Less obvious is the potential effect of humoral mediators
of blood pressure on the artery wall, as, for example, Angiotension
II (9). Since some antihypertensive drugs lead to increased levels
of these mediators, such drug regimens may augment rather than
ameliorate the atheorgenic effect of hypertension. The beneficial
effects of antihypertensive drug therapy on stroke and congestive
heart failure are not in question, but whether such therapy reduces
coronary heart disease incidence is still doubtful. Hypertension
also may affect thrombosis as well as atherogenesis.

Diabetes Mellitus

Cardiovascular disease, particularly atherosclerotic disease,
remains the major health hazard for the diabetic. The atherogenic
effect of diabetes has not been linked to the capillary basement
membrane thickening characteristic of diabetes. Both vascular
lesions may have as a common basis a fundamental defect affecting
connective tissue, but such a link is speculative. Diabetics
have higher serum lipids levels, especially of triglycerides, than
do nondiabetics but the differences do not account for the increased
risk of atherosclerotic disease. Diabetes reduces greatly the
sex differential in mortality from coronary heart disease, but
does not change the sex differential in angina pectoris (10). A

diabetic effect on the terminal episode would be consistent with this observation. Neither insulin nor oral hypoglycemic agents protect diabetics from the increased risk of atherosclerotic disease, and the findings of the well known UGDP study indicate that oral hypoglycemic drugs increase the probability of cardio-vascular death for the diabetic (11). As with other complex metabolic diseases, it seems likely that diabetes also may influence thrombosis.

Cigarette Smoking

As the association between cigarette smoking and atheroscler-otic disease was developed in epidemiological studies, there was initial uncertainty whether cigarette smoking accelerated athero-genesis or whether it only predisposed to the terminal episode by precipitating thrombosis or arrhythmia. It now appears certain that cigarette smoking augments atherogenesis in the coronary arteries and the abdominal aorta (12), and it probably has a similar effect on the peripheral arteries. The experience of those who stop smoking suggests that it also affects the terminal occlusive episode since the risk of ex-smokers begins to drop more rapidly after cessation than we would expect from regression of advanced atherosclerosis alone (13).

We do not know what component of cigarette smoke is respon-sible for the acceleration of atherosclerosis nor the hypothe-sized effect on thrombosis. Nicotine appears innocuous, at least with regard to atherogenesis. Carbon monoxide is widely suspected but its role is not proven. Cigarette smoke contains about 3,000 identified chemicals and probably more unidentified ones, and therefore many possibilities remain.

Of all the risk factors, cigarette smoking seems the most likely to be thrombogenic as well as atherogenic. Scattered reports indicate that it affects several coagulation tests. A promising new lead is that a tobacco glycoprotein activates Factor XII (14).

Family History

Familial aggregation of atherosclerotic disease has long been recognized, but only a small beginning has been made in iso-lating the strictly genetic basis for this aggregation in contrast to the common environment shared by family members. The only specific progress has been in identifying genetic hyperlipidemias. Genetic bases for hypertension and diabetes are suspected. Un-doubtedly, a portion of the residual variability in atherosclerosis not explained by the known risk factors lies in unidentified

genetic traits, perhaps programmed characteristics of the artery
wall. Genetically determined variations in susceptibility to
atherosclerosis have been demonstrated in pigeons (15) and undoubtedly exist in humans as well.

In view of the numerous genetic defects in the coagulation
system and the presumed important role of thrombosis in atherosclerotic disease, it is remarkable that no genetic coagulation
abnormality has been found associated with atherosclerotic disease.

Obesity

The role of obesity in atherosclerotic disease remains
uncertain, despite nearly universal recommendations that obesity
should be avoided in order to reduce risk of atherosclerotic
disease. Obesity appears well established as a risk factor for
hypertension and diabetes, and undoubtedly influences atherosclerosis indirectly through these mechanisms; but in their absence, no
clear association of obesity with either atherogenesis or with
atherosclerotic disease has been demonstrated.

Physical Activity

Many benefits are derived from moderate regular physical
activity, and it has been widely recommended for preventing
atherosclerotic disease. There is some evidence that extreme
physical activity is associated with less risk of coronary heart
disease (16), but the level of activity required is difficult to
attain in our society. No association of lack of physical activity with atherosclerotic lesions has been demonstrated.

Personality Type

Despite continued demonstrations of an association between
certain personality types and coronary heart disease, the relationship remains highly controversial and has received only
limited serious attention from investigators (17).

CONCLUSION

When combined in the multiple logistic equation with which
most of the large epidemiological studies have been analyzed, it
is possible to define a group of high risk individuals among whom
about half the future cases of coronary heart disease will develop.
However, individuals classified as non-high risk will contribute

the other half (18). There are less data on other forms of atherosclerotic disease, but the proportion of cases "explained" by the
established risk factors is probably no higher than that for coronary heart disease. What accounts for the remaining variance?

The most likely explanation is that there are unrecognized or
unmeasured risk factors. One of these, described briefly above,
is the susceptibility of the artery wall to the other causative
agents or intervening variables -- that is, its response to hypercholesterolemia, hypertension, or cigarette smoking. Since we do
not know the nature of this ill-defined, hypothetical susceptibility, there is no way to measure it. Even if we knew what it was,
it would be difficult to measure in inaccessible sites such as
the coronary arteries.

The uncertain or controversial risk factors, which are not
used in the multiple logistic equation because their effect is not
statistically significant as currently measured, also may account
for a portion of the remaining variance. Better methods of measuring other suspected risk factors may lead to some improvement
in the predictive power of the equation and consequently to some
reduction in the unexplained variance.

Finally, there may exist risk factors that so far have not
been recognized and therefore are not measured. Whatever the risk
factors for thrombosis are, they are likely both to augment atherogenesis and to predispose to terminal thrombosis, and therefore
are likely to be risk factors for the atherosclerotic diseases.
Identification of measurable characteristics associated with probability of thrombosis would make possible testing their relationship to atherosclerotic disease.

REFERENCES

1. McGill, H.C., Jr. (1968) The Geographic Pathology of Athero-
    sclerosis, Williams & Wilkins, Baltimore, 193 pp.

2. Bierman, E.L., and Ross, R. (1977) in Atherosclerosis Reviews,
    Vol. 2, (Gotto, A.M. and Paoletti, R., Eds.), Raven Press,
    New York, pp. 79-111.

3. McGill, H.C., Jr., and Stern, M.P. (1978) in Atheroclerosis
    Reviews, Vol. 3, (Gotto, A.M. and Paoletti, R., Eds.), Raven
    Press, New York.

4. Inter-Society Commission for Heart Disease Resources. (1970)
    Circulation 42, A-55-A-95.

5. Goldstein, J.L., and Brown, M.S. (1975) Arch. Pathol. 99, 181-184.

6. Rifkind, B.M. (1977) in Atheroclerosis Reviews, Vol. 2, (Gotto, A.M. and Paoletti, R., Eds.), Raven Press, New York, pp. 67-78.

7. Gordon, T., Castelli, W.P., Hjortland, M.C., Kannel, W.B., and Dawber, T.B. (1977) Am. J. Med. 62, 707.

8. Solberg, L.A., and McGarry, P.A. (1972) Atherosclerosis 16, 141-154.

9. Hollander, W. (1973) Circulation 48, 1112-1127.

10. Gordon, T., and Shurtleff, D. (1973) An Epidemiological Investigation of Cardiovascular Disease, Section 29, DHEW Publication No. (NIH) 74-478, Washington, D.C.

11. The University Group Diabetes Program. (1970) Diabetes 19, Suppl. 2, 787-830.

12. Strong, J.P., and Richards, M.L. (1976) Atheroscl. 23, 451-476.

13. Gordon, T., Kannel, W.B., McGee, D., and Dawber, T.R. (1974) Lancet 2, 1345-1348.

14. Becker, C.G., and Dubin, T. (1977) J. Exp. Med. 146, 457-467.

15. Wagner, W.D., Clarkson, T.B., Feldner, M.A., and Pritchard, R.W. (1973) Exp. Mol. Pathol. 19, 304-319.

16. Paffenbarger, R.S., Jr., and Hale, W.E. (1975) N. Engl. J. Med. 292, 545-550.

17. Jenkins, C.D. (1976) N. Engl. J. Med. 294, 987-994; 1033-1038.

18. Stamler, J., and Epstein, F. (1972) Prov. Med. 1, 27-48.

RELATIONSHIP OF RISK FACTORS FOR ATHEROSCLEROSIS
TO ARTERIAL THROMBOSIS

J.R.A. Mitchell
Department of Medicine
Nottingham University
Nottingham, England

"Those who have dissected or inspected many bodies
have at least learned to doubt; when others, who
are ignorant of anatomy and do not take the trouble
to attend to it are in no doubt at all."
(Morgagni, 1761)

In old mathematics, the golden rule for manipulating numbers
was to ensure that they all had a common denominator. So too with
words, in that they must have a common root if they are to be manipulated. Close scrutiny of the topic which was assigned to me
shows that each component of my title has a different base, so
we must recognize this and try to compensate for it.

By common usage, a "risk factor" is some attribute of a living person (such as being a man, being obese, being a smoker or
being hyperlipidemic) which is associated with an increased likelihood of developing some marker event. In the field of vascular
disease, these marker events are essentially clinical syndromes
(sudden death, myocardial infarction, stroke, etc.) rather than
pathological processes. The majority of large-scale, prospective,
risk-factor-identifying studies have used clinical markers (history, physical examination, and tests available on an appropriate
scale in the chosen location) since they could not use pathological indices of disease in survivors of the events, and were usually unable to do so in the bulk of those who died.

"Atherosclerosis" on the other hand, is a disease of blood
vessel walls which cannot be measured in life, save by tests whose
unpleasant nature, cost and limited availability preclude their

use in large population studies. "Atherosclerosis" is thus a condition which can usually only be identified after death, and even
then it can only be quantitated if the investigator recognizes
the need for precision in terminology and accuracy in measurement
(1). If one studies "atherosclerosis" as revealed at post-mortem
it is extremely unlikely that information about risk factors will
already be available; if it is not, it cannot be gained retrospectively, i.e., if an individual has never had his blood pressure
measured in life, no post-mortem study however careful can correlate atherosclerosis with hypertension.

"Thrombosis" is also a pathological process which can be con-
fidently recognized at post-mortem, but which can only be inferred
in life by identifying clinical events which are universally
accepted as being due to thrombosis, and which can never be due
to anything else. As we shall see, this is a situation which is
not matched in practical medicine.

My title thus contains words which have little in common,
and we need to ask questions, rather than to answer them:

1. Are there such things as "risk factors" for "atherosclerosis" or are there only "risk factors" for clinical events? If
so, the relation between "risk factors" and "atherosclerosis" will
then depend on the link between atherosclerosis and the marker
events. As risk factors are defined in the living while atherosclerosis is defined in the dead, definitive studies linking the
two together are rare.

2. What consequences stem from atherosclerosis? Does atherosclerosis ever produce clinical events directly or does it only
lead to death and disability by producing thrombosis? Does atherosclerosis actually produce thrombosis or does thrombosis produce
atherosclerosis? What clinical consequences can be labeled as
being due to thrombosis?

3. If thrombosis, atherosclerosis, and clinical events bear
an uncertain relationship to each other, then may each one have
its own set of risk factors? The search for risk factors for
thrombosis as such goes back to Rokitansky's belief that a "crasis
in the blood" precedes thrombosis (2). All the studies on coagulation, platelet behavior, and fibrinolysis represent attempts to
identify risk factors for thrombosis which offer better predictive
value than conventional, event-determined ones. Are there any
tests which will predict an individual's chances of developing
arterial thrombosis so that these can be used as risk-markers for
thrombosis?

There are no answers to the majority of these questions, but to illustrate our urgent need to increase precision in speech, writing and thought, I propose to examine one topic from each of the widely-used but ill-defined concepts embodied in my title.

A. "RISK FACTORS"

For many people, the use of the word "factor" has come to imply a causal association. Since many of the attributes are amenable to change, it has led the unwary to assume that modifying a risk factor will thereby modify the risk. Thus the association between hypercholesterolemia and an increased risk of cardiovascular death has led theoreticians (3) to calculate how many lives would be saved if lipid levels were reduced. The fallacy in this calculation is that association does not indicate causation. Generations of Irishmen have eaten a lot of potatoes and have also been at high risk from tuberculosis so it is possible to argue that potatoes cause tuberculosis. It is also possible that both observations spring from some hidden underlying attribute such as poverty. In present-day terms, we could test the causal hypothesis by mounting a primary intervention trial in which one would modify the "risk factor" by limiting potato intake in part of the population and would observe the effect of this on tuberculosis. If modifying the risk factor reduced the risk, then a causal link would have been established; if it did not, then one must substitute "risk marker" for "risk factor" since it is indicative, rather than causal.

If we examine the major risk factors which have been described in respect of the clinical events grouped together as coronary heart disease (sudden death, myocardial infarction, onset of angina pectoris) we can characterize them according to the effect on mortality which has been observed when they have been modified. We find that reduction of systemic arterial pressure (4) and of serum lipids (5) do not appear to reduce risk, whereas cessation of cigarette smoking does (6). If this enables us to characterize hypertension and hyperlipidemia as "markers" or "indicators" while retaining cigarette smoking as a true risk factor, this could influence our search for links between these risk attributes and pathological events such as thrombosis and atherosclerosis. If hypertension and hyperlipidemia are epiphenomena then we perhaps should invest less effort in studying the ways in which they might have caused disease and concentrate our resources instead on the way in which cigarette smoking alters vessel or blood properties. Thus to search for tests which will show how serum lipids affect platelet behavior may be quite fruitless since neither the serum lipids nor platelet behavior has been shown to be directly involved in the clinical situations from which the risk factor concept has derived.

Moreover, risk factors tend to vary in power in different
clinical events which nevertheless share a common pathology. Thus
cerebral infarction is thought to originate from thrombosis of the
brain supply arteries in association with atheroma, and transmural
myocardial infarction derives from coronary artery thrombosis in
association with atheroma. If the risk factors operated through
pathological processes then coronary and cerebral risk factors
should be the same since atheroma and thrombosis are common to both
clinical events. In reality, the "big three" for the heart turn
out not to be equally powerful for the brain, where cigarette smoking and hyperlipidemia show reduced predictive power while the link
with hypertension becomes stronger (7). In searching for links between risk factors and pathological processes is it possible that
thrombosis and atheroma differ in different territories and that
different pathogenetic mechanisms must be sought? Alternatively,
is it only the clinical markers which differ? If so, we should be
able to identify true risk factors which should be identical for
atheroma and thrombosis, wherever they occurred.

B. PATHOLOGICAL PROCESSES UNDERLYING CLINICAL EVENTS

By common usage, three clinical events (myocardial infarction,
sudden death, and angina pectoris) have been grouped together as
"coronary heart disease" and a wide variety of pathology-derived
terms and ill-defined terms have been loosely applied to the group
("coronary artery disease," "ischemic heart disease," "coronary
atherosclerosis," "atherosclerotic heart disease," etc.) After
many years of debate in which workers have held forceful but dia-
metrically opposing views on the pathological processes underlying
the clinical events (that massive myocardial necrosis is caused by
thrombotic coronary occlusion (1); that necrosis causes coronary
thrombosis (8); or that the necrosis is metabolic and is unrelated
to events in the coronary tree (9)) we can begin to see that the
reason for the conflict is that the workers are talking about different problems. Thus we can find a measure of agreement that the
clinical syndrome of myocardial infarction (chest pain, Q waves and
ST-T changes on ECG, cardiac enzyme elevation) is brought about by
thrombotic occlusion of a coronary artery, usually in association
with coronary atherosclerosis which is of more than average severity (10). Unheralded sudden death, on the other hand, is clearly
a different process, in that if its victims are resuscitated, they
do not go on to develop the features of myocardial infarction, and
their subsequent outcome is also very different from the relatively
favorable prognosis observed in infarct survivors (11). This clinical diversity is matched by pathological dissimilarity, in that
it is now generally agreed that myocardial necrosis and thrombotic
occlusion will not be found in patients with unheralded sudden
death, but that atheroma of much more severe degree than the rest
of the population will be present (12).

Table 1.   Information Needed to Link Real Events to Pathological
           Processes

Real event	Coherent sub-groups	Part played by	
		Atherosclerosis	Thrombosis
	(Transmural necrosis	+	+++
	(Sudden death	+++	o
Heart attack	(Heart failure/		
	dysrhythmia	?	?
	(Angina	+	+
	(Hemorrhage	o	o
	(Infarction-thrombotic	+	+++
Stroke	(-embolic	++	++
	(TIA	+++	+
Gangrene/	(Occlusion	+	++
claudication	(Embolization	+	+
DVT/PE	(Clinical diagnosis	o	+++
	(Test-aided diagnosis	o	+++

     Thus we can only begin to make sense out of apparently con-
flicting observations when we recognize that words like "coronary
artery disease" are getting in the way of our studies, rather than
helping them. I have set out in Table 1 what we ought to do for
some of the real clinical events which we use as markers; namely,
to divide the clinical events into coherent sub-groups which can
be manipulated, and then to assign pathogenetic mechanisms to each
sub-group. Only then can we link the "risk-markers" for the events
to the pathological processes such as atheroma and thrombosis.

     Table 1 is illustrative, and not definitive, since the infor-
mation needed to complete the pathological columns is not available
for most of the subgroups. Thus in the heart disease area, transmural necrosis and sudden death are now well documented, whereas
angina, being a non-fatal condition, is not. As heart-failure and
dysrhythmias can have diverse causes which are unrelated to atheroma and thrombosis, they clearly constitute a poor marker-event
for the processes which we wish to study. Their presence in the
list is useful, since it provides a valid illustration of the problems which we will encounter in the next clinical marker group,
which is "stroke."

It is easy to perceive that a stroke has occurred, in that a previously intact individual suddenly develops a neurological deficit. The first task is however to separate out "strokes" which are not due to cerebrovascular disease (bleeding into a tumor, post-epileptic paralysis, hemiplegic migraine, hypoglycemia, etc.) In this respect then, stroke resembles "heart failure/dysrhythmias" in that it can be due to the events which we wish to study, but it has other, unrelated causes. Even when we have excluded non-vascular "stroke" we can then find that there are three very different subgroups to try and differentiate (13). In group 1, the neurological deficit is due to destructive bleeding, which does not of course arise from atheroma and thrombosis, but from miliary aneurysms in the brain substance. Group 2 is cerebral infarction due to cerebral artery occlusion and must immediately be subdivided into thrombosis in situ, whether of intra-cranial or neck vessels, and embolization by diverse materials coming from diverse sources. Group 3 is transient neurological deficit, but unless this is defined very carefully, overlap with groups 1 and 2 will occur. Some workers insist that "transient" must be of less than an hour's duration, while others permit an attack to last up to 24 hours. These variations in definition must mean that attempts to clarify "risk factors" and "pathogenetic mechanisms" in TIA's will be doomed to failure.

The dismal truth is that at the bedside, the very real and clear-cut event of a "stroke" cannot even be assigned to a bleeding or to an occlusive subgroup with any degree of confidence. Clinical signs, including examination of the cerebrospinal fluid, can seldom differentiate between intra-cerebral hemorrhage and cerebral infarction. Apparently precise terms, used in major risk-factor studies, are not as precise as their readers would imagine. Thus the Framingham-derived term "atherothrombotic brain infarction" or "ABI" (14) simply means "stroke with non-hemorrhagic CSF" and this group therefore includes patients with intra-cerebral hemorrhage which has not broken through into the CSF. Study of such a group for various attributes which could indicate a propensity to "atherothrombotic" disease would be doomed to failure because the group would be diluted by patients with a totally different problem.

Thus the information which we need to enter for cerebral infarction on Table 1 is not yet available. All we can say is that the site of infarction is more closely linked to the presence and location of thrombotic occlusion than to the site and severity of atherosclerosis (15), that embolic cerebral occlusion and infarction accounts for some 60-70% of all infarcts (16, 17), and that transient ischemic attacks, although thought by many to arise from emboli triggered off by supply-vessel atherosclerosis, show quite different disease patterns in these neck vessels from patients with completed strokes (18). As I have done in Table 1, we thus need

to keep them separate and distinct in word and thought until we can
enter appropriate symbols in the "mechanism" columns.

The situation in peripheral vascular disease is no less con-
fusing and for completeness we should point out that thrombosis
arises in veins without any wall disease such as atherosclerosis
to trigger it. Moreover we need to keep the various ways of reveal-
ing venous thrombosis and embolization (clinical, isotopic, angio-
graphic, etc.) separate because they may all identify different
subsets from the total group.

Perhaps discussion at the meeting will have enabled precise
figures to be inscribed against each of the columns in the Table,
so that we will be able to write "myocardial infarction - atheroma
15%, thrombosis 85%; sudden death - atheroma 100%; thrombosis 0%;
hemorrhagic stroke - atheroma 0%; thrombosis 0%" and so on. I
think this is unlikely, because what we lack is facts.

C. THE SEARCH FOR THE CRASIS IN THE BLOOD

In the so-called "Virchow Triad" we have total theoretical
coverage of all the possible mechanisms by which thrombosis might
arise, without any of them being known. If one takes the triad at
face value and accepts that an unknown blend of vessel wall, blood
flow and blood behavioral factors may generate a thrombus, then
this has implications for the value of tests of blood behavior in
"risk factor" identification.

If we postulate that diseased vessel walls tell the passing
blood to form a thrombus, then the nature and durability of this
message will determine whether a blood sample from another site,
such as an arm vein, will reveal it. If the message is locally
powerful but ephemeral, then the distant blood will not contain
it, whereas if all the blood which has traversed the message-pro-
ducing site is permanently changed, then a distant sample will
reveal it. Moreover the blood components which are capable of
receiving the message may respond to it by producing a thrombus
leaving the components which do not respond to the message to be
sampled. Thus in a situation where "receptive platelets" are involved, the tests of platelet behavior at a distant site would show
reduced platelet activity. Thus in an "atherogenic" model where
the vessel wall calls the tune, blood at a distant site could be
totally normal if the message is a local one; it could be abnormal
if the message produces a generalized activation of some blood property; or it could even show reduced activity, if all the active
components are busy being active elsewhere, leaving the inactive or
lazy components to be sampled.

If _flow_ holds the key to thrombus formation, then there will be no local messenger in a chemical sense, and the chances of detecting changes in sampled blood at a distant site will be determined by the impact which flow produces upon the circulating blood.

Finally, let us suppose that thrombosis is due to an _abnormality of the circulating blood_ and that all other processes, including atheroma, derive from blood-triggered thrombus formation. Then it might be argued that a blood sample should provide all the clues which we need. Four difficulties still remain:

1. What Blood Property Should We Study?

A well developed arterial thrombus contains masses of adherent platelets surrounded by polymorphonuclear leucocytes and by coarse fibrin strands (1). It is tempting to look at the _participants_ in thrombus formation and to label them as the _prime movers,_ but this may be fallacious. An aerial photograph of most English cities on a Saturday afternoon would reveal densely packed masses of human beings and we might assume that some abnormality of behavior had caused them to aggregate. Close scrutiny would however reveal 22 individual highly colored particles with an ever smaller particle passing between them and we would then realize that the larger aggregates were showing a normal behavior pattern in response to a hitherto undetected stimulus. Thus the search for intrinsic abnormalities of platelets and clotting behavior may be fruitless since these known components of a thrombus may be responding normally to some unknown abnormal message.

2. What Are We Looking For?

In the bone marrow, the embryo platelets adhere together to comprise the megakaryocyte; in the circulating blood they probably wander around as single cells and yet when we meet them in a thrombus, they have reverted to their "foetal" state of adherence to each other. When one looks at a thrombus it is tempting to imagine that some abnormal activity has developed which has produced adherence (i.e., that the equivalent of a glue has been formed). Might not the abnormality be the mirror-image of this, in that the normal individual circulating platelets possess an anti-glue, so that it is the loss of this property, rather than the arrival of a glue which constitutes the abnormality?

In the clotting system too there are checks and balances in the shape of reactions which favor fibrin formation while others hinder it. Moreover fibrin itself can be removed by the fibrinolytic system, but we must be alert to the lack of evidence for a

physiological role for this system. That shed blood, suitably
diluted and buffered will lyse its fibrin clots is universally accepted; that the infusion of pharmacological amounts of lytic activators can enhance fibrin dissolution is accepted and that in certain pathological states, abnormal lysis can occur is also accepted.
This does not prove however that the reader of these words is being
kept in a physiologically fluid state by the forces of good
(fibrinolysis) triumphing over the forces of evil (clot or thrombus
formation). Pathological processes seldom arise as the simple
converse of physiological processes.

3. How Should We Measure It?

We must avoid the tacit assumption that measurable in vitro
activities truly reflect the in vivo state. In the platelet field
we speak glibly of "platelet function tests" and thereby imply that
the ability of platelets to aggregate in the presence of adenosine
diphosphate (ADP), for example, is one of their natural functions.
From there it is but a short step to the assumption that because a
platelet aggregate can be produced in a test tube by ADP, so a
thrombotic mass of platelets has been initiated by ADP. We can
then come to believe that agents which prevent ADP aggregation in
vitro will ipso facto be antithrombotic. This must however be
proved by clinical trials and if it cannot be proved then our basic
assumptions are probably wrong.

We should therefore stop talking of "platelet function" and
talk instead of "platelet behavior." This would remind us that the
tricks which these cells can be persuaded to do under totally unphysiological conditions do not necessarily occur in the circulating
blood since abnormal calcium concentrations and citrate may be
directly responsible for some of the so-called "platelet functions"
(19, 20).

4. On Whom Should We Make Measurements?

Two groups of subjects could be examined. First, we could
study the survivors of event-markers such as myocardial infarction
or stroke. If we study them early in their illness we risk confus-
ing the non-specific consequences of their illness (which may
merely be the platelet or coagulation test reflections of secondary events such as an elevation of the plasma fibrinogen) with
its causes. If we wait until the acute illness has subsided, we
are then left with a highly selected survivor population and we can
easily mislead ourselves. If one found an excess of Blood Group A
patients in the long-term survivors of heart attacks, this might
mean that the Group A individuals in the community had an increased

Table 2. Blood Properties and Risk Factors

Hyperlipidemia	Platelet electrophoresis - Hampton and Gorlin (25)
	Platelet sedimentation and ultra-structure - Saleh and Hashim (26)
Fat feeding	Platelet survival and coagulation - Mustard and Murphy (27)
	Filtraggometer - Hornstra et al. (28)
	Heparin neutralizing activity - O'Brien et al. (29, 30)
	Aggregation - Baghurst (31)
Sucrose feeding	Platelet adhesiveness - Szanto and Yudkin (32)

Table 3. Blood Properties and Risk Factors

Smoking	Platelet survival - Mustard and Murphy (33)
	Platelet stickiness - Ashby et al. (34)
	Platelet adhesiveness - Murchison and Fyfe (35)
	Platelet aggregation and electrophoresis - Hawkins (36)
	Platelet behavior lysis and coagulation - Meade et al. (22-24)
Oral contraceptives	Coagulation and platelet aggregation - Poller (37)
	Platelet electrophoresis - Hampton and Mitchell (38)
	Platelet behavior lysis and coagulation - Meade et al. (22-24)
Exercise	Platelet aggregation - Warlow and Ogston (39)
	Platelet adhesion - Pegrum et al. (40)
"Stress"	Platelet aggregation - Gordon et al. (41)

risk of developing the disease, or that being group A increased an individual's chance of surviving a heart attack. Thus we would be left in doubt, from survivor studies, whether an attribute enhanced the likelihood of developing a disease or protected those who did develop it.

If, on the other hand, one embarks on a thrombotic Framingham-type study, the magnitude of the task is daunting, since very large numbers need to be studied over a prolonged period to yield a small group of previously well individuals who go on to develop the index events, so that their attributes on entry can be compared with the unaffected individuals. If one accepts that high serum lipids, cigarette smoking and arterial hypertension can be used to identify a group who are at high risk from heart attack, then we should note that only 8% of that group will develop a heart attack during a 10-year follow-up period (21). If blood tests for thrombosis were to be based on this type of group, then 100 people would need to be tested and followed for 10 years so that the 8 who developed the index disease could be compared with the 92 who did not. If the tests used had a wide range of within-patient variability, then the numbers which need to be studied to reveal true between-patient differences are enormous. Nevertheless, such studies are under way, and in North London, Meade and his colleagues (22-24) have measured a wide variety of hematological characteristics in people who were healthy at the time of assessment: we must now wait and see what predictive power these various measurements will have.

In contrast to these very long-term prospective studies, a wide variety of blood properties have been scrutinized in patients or in situations where enhanced risk of heart attack is postulated. To allow the reader to evaluate these studies against the general background requirements which I have been describing, I have listed representative examples in Tables 2 and 3. What emerges is that at the present time we have no test of blood behavior which will pick out individual patients who have thrombosed, who are thrombosing or who are about to thrombose.

SUMMARY

Risk factors are defined in the living by the occurrence of subsequent clinical events and many of them may be risk markers rather than causal factors. Atherosclerosis, however, can only be defined and measured in the dead so information about conventional risk factors cannot usually be obtained in retrospect. The mechanism of thrombus production is unknown and at the present time no test of coagulation or blood cell behavior can be used to predict a thrombotic tendency.

The pathological basis for the majority of clinical events which are used to identify risk-markers (sudden death, myocardial infarction and stroke) is not sufficiently precise for us to decide whether the risk-markers are linked to atherosclerosis, to thrombosis or to the clinical events themselves.

Only when these gaps in our knowledge have been filled shall we be able to link risk factors, atherosclerosis and arterial thrombosis.

REFERENCES

1. Mitchell, J.R.A., and Schwartz, C.J. (1965) Arterial Disease Blackwell Scientific, Oxford.

2. Rokitansky, C. (1852) A Manual of Pathological Anatomy, Sydenham Society, London.

3. Whyte, H.M. (1975) Lancet 1, 906-910.

4. Breckenridge, A., Dollery, C.T., and Parry, E.H.O. (1970) Quart. J. Med. 39, 411-429.

5. Dayton, S., and Pearce, M.L. (1970) Lancet 1, 473-474.

6. Gordon, T., Kannel, W.B., McGee, D., and Dawber, T.R. (1974) Lancet 2, 1345-1348.

7. Housley, E. (1976) in Stroke (Gillingham, F.J., Mawdsley, C. and Williams, A.E., Eds.) Churchill Livingstone, Edinburgh, pp. 251-262.

8. Spain, D.M., and Bradess, V.A. (1960) Am. J. Med. Sci. 240, 701-710.

9. Baroldi, G., Radice, F., Schmid, G., and Leone, A. (1974) Am. Heart J. 87, 65-75.

10. Chandler, A.B., Chapman, I., Erhardt, L.R., Roberts, W.C., Schwartz, C.J., Sinapius, D., Spain, D.M., Sherry, S., Ness, P.M., and Simon, T.L. (1974) Am. J. Cardiol. 34, 823-832.

11. Cobb, L.A., Baum, R.S., Alvarez, H., and Schaffer, W.A. (1975) Circulation 51-52, Suppl. III, 223-228.

12. Schwartz, C.J., and Gerrity, R.G. (1975) Circulation 51-52, Suppl. III, 18-26.

13. Mitchell, J.R.A. (1976) in Stroke (Gillingham, F.J., Mawdsley,
     C. and Williams, A.E., Eds.) Churchill Livingstone, Edinburgh,
     pp. 301-316.

14. Kannel, W.B., Wolf, P.A., Verter, J., and McNamara, P.M. (1970)
     JAMA 214, 301-310.

15. Battacharji, S.K., Hutchinson, E.C., and McCall, A.J. (1967)
     Br. Med. J. 2, 270-274.

16. Adams, R.D., and Vandeer Eecken, H.M. (1953) Ann. Rev. Med. 4,
     213-252.

17. Lhermitte, F., Gautier, J.C., and Derousne, C. (1970) Neurology
     20, 82-88.

18. Harrison, M.J.G., and Marshall, J. (1976) Br. Med. J. 1, 205-
     207.

19. Macfarlane, D.E., Walsh, P.N., Mills, D.C.B., Holmsen, H., and
     Day, H.J. (1975) Br. J. Haematol. 30, 457-463.

20. Heptinstall, S. (1976) Thromb. Diath. Haem. 36, 208-220.

21. Report of Intersociety Commission for Heart Disease Resources
     (1970) Circulation 42, A-55.

22. Meade, T.W. (1973) Thromb. Diath. Haem. Suppl. 54, 317-320.

23. Meade, T.W., Brozovic, M., Chakrabarti, R., Howarth, D.J.,
     North, W.R.S., and Stirling, Y. (1976) Br. J. Haematol. 34,
     353-364.

24. Meade, T.W., Chakrabarti, R., and North, W.R.S. (1977) Br. Med.
     J. 1, 837.

25. Hampton, J.R., and Gorlin, R. (1972) Br. Heart J. 34, 465-471.

26. Saleh, J.W., and Hashim, S.A. (1974) Circulation 50, 880-886.

27. Mustard, J.F., and Murphy, E.A. (1962) Br. Med. J. 1, 1651-1655.

28. Hornstra, G., Lewis, B., Chait, A., Turpeinen, O., Karvonen,
     M.J., and Vergroesen, A.J. (1973) Lancet 1, 1155-1157.

29. O'Brien, J.R., Etherington, M.D., and Jamieson, S. (1976)
     Lancet 1, 878-880.

30. O'Brien, J.R., Etherington, M.D., Jamieson, S., Vergroesen, A.J., and Ten Hoor, F. (1976) Lancet 2, 995-997.

31. Baghurst, K.I., Raj, M.J., and Truswell, A.S. (1977) Lancet 1, 101.

32. Szanto, S., and Yudkin, J. (1969) Postgrad. Med. 45, 602-607.

33. Mustard, J.F., and Murphy, E.A. (1963) Br. Med. J. 1, 846-849.

34. Ashby, P., Dalby, A.M., and Millar, J.H.D. (1965) Lancet 1, 158-159.

35. Murchison, L.E., and Fyfe, T. (1966) Lancet 2, 182-184.

36. Hawkins, R.I. (1972) Nature 236, 450-452.

37. Poller, L., Priest, C.M., and Thomson, J.M. (1969) Br. Med. J. 4, 273-274.

38. Hampton, J.R., and Mitchell, J.R.A. (1974) Thromb. Diath. Haem. 31, 204-244.

39. Warlow, C.P., and Ogston, D. (1974) Acta. Haemat. 52, 47-52.

40. Pegrum, G.D., Harrison, K.M., Shaw, S., Haselton, A., and Wolff, S. (1967) Nature 213, 301-302.

41. Gordon, J.L., Bowyer, D.E., Evans, D.W., and Mitchinson, M.J. (1973) J. Clin. Path. 26, 958-962.

POSSIBLE EFFECTS OF RISK FACTORS ON FIBRINOLYSIS

Hau C. Kwaan

Northwestern University Medical School
and Veterans Administration Lakeside Hospital
Chicago, Illinois

The hypothesis that atheromatous plaques originate as intimal collections of blood components was first advanced by Rokitansky (1). This hypothesis has since been revived by Duguid (2) and others (3, 4). Recent findings in support of this concept include the demonstration that the intimal deposits may consist of platelets as well as fibrin. The presence of high thromboplastic activity in the intimal layer of blood vessels, especially arteries (5), provides a mechanism for fibrin or platelet deposition. Additionally, any increase in the coagulability of the circulating blood would facilitate the process. On the other hand, fibrinolytic activity is high in the vascular intima, though less active in arteries than in veins, and could be important in the removal of mural thrombi.

The balance between thrombogenic and thrombolytic activity could be disturbed in states wherein the fibrinolytic process is impaired, either locally by damage to the intima, or systemically, by inhibition of circulating fibrinolytic activity. Pathologic conditions as well as variations in the normal physiologic state may influence circulating fibrinolytic activity. Many of these conditions are also considered to be risk factors for atherogenesis. A list of those factors that inhibit fibrinolysis is shown in Table 1, while those potentiating fibrinolysis are listed in Table 2.

Age. In a study of 2,000 men between the ages of 40 and 60, Papilian and Nita (6) found that the spontaneous plasma fibrinolytic activity was significantly less than that seen in men between the ages of 18 and 25. They believed that the lowered fibrinolytic activity was due to higher "anti-plasmin" activity in the elderly

Table 1.   Risk Factors Inhibiting Fibrinolysis

Increasing age
Cigarette smoking
Obesity
Hypercholesterolemia
Hypertriglyceridemia
Diabetes mellitus
Hypertension

subjects. They found that firm and non-lysable opaque clots could
be produced from the plasma of 20% of the elderly group and from
plasma of only 8% of the younger group. When the elderly subjects
were followed over a period of 3 years (7), the antiplasmin activity remained high in over 55% of the subjects.

Cigarette Smoking. Billimoria, et al. (8) found that euglobu-
lin lysis times were significantly longer in heavy smokers than in
non-smokers, particularly among the female subjects. These data
are at variance with those reported by Korsan-Bengtsen et al. (9)
who did not find any difference in the plasma fibrinolytic activity
between smokers and non-smokers. Cigarette smoking was shown to
accelerate in vitro thrombosis in the Chandler loop (10) and to
increase platelet aggregation acutely in man (11, 12) and chronically in experimental animals (13).

Obesity. Using a wide range of methods for the assay of fibrinolytic activity, Grace et al. (14) found that the blood fibrinolytic activity decreased with increasing body fatness. Obesity was
found to be associated with normal plasminogen and increased fibrinogen levels. Bennett (15) considers the low activity in obesity
due to decreased production of plasminogen activator rather than
excessive inhibition.

Hyperlipidemia. While investigating the possibility that reduced fibrinolysis in obesity might be due to abnormalities of
lipid and carbohydrate metabolism, Grace et al. (14) as well as
Korsan-Bengtsen et al. (9) found a significant negative correlation
between fibrinolytic activity and plasma triglyceride and free
fatty acid levels, but these relationships became insignificant
when the effect of obesity was taken into account. On the other
hand, increased thromboembolic disease in a family with Type IV
hyperlipoproteinemia was attributed by Anderson (15) to reduced
fibrinolysis. An increase in the pre-B-lipoprotein fraction in the
plasma of heavy smokers was thought to be responsible for reduced
fibrinolysis in these subjects.

Diabetes Mellitus. A picture of hypercoagulability, associated with increased activity of various clotting factors (16, 17), an increased turnover of fibrinogen (18), and impaired fibrinolytic activity is seen in diabetes mellitus. In addition to a lowered spontaneous plasma fibrinolytic activity (19), diabetic subjects were found to have impaired release of plasminogen activator from the blood vessel wall (20). These changes were more marked when obesity and retinopathy were present. The decreased fibrinolysis may be partly due to increased activity of alpha-1-antitrypsin and alpha-2-macroglobulin, both being inhibitors of plasmin and plasminogen activator (21).

Since atherosclerosis as well as thromboembolic complications is a major cause of morbidity in diabetes, the changes in the hemostatic mechanism in these patients become the object of much investigation. In addition to the above-mentioned abnormalities in fibrinolysis, increased platelet adhesiveness (22, 23) and sensitivity to aggregation by various agents have been reported (24-26). A plasma factor that can enhance ADP-induced aggregation was found in diabetic subjects, particularly those with retinopathy and nephropathy (25). A review of these findings in diabetes has been published (26).

Potentiation of Fibrinolytic Activity. A number of risk factors that may potentiate circulating fibrinolytic activity are listed in Table 2. The effect of these factors, however, is short-lived. As such, these factors are considered a minor influence in body fibrinolytic activity and probably play no part in atherogenesis.

Exercise. The effect of exercise is bimodal. While active exercise is associated with a prompt rise in the plasma fibrinolytic activity (28), this effect is also short-lived. On the other hand, if exercise is carried out under ischemic conditions, the development of fibrinolytic activity is impaired (29). These observations could have significant implications, since they may be applicable to ischemic myocardium. The fibrinolytic response to exercise is also impaired in type IV hyperlipoproteinemia (30).

Local Fibrinolytic Activity at Vessel Wall. While most of the above mentioned factors affect the circulating fibrinolytic activity only transiently, local fibrinolytic activity in the vessel wall can be chronically affected. In diabetes mellitus, a failure of release of plasminogen activator from the vessel wall has been observed (20). If such local plasminogen activator possesses a physiologic function in the resolution of thrombi (31-33), any injury to the vascular intima would provide a local condition favorable to mural thrombus formation. The findings of high thromboplastic activity in the arterial intima by biochemical (5) and immunofluorescent techniques (34) supports this hypothesis. When

Table 2. Risk Factors Potentiating Fibrinolysis

Acute anxiety
Physical exercise
Coffee
Alcohol
Miscellaneous foods

histochemical studies were carried out on atherosclerotic vessels, it was observed that the endothelium covering an atherosclerotic plaque was richer in fibrinolytic activity than the normal endothelium (35). The author speculated that such activity could inhibit thrombosis on an atheromatous plaqte. Thus, the incidence of thrombosis in atheromatous vessels might be much greater if increased local fibrinolysis did not exist.

Effect of Inhibition of Fibrinolysis on Experimental Atheroma Formation. Several studies on the effect of inhibition of fibrinolysis on the experimental production of atherosclerosis have been reported (36-38). When experimental animals were fed an atherogenic diet, the addition of an inhibitor of fibrinolysis, epsilon aminocaproic acid or a purified preparation of a trypsin inhibitor derived from peanuts, resulted in enhancement of aortic intimal hyperplasia along with an acceleration in atherogenesis and atheroma formation.

CONCLUSION

Evidence presented in this paper indicates that fibrinolytic activity may be impaired locally or systemically by various factors that are associated with a high risk for atherogenesis. Experimental atherogenesis was also observed to be enhanced by the administration of various inhibitors of fibrinolysis. It would seem that these findings tend to support the hypothesis of Rokitansky. However, direct evidence of a protective role for fibrinolysis is lacking. An experimental model for the study of the effect of a long-term enhanced fibrinolytic state on atherogenesis is not presently available.

REFERENCES

1. von Rokitansky, C. (1852) Manual of Pathological Anatomy, Vol. 3, Sydenham Soc., London, p. 261.

2. Duguid, J.B. (1946) J. Path. Bact. 58, 207-212.

3. Morgan, A.D. (1962) Cardiologia 40, 77-96.

4. Astrup, T. (1964) Minnesota Med. 47, 373-382.

5. Astrup, T., and Buluk, K. (1963) Circulation Res. 13, 253-256.

6. Papilian, M., and Nita, I. (1975) Rev. Roum. Med. - Med. Int. 13, 95-103.

7. Papilian, M., and Nita, I. (1975) Rev. Roum. Med. - Med. Int. 13, 271-282.

8. Billimoria, J.D., Pozner, H., Metselaar, B., Best, F.W., and James, D.C.O. (1975) Atheroscl. 21, 61-76.

9. Korsan-Bengtsen, K., Wilhelmsen, L., and Tibblin, G. (1972) Thromb. Diath. Haemorrh. 28, 99-108.

10. Engelberg, H. (1965) JAMA 193, 1033-1035.

11. Levine, P.H. (1973) Circulation 48, 619-623.

12. Mustard, J.F., and Murphy, E.A. (1963) Br. Med. J. 1, 846-849.

13. Moschos, C.B., Ahmed, S.S., Lahiri, K., and Regan, T.J. (1976) Atheroscl. 23, 437-442.

14. Grace, C.S., and Goldrick, R.B. (1968) J. Atheroscl. Res. 8, 705-719.

15. Andersen, P. (1976) Acta Med. Scand. 200, 289-291.

16. Egeberg, O. (1963) Scand. J. Clin. Lab. Invest. 15, 533-538.

17. Valdorf-Hanson, F. (1967) Acta Med. Scand. Suppl. 476, 147-157.

18. Ferguson, J.C., Mackay, N., Philip, J.A.D., and Sumner, D.J. (1973) Brit. J. Haemat. 25, 545.

19. Fearnley, G.R., Chakrabarti, R., and Avis, P.R. (1963) Br. Med. J. 1, 921-923.

20. Almer, L., and Nilsson, I.M. (1975) Acta Med. Scand. 198, 101-106.

21. Ganrot, P.O., Gydell, K., and Ekelund, H. (1967) Acta Endocrin. 55, 537-544.

22. Shaw, S., Pegrum, G.D., Wolff, S., and Ashton, W.L. (1967) J. Clin. Path. 20, 845-847.

23. Hellem, A.J. (1971) Acta Med. Scand. 190, 219-295.

24. Heath, H., Brigden, W.D., Canever, J.V., Pollock, J., Hunter, P.R., Kelsey, J., and Bloom, A. (1971) Diabetologia 7, 308-315.

25. Kwaan, H.C., Colwell, J.A., and Suwanwela, N. (1972) J. Lab. Clin. Med. 80, 236-246.

26. Sagel, K., Colwell, J.A., Crook, L., and Laiminis, M. (1975) Ann. Int. Med. 82, 733-738.

27. Kwaan, H.C. (1977) in The Significance of Platelet Function Tests in the Evaluation of Hemostasis and Thrombotic Tendencies (Day, H.J., Zucker, M.B. and Holmsen, H., Eds.). In press.

28. Biggs, R., Macfarlane, R.G., and Pilling, J. (1947) Lancet 1, 402-207.

29. Kwaan, H.C., Lo, R., and McFadzean, A.J.S. (1958) Clin. Sci. 17, 361-368.

30. Epstein, S.E., Rosing, D.R., Brakman, P., Redwood, D.R., and Astrup, T. (1970) Lancet 2, 631-634.

31. Kwaan, H.C., Lo, R., and McFadzean, A.J.S. (1957) Clin. Sci. 16, 241-253.

32. Kwaan, H.C., Lo, R., and McFadzean, A.J.S. (1958) Br. J. Haem. 4, 51-62.

33. Kwaan, H.C. (1969) in Dynamics of Thrombus Formation and Dissolution (Johnson, S.A. and Guest, M.M., Eds.) Lippincott, Philadelphia, pp. 340-349.

34. Kwaan, H.C. (1969) in Dynamics of Thrombus Formation and Dissolution (Johnson, S.A. and Guest, M.M., Eds.) Lippincott, Philadelphia, pp. 116-120.

35. Kwaan, H.C., and Astrup, T. (1967) Circ. Res. 21, 799-804.

36. Kwaan, H.C., and Astrup, T. (1964) Arch. Path. 78, 474-482.

37. Naimi, S., Loncin, H., Wilgram, G.F., and Proger, S. (1962) Abstracts of IV World Congress of Cardiology, Mexico, p. 258.

38. Coccheri, S. (1962) Boll. Soc. Ital. Biol. Sper. 38, 64-68.

HYPERCHOLESTEROLEMIA AND PLATELETS

Robert S. Lees and Angelina C.A. Carvalho

Arteriosclerosis Center
Massachusetts Institute of Technology
Cambridge, Massachusetts

Many lines of evidence have linked the circulating plasma lipoproteins with thrombosis, and both with atherosclerosis. Many theories of atherogenesis include mural thrombosis as one of the inciting factors, or the sole inciting factor, for atherosclerotic plaque formation. Clinically, elevated plasma lipids and increased concentrations of circulating lipoproteins have been known for years to predispose to early and severe atherosclerosis and its thrombotic complications. Familial hypercholesterolemia (Type II hyperlipoproteinemia) in particular, especially in the homozygous state, is associated with a very high incidence of premature, severe, and often generalized atherosclerosis (1). Over the past 7 years, we have studied the relationships among hyperlipoproteinemia, platelet function, soluble coagulation parameters, and clinical evidence of atherosclerosis and thrombosis. Our results suggest that patients with Type II hyperlipoproteinemia have a particular predisposition to thrombosis because of increased platelet function, both in comparison with normal subjects, and with patients with other forms of hyperlipoproteinemia. Laboratory studies suggest that these differences may be mediated through alterations in platelet fatty acid metabolism in hypercholesterolemia, particularly in thromboxane formation from arachidonate. In this paper, we shall review our data on platelet function in hyperlipoproteinemia.

METHODS AND MATERIALS

Subjects

Seventy-five subjects have formed the basis of our investigations. Of these, 26 were normal, 35 had Type II hyperlipopro-

teinemia and 14 had Type IV hyperlipoproteinemia. All of the
subjects with Type II and most of those with Type IV hyperlipoproteinemia had at least 1 blood relative with documented hyperlipoproteinemia or xanthomatosis. Each patient had a medical
history and physical examination, with particular attention to
previous atherosclerotic complications, present symptomatic state
of atherosclerosis, and the presence or absence of stigmata of
hypercholesterolemia. All patients had electrocardiograms. In
many patients coronary, cerebral, or peripheral angiograms were
available. Finally, many were followed for periods of 5 years or
longer and the incidence of atherosclerosis and its thrombotic
complications observed. All patients had fasting blood lipid
estimations (2) on at least 2 occasions, and all had qualitative
assessment of the plasma lipoprotein pattern by paper electrophoresis (3, 4). Many had quantitative lipoprotein estimations
by the technique of preparative ultracentrifugation and polyanion
precipitation (2). The normal subjects had fasting plasma lipids
and lipoprotein electrophoreses which were within normal limits.
All subjects had no medications for at least 15 days before
platelet and coagulation studies, except when specific therapeutic agents were under investigation. Nearly all of the patients
with hyperlipoproteinemia were on low cholesterol diets, with
varying adherence; the normal subjects were on free diet. As a
crude estimate of the relationship between laboratory findings
and atherothrombotic events, the incidence of clinical events involving thrombosis or embolism in the patient groups with Type II
and Type IV hyperlipoproteinemia was compared retrospectively by
dividing the number of events for each patient by the number of
months of patient follow-up in our clinic, to obtain the number
of events per month (5). Cerebral thrombosis or embolus, acute
myocardial infarction, peripheral arterial thrombosis and embolus,
and thrombophlebitis were considered as thromboembolic events.

   Blood sampling. Venous blood was collected with a silicon-
ized needle and plastic syringes. Nine volumes of blood were added
to 1 volume of 3.8% sodium citrate (final concentration 0.013M)
in plastic tubes.

   Preparation of platelet rich and platelet poor plasma. Blood
samples were centrifuged at 23° for 10 minutes at 100g; the resulting platelet rich plasma (PRP) had a platelet count by Coulter
counter of 180,000-330,000/μ liter. The remaining blood was centrifuged at 3000g for 15 minutes at 4°. The platelet count of the
resulting platelet poor plasma (PPP) was less than 20,000/μ liter.

   Platelet aggregation studies. Platelet aggregation was studied at 37° according to a modification (6) of the method of Born
(7). The details of the assay are published elsewhere (6, 8).
The aggregating agents studied included ADP (which was stored
frozen at a concentration of $5 \times 10^{-4}M$ in 0.1M sodium phosphate

buffer, pH 6.8, containing 0.15M NaCl), L-epinephrine (2.5×10^{-3}M), and acid soluble calfskin collagen (5.5 µg/ml).

Platelet nucleotide release was studied by a modification (6) of the procedure of Wolfe and Shulman (9).

Platelet lipid analysis. Washed platelets were extracted with redistilled chloroform:methanol (2:1), and the phases split with dilute aqueous sulfuric acid (1:2000). The upper phase was discarded. After removal of the solvents from the lower phase by drying under nitrogen, cholesterol and triglycerides were determined by Auto Analyzer (3) and phospholipid classes were separated by thin layer chromatography, as described by Skipski et al. (11). Prostaglandin and thromboxane production by platelets was determined as described elsewhere (12).

RESULTS

In comparison with normal subjects, patients with Type II hyperlipoproteinemia had platelets which were more sensitive to aggregation with ADP, epinephrine and collagen (Figure 1). Platelets from patients with Type IV had slight hypersensitivity to epinephrine but their response to ADP and collagen was unremarkable. Similarly, nucleotide release in response to these aggregating stimuli was greater than normal for Type II platelets, but not significantly different from normal for platelets from Type IV subjects (Figure 2). The phospholipid content of the Type II and Type IV patients' platelets was greater than normal, but so was their cholesterol content, so that the free cholesterol:phospholipid ratios were not significantly different from normal (Table 1). When the individual phospholipids were examined, their relative concentrations were not greatly altered: a mild relative increase in phosphatidyl inositol in both Type II and Type IV platelets (Table 2) was the most striking difference from normal (p<0.01).

When incubated with an excess of ^{14}C-arachidonic acid, platelets from Type II subjects converted much more of it to thromboxane A_2 at 30 seconds than did normal platelets; after 5 minutes of incubation, thromboxane A_2 concentration, although much lower than at 30 seconds, was twice as high in Type II as in normal platelets. The platelets from Type IV subjects showed only an increase in HETE production after 5 minutes of incubation.

DISCUSSION

Our results demonstrate that platelets from subjects with Type II hyperlipoproteinemia are different from normal in a number of respects. Their response to standard aggregating stimuli is

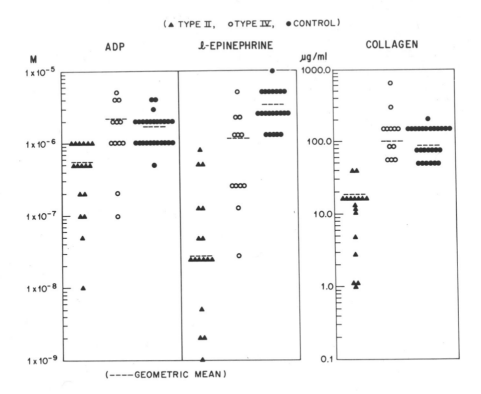

Figure 1. Platelet Aggregation in Patients with Type II Hyperlipoproteinemia. The ordinate represents the minimum concentrations
(logarithmic scale) necessary for full response to each aggregating
agent. The dashed lines represent the geometric mean for each
group. (Reprinted from Reference 6 by permission of the New England
Journal of Medicine.)

abnormal and reflects increased in vitro sensitivity to aggregation.
Platelet nucleotide release is also abnormally increased to a remarkable degree. Platelet content of both cholesterol (which is essentially all free cholesterol) and total phospholipids is increased,
but the free cholesterol:phospholipid ratio is not different from
normal. Although the percentage concentration of phosphatidyl
inositol is somewhat increased in Type II platelets, it is also
increased in platelets from patients with Type IV hyperlipoproteinemia, which do not behave abnormally, except for slight hypersensitivity to epinephrine.

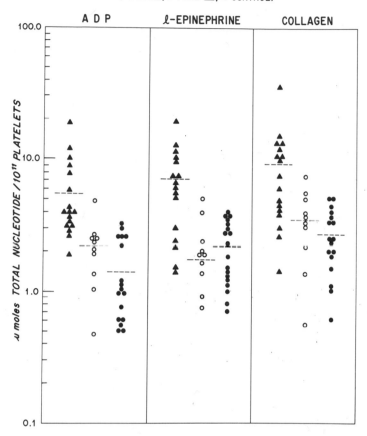

Figure 2. Platelet Nucleotide Release in Hyperlipoproteinemia.
The ordinate represents the concentration of total nucleotides
released. Adenosine diphosphate, 1-epinephrine and acid-soluble
collagen were employed at concentrations designated in the Methods
section. The dashed lines represent the geometric mean for each
group. (Reprinted from Reference 6 by permission of the New England Journal of Medicine.)

    We conclude from these data that the platelet hypersensitivity
to aggregation which is characteristic of Type II hyperlipropro-
teinemia is probably not due to any gross abnormality of platelet
lipid composition.

    Two reservations must be expressed about overinterpretation
of our data, however. With regard to the hypersensitivity of

Table 1. Platelet Free Cholesterol:Phospholipid Ratio

Normal Subjects	Type II Patients	Type IV Patients
	Mean ± standard deviation	
0.54 ± 0.07	0.58 ± 0.12	0.52 ± 0.11

Table 2. Relative Platelet Phospholipid Concentration

	Type II	Type IV
	Percent of normal	
Unidentified Polar Phospholipids	100	115
Lysolecithin	100	100
Sphingomyelin	85	100
Lecithin	100	100
Phosphatidyl Inositol	125	125
Phosphatidyl Serine	100	90
Phosphatidyl Ethanolamine	100	100

platelets from patients with hypercholesterolemia, these data are
based on in vitro assays and extrapolation to the in vivo situation
is potentially hazardous. On the other hand, Steele and Rainwater
have recently performed platelet kinetic studies in otherwise
healthy human subjects with hypercholesterolemia and shown that
platelet survival is decreased (13). Furthermore, the incidence
of apparently thrombotic clinical events (as defined under Methods)
was more than twice as great in our Type II than in our Type IV
patients (5). Lastly, Type II patients have evidence of prekal-
likrein activation and high levels of circulating soluble fibrin
complexes, other findings which are consistent with platelet-
mediated activation of the intrinsic coagulation system (5, 14).

The second reservation is with regard to the lipid composition of Type II platelets. We have not specifically isolated and
analyzed the platelet membranes to determine whether their composition and cholesterol:phospholipid ratio differs from normal.

As Dr. Colman will tell us later in the Workshop, this may be the case.

Because the changes we observed in platelet lipid composition did not appear to be an adequate explanation for the observed changes in function, we studied the metabolism of arachidonic acid in search of a mechanism by which platelets from hypercholesterolemic subjects might be rendered hypersensitive to aggregation. Platelet aggregation is known to be mediated by cyclic derivatives of arachidonic acid, particularly thromboxane A$_2$ (15). Furthermore, plasma cholesterol esters contain linoleic acid, the metabolic precursor of arachidonic acid, as their major fatty acid, and the plasma concentration of cholesterol esters is, of course, elevated in Type II hyperlipoproteinemia. Our analyses of platelet fatty acid composition are still in progress. However, when an excess of radiolabeled exogenous arachidonic acid was added to platelet suspensions, platelets from hypercholesterolemic patients produced significantly more thromboxane A$_2$ than did either normal or Type IV patients' platelets. These preliminary findings suggest to us that the hypersensitivity of platelets from Type II patients may be mediated by increased production of thromboxane A$_2$. Whether this is secondary to an adaptive increase in the enzymes leading to thromboxane production because of greater substrate availability in vivo, or is an inherited defect, remains to be determined.

In summary, platelet lipid composition and platelet function in patients with Type II hyperlipoproteinemia are both abnormal. Comparison with platelets from patients with Type IV hyperlipoproteinemia suggests that the functional differences are not due to gross changes in platelet lipid composition. Preliminary data suggests, in contrast, that the platelet hypersensitivity of Type II hyperlipoproteinemia is mediated via abnormalities in platelet metabolism of arachidonic acid and its derivatives.

REFERENCES

1. Lees, R.S., Wilson, D.E., Schonfeld, G., and Fleet, S. (1973) Prog. Med. Genetics 9, 237-290.

2. Hatch, F.T., and Lees, R.S. (1968) Adv. in Lipid Res. 6, 1-68.

3. Lees, R.S., and Hatch, F.T. (1963) J. Lab. Clin. Med. 61, 518-528.

4. Fredrickson, D.S., and Lees, R.S. (1965) Circulation 31, 321-327.

5. Carvalho, A.C., Lees, R.S., Vaillancourt, R.A., and Colman, R.W. (1977) Circulation 56, 114-118.

6. Carvalho, A.C., Colman, R.W., and Lees, R.S. (1974) N. Engl. J. Med. 290, 434-438.

7. Born, G.V.R. (1962) Nature (Lond.) 194, 927-929.

8. Carvalho, A.C., Colman, R.W., and Lees, R.S. (1974) Circulation 50, 570-574.

9. Wolfe, S.M., and SHulman, N.R. (1970) Biochem. Biophys. Res. Comm. 41, 128-234.

10. Bartlett, G.R. (1959) J. Biol. Chem. 234, 466-468.

11. Skipski, V.P., Peterson, R.F., and Barclay, M. (1964) Biochem. J. 90, 374-378.

12. Bizios, R., Wong, L.K., Vaillancourt, R., Lees, R.S., and Carvalho, A.C. (1977) Thrombosis and Haemostasis 38, 228.

13. Steele, P., and Rainwater, J. (1977) Circulation 56 (III), 120.

14. Carvalho, A.C., Lees, R.S., Vaillancourt, R.A., Cabral, R.B., Weinberg, R.M., and Colman, R.W. (1976) Thromb. Res. 8, 843-857.

15. Hamberg, M., Svenson, J., and Samuelsson, B. (1975) Proc. Nat. Acad. Sci. USA 72, 2994-2998.

PILOT EPIDEMIOLOGICAL STUDIES IN THROMBOSIS

James M. Iacono and Rita M. Dougherty
Lipid Nutrition Laboratory
Nutrition Institute, ARS
U.S. Department of Agriculture
Beltsville, Maryland USA

Rodolfo Paoletti and Claudio Galli
Istituto di Farmacologia e di Farmacognosia
Universita di Milano
Milan, Italy

Angelina C.A. Carvalho
Special Clotting Laboratory
Massachusetts General Hospital
Boston, Massachusetts USA

Anna Ferro-Luzzi
Istituto Nazionale della Nutrizione
Via Lancisi
Rome, Italy

Donald G. Therriault and Gary J. Nelson
Division of Blood Diseases and Resources
National Heart, Lung, and Blood Institute
National Institutes of Health
Bethesda, Maryland USA

Ancel Keys
School of Public Health
University of Minnesota
Minnesota, Minnesota USA

The role of nutrition in haemostasis and thrombosis is still relatively undefined. Recently, however, there has been modest activity in the study of the relationship between dietary fats and thrombosis (1). Present knowledge is limited and there is a question as to whether or not ingested dietary fats alter the mechanism of coagulation to a degree that would induce a hypercoagulable state.

In an early report, Thomas and Hartroft (2) related nutrition to the clotting mechanism. They induced spontaneous thrombosis in rats by feeding them a diet that was rich in saturated fat and cholesterol and included thiouracil and cholic acid. Hartroft and O'Neal (3) found that rats fed diets supplemented with cocoa butter or butter developed thrombi, generally in the cardiac cavities and coronary arteries, but rats fed plant oils, such as cottonseed or corn oil, did not. Other investigators have made similar observations in rats (4-6), rabbits (7), and pigs (8-9). From the many studies of animals, Renaud and Gautheron (10) concluded that diets with high contents of saturated fat appeared to predispose animals to thrombosis.

The purpose of this study was to investigate the influence of dietary fats on the lipids of plasma, red blood cells, and platelets and to determine the relationship between any changes detected and the functional activity of platelets. A study also was made of the conversion of arachidonic acid to prostaglandin derivatives in platelets. Rural areas in three countries were selected for a pilot study in thrombosis as related to the kinds and levels of dietary fats and to the rates of mortality from coronary heart disease (11). The study was conducted on farmers in the vicinities of Canino, Italy; Nurmijarvi, Finland; and Beltsville, Maryland, USA. This is a preliminary report of one phase of the study and is not intended to be complete in terms of presentation and interpretation of the data.

PROCEDURES AND METHODS

Selection of Subjects

General. The Italian part of the study took place at Canino in the Province of Viterbo, 100 km north of Rome in the spring of 1976. The area had a population of 5,000 and was located in an agricultural district of medium income level. The main product of the locality is olive oil. Census lists were used to identify the inhabitants in the correct age group with the preferred occupation and medical history. The subjects were interviewed about their drinking, smoking, and eating habits. The general health of each was evaluated by medical examination. Rejection rate was high, mainly because of smoking habits. Twenty-four subjects were finally selected for the dietary survey, and blood samples were taken from 20 of them.

The Finnish part of the study took place at Nurmijarvi County, 37 km northeast of Helsinki during the summer of 1976. The population of the area was about 18,500. Of these, about 15% were employed in agricultural or forestry-related jobs. From census lists, names were selected on the basis of age and occupation as possible subjects. After contact by telephone, 40 subjects were chosen for further screening, and 29 subjects were selected. Blood samples were taken from 21 subjects.

The American phase of the study took place north of the Washington, D.C. metropolitan area in late autumn of 1976. The subjects were located on farms 45 to 75 km from the Beltsville Agricultural Research Center, near the towns of Ellicott City, Damascus and Frederick. Of the population of the Washington area, only 0.5% worked on farms; this area was chosen for its accessibility. By initial screening with the aid of USDA County Agents, Farm Bureau Directories and Cooperative Farm Credit Associations, possible subjects were identified. Of 43 eligible subjects, 21 were chosen, and blood samples were taken from all.

Dietary survey. In view of the specific purpose of the study and the need for reliable and precise data on individual nutrient intakes (12-14), specifically of fatty acids, a method of survey that would guarantee a high degree of standardization was essential. Therefore a precise weighing method (15) was adopted.

All foods eaten by the subjects during 7 consecutive days were weighed before cooking and also immediately before consumption. For combinations of ingredients, each ingredient was weighed before cooking, and the individual portions were weighed after cooking. Weights of leftovers were subtracted from the original weights of cooked portions. Care was taken to insure that foods eaten away from home were reported.

Hematology and chemical analyses. Blood was collected by the same investigator in each of the three locations. Platelets, red blood cells, and plasma were prepared by standardized procedures. Platelet aggregation was studied in aggregometers (PAP-2), provided by BioData Corp. (Hatboro, PA), according to a modification of the method of Born (16). Platelet ^{14}C-serotonin release was measured after platelet-rich plasma was incubated with 0.8 μ Ci of ^{14}C-serotonin for 25 minutes at 37° according to the method of Jerushalmy and Zucker (17). Protein, cholesterol, triglyceride, and phospholipid were determined by standard methods (18-23). Thin-layer chromatography (24-25) was used to separate lipid classes (26) and fatty acid methylesters of lipid fractions were prepared (27-28) and analyzed by gas-liquid chromatography. The conversion of arachidonic acid in platelets (29-31) was also studied.

RESULTS AND DISCUSSION

Anthropometry and dietary survey. The physical character-istics of the subjects showed that average heights of the American and Finnish farmers were about the same (Table 1), but the range was wide (160 to 194 cm) for the latter. The Italian subjects were the shortest and also weighed the least.

Table 1. Physical characteristics and blood pressures of the subjects in the three experimental areas[1,2]

	Area		
	Canino	Nurmijarvi	Beltsville
Age, yrs	$43.0 \pm 1.9^{a,b}$	42.9 ± 0.4^{a}	44.2 ± 0.3^{b}
Weight, kg	74.3 ± 1.8^{a}	81.3 ± 2.5^{b}	83.9 ± 2.8^{b}
Height, cm	167.9 ± 1.1^{a}	176.3 ± 1.8^{b}	176.5 ± 1.4^{b}
Body Fat, %[3]	23.5 ± 0.8^{a}	21.7 ± 1.1^{a}	30.0 ± 0.7^{b}
Blood Pressure, mm Hg			
Systolic	125.3 ± 1.7^{a}	136.2 ± 2.6^{b}	123.6 ± 1.2^{a}
Diastolic	79.7 ± 1.9^{a}	90.4 ± 1.4^{b}	78.0 ± 1.3^{a}

[1] Each value represents the mean $\pm$ SEM of n = 24 in Canino; n = 29 in Nurmijarvi; and n = 21 in Beltsville.

[2] Within a line, means not sharing a common letter superscript are significantly different (P<0.05).

[3] Durnin, J., and Womersley, J. (1974), Br. J. Nutr. 32, 77.

COMPOSITION OF DIETS

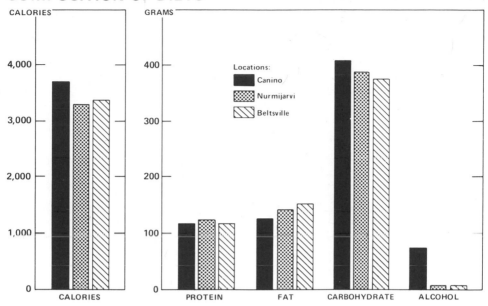

Figure 1. Average daily intakes. Each bar represents the mean intake for 7 consecutive days per subject; n = 168 in Canino; n = 203 in Nurmijarvi; and n = 147 in Beltsville.

The farmers from Beltsville weighed more than the other groups and this was clearly reflected in their total body fat of 30% (32). For Finnish and Italian farmers, body fat was 22 and 24% respectively, values which are within the ranges observed in most technologically developed countries for their age group. Systolic and diastolic blood pressures were highest for the Finnish farmers.

Average daily intakes of energy, protein, fat, carbohydrate and alcohol for the three groups of subjects are shown in Figure 1. Total protein intakes were about 120 grams per day in the three localities. Values usually are similar in developed countries, and greatly exceed the RDA's. The total fat intake was lowest, 129 grams per days, in the Italian diet and highest, 151 grams per day, in the USA diet. The daily intake of fat by the Finnish farmers, 144 grams per day, was slightly less than the intake by the Americans.

One unique aspect of the Italian diet was the high alcohol intake, 73 grams per day, as opposed to 5 grams per day for the other two groups. Most of the excess calories consumed by the

CALORIES FROM DIETS

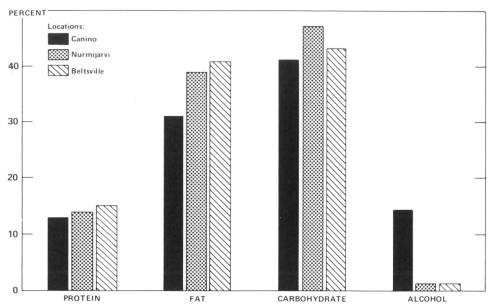

Figure 2. Percent of energy derived from different sources in the diets.

Italian farmers could be attributed to their high alcohol intake. Energy intake was highest for Italians, 3690 calories, and was lower for Finns and Americans, 3293 and 3354 calories, respectively. Energy intake, in calories per kg body weight, was 50 for Italians and 41 and 40 for the Finns and Americans, respectively.

Fat provided 32% of the total caloric intake in Canino and about 40% in both Finland and the USA (Figure 2). Total intake of saturated fatty acids was highest in the Finnish diet (80 g/day), lowest in the Italian diet (32 g/day), and intermediate in the American diet (59 g/day). Total intake of unsaturated fatty acids averaged 84, 77 and 57 grams per day, respectively, for American, Italian and Finnish farmers (Figure 3). Total saturated fatty acids contributed 7.8%, 12.8% and 15.7% of total energy, respectively, in Canino, Nurmijarvi and Beltsville. Unsaturated fatty acids contributed a similar amount, 20%, of total energy to the diets in Canino and Beltsville, and 16% to diets in Nurmijarvi. Monoenoic fatty acids represented 15.8% and 16.1% of total calories in Canino and Beltsville and slightly less (14%) in Nurmijarvi. In the Italian diet the primary monoenoic fatty acid was oleic acid, whereas, in the American diet the monoenoic acids

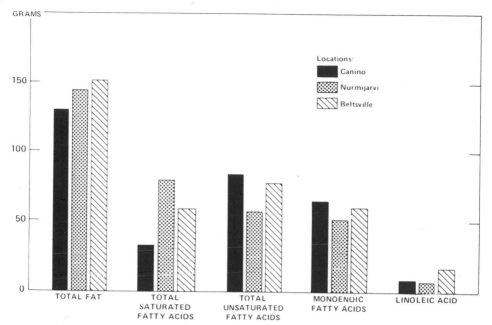

Figure 3. Fatty acid composition of diets. (See Figure 1 for numbers of observations.)

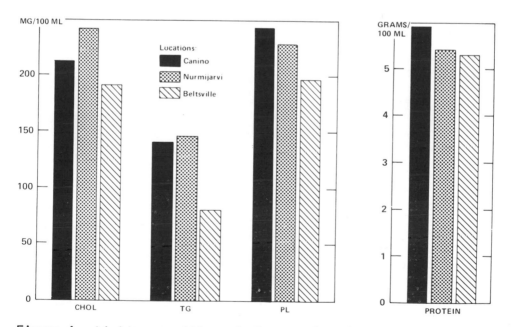

Figure 4. Lipid composition of plasma. Each bar represents the mean of 20 subjects in Canino, 21 subjects in Nurmijarvi and 21 subjects in Beltsville.

were a mixture of oleic and elaidic acids. The elaidic acid was
provided by margarines. The energy derived from linoleic acid was
lowest in Nurmijarvi at 1.7% and highest in Beltsville at 4.4%.

Analyses of the composited diets to determine their lipid
composition showed that actual values were essentially the same
as calculated values, except for oleic acid in the Italian diet.
That actual value was strikingly higher (55.7%) than the calculated value.

Lipids in plasma, red blood cells and platelets. Plasma
lipids are summarized in Figure 4. Plasma protein levels were
within the normal range for the three areas studied but were highest in the samples from Canino. Total cholesterol in plasma was
highest in Finnish (241 mg%), lowest in American (191 mg%), and
intermediate in the Canino samples (213 mg%). The high total
cholesterol level in the plasma samples from Finland reflected
the high saturated fat content of the Finnish diet. The high
polyunsaturated fat intake by the Americans in this study might
explain their low plasma cholesterol levels. Plasma triglyceride
values were similar for subjects in Canino and Nurmijarvi, and
exceeded the values for subjects in Beltsville. Levels of plasma
phospholipids were lower for the American group than for the
other two groups.

The distribution of phospholipids in platelets was variable
(Figure 5). For sphingomyelin (SPH) and phosphatidylinositol (PI)
fractions of platelets, the levels were lower in samples from
Nurmijarvi than in samples from Canino and Beltsville. In platelets, phosphatidylcholine (PC) was lowest in samples from Beltsville and phosphatidylethanolamine (PE) was highest in those from
Nurmijarvi and lowest in those from Canino. The phosphatidylserine
(PS) fraction of platelets did not differ significantly among
samples from the three areas. Differences among classes of phospholipids, except for PS, have been observed in dietary studies;
however, significant differences in PS have not been observed
(33-35) in either man or animals.

The differences in the fatty acid composition of cholesterol
esters and PC in plasma generally reflected differences in the
fatty acid composition of the diets in the three areas (Figure
6). The saturated fatty acids were highest in cholesterol esters
in the plasma samples from Nurmijarvi. The amounts of monounsaturated fatty acids in the cholesterol esters and PC of plasma from
Canino reflected the high level of 18:1 in the Italian diet. The
polyunsaturated fatty acids were highest in the cholesterol esters
and PC of plasma and in the diets of the Beltsville subjects.

The fatty acid composition of the glycerophospholipids of
red blood cells (Figure 7) also was influenced by diet. Levels

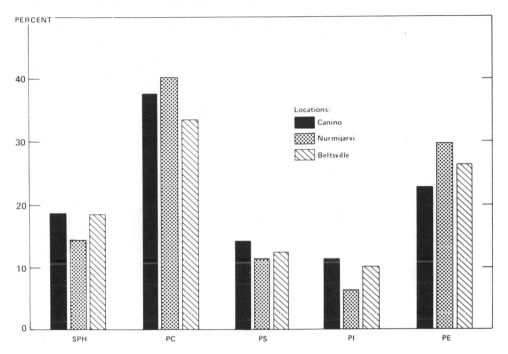

Figure 5. Distribution of phospholipids in platelets. (See
Figure 4 for numbers of observations.) Sph - sphingomyelin, PC -
phosphatidylcholine, PS - phosphatidylserine, PI - phosphatidylinositol, and PE - phosphatidylethanolamine.

of total saturated fatty acids were highest in PC, PS and PE of
red blood cells from Nurmijarvi where the dietary intake of
saturated fat was highest. Total monounsaturated fatty acids were
highest in the glycerophospholipids of red blood cells in the
samples from Italians and also were highest in the Italian diets.
The influence of the high intake of dietary polyunsaturated fatty
acids of the farmers near Beltsville was reflected in the polyunsaturated fatty acids in the glycerophospholipids of their red
blood cells.

     Fatty acid analysis of the glycerophospholipids in platelets
(Figure 8) showed that in PC and PS levels of saturated fatty
acids were higher for samples from Nurmijarvi than for those from
Canino and Beltsville. In all glycerophospholipids of platelets,
monounsaturated fatty acids were highest in samples from Canino.

Phosphatidylcholine

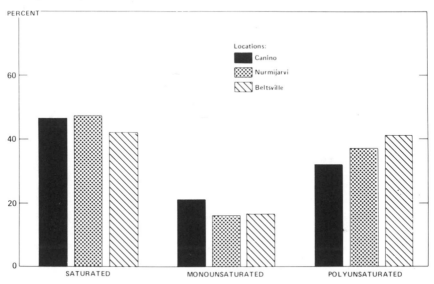

Cholesterol Esters

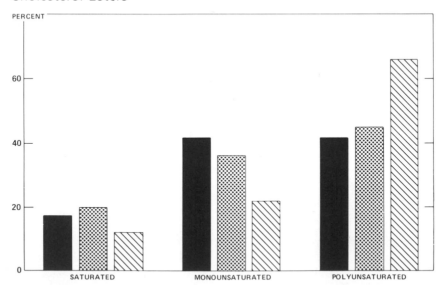

Figure 6. Major fatty acid groups in phosphatidylcholine and cholesterol esters of plasma.

Phosphatidylcholine

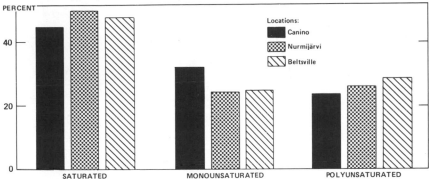

Phosphatidylserine

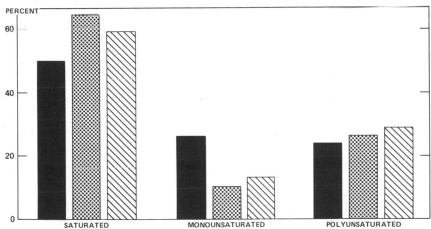

Phosphatidylethanolamine

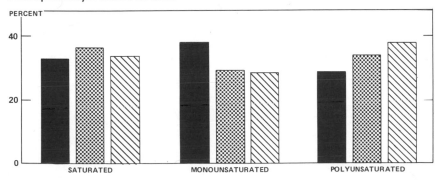

Figure 7. Major fatty acid groups in the glycerophospholipids of red blood cells.

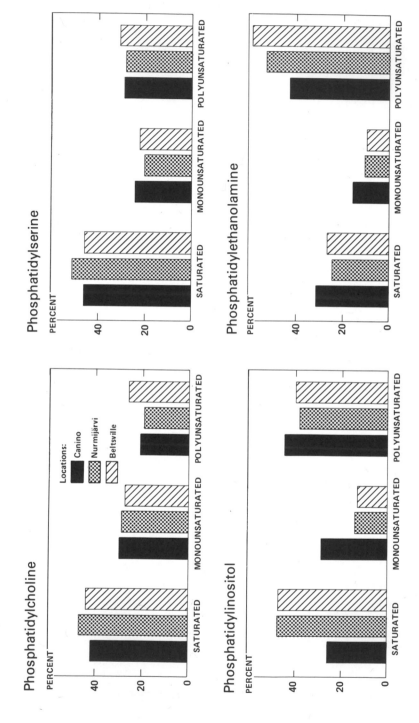

Figure 8. Major fatty acid groups in the glycerophospholipids of platelets.

Polyunsaturated fatty acids of the n-6 series were generally highest in the glycerophospholipids of platelets in samples from Beltsville.

The fatty acid patterns of plasma, red blood cell and platelet glycerophospholipids generally reflected the predominant fatty acids present in the diets.

Hematology. Responses of platelets from the three groups of subjects to aggregating agents are shown in Figure 9. All thresholds were determined on samples of platelet-rich plasma that had identical platelet counts. The amount of ADP required to produce similar platelet responses (% Transmittance) did not differ among areas. Threshold concentrations of epinephrine, collagen and thrombin did differ among areas. The platelets of the subjects from Nurmijarvi were most hypersensitive to epinephrine and thrombin and were least hypersensitive to collagen. Those findings agree, in general, with published data (36-40).

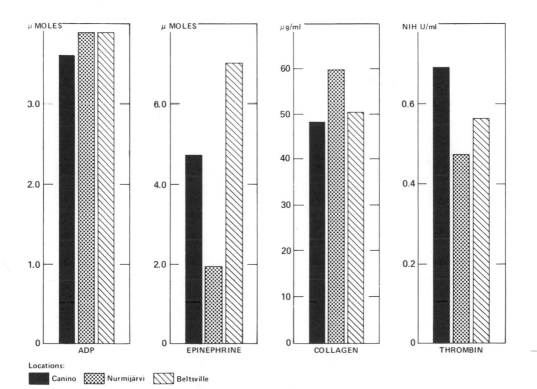

Figure 9. Threshold concentrations for aggregation of platelets. (See Figure 4 for numbers of observations.)

To obtain equivalent aggregation and ^{14}C-serotonin release, platelets from all three groups required similar concentrations of ADP (Figure 10). Less epinephrine was required by the samples from Nurmijarvi than was required by platelets from Canino and Beltsville to release equivalent amounts of ^{14}C-serotonin. Similar concentrations of collagen were required for total release by platelets from Canino and Nurmijarvi. Platelets from the Beltsville subjects were more hypersensitive to collagen than platelets from Nurmijarvi, but they did not differ from the samples from Canino. The platelets from the Beltsville group were more hypersensitive to thrombin than those from Canino.

Arachidonic acid conversion. The purpose of this part of the study was to investigate the formation of metabolic products, which arise in platelets from arachidonic acid (20:4), and have recently been correlated with the processes of platelet adhesion, aggregation and release. The phospholipids of platelets are very rich in 20:4, and phospholipase A_2 (PLA$_2$) in platelets (41) is

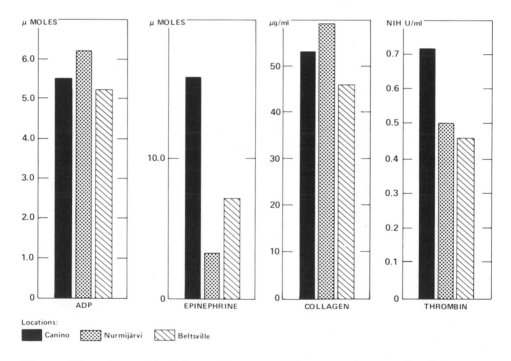

Figure 10. Concentrations of aggregating agents required for release of equal amounts of ^{14}C-serotonin from platelets. (See Figure 4 for numbers of observations.)

Table 2. Conversion of arachidonic acid to thromboxane[1] and products of lipoxygenase activity[2], and total conversion of arachidonic acid[3] after TLC and radioscanning of TLC zones[4,5]

	Area		
	Canino	Nurmijarvi	Beltsville
Thromboxanes[1]	34.3 + 1.9	33.2 + 1.4	33.7 + 1.5
Lipoxygenase products[2]	40.8 + 1.1[a]	48.8 + 0.9[b]	41.0 + 1.5[a]
Total conversion[3]	74.8 + 1.3[a]	80.6 + 1.3[b]	73.5 + 1/1[a]

[1]Thromboxanes = $\dfrac{\text{area of thromboxane} \times 100}{\text{Total area of peaks}}$

[2]Lipoxygenase products =

$\dfrac{\text{Total area of peaks - [area of 20:4 + area of thromboxanes]} \times 100}{\text{Total area of peaks}}$

[3]Total conversion of 20:4 =

$\dfrac{\text{Total area of peaks - area of 20:4} \times 100}{\text{Total area of peaks}}$

[4]Each value represents the mean + SEM of n = > 6 in Canino; n = > 12 in Nurmijarvi; and n = > 11 in Beltsville.

[5]Within a line, means not sharing a common letter superscript are significantly different ($P<0.05$).

activated during the sequence of events leading to aggregation. The availability of 20:4 appears to be a limiting factor in the activation of the prostaglandin system.

Platelets contain enzymes that convert 20:4 into cyclic endoperoxides, prostaglandins (E_2, $F_{2\alpha}$ and D) and thromboxanes (TXA_2 and TXB_2). Thromboxane A_2 is labile ($T_{\frac{1}{2}}$ = 30 seconds) and may be responsible for the contraction of the platelet microtubular system that facilitates the process of exocytosis by the cell.

Table 2 shows the values for total conversion of arachidonic acid for the formation of thromboxanes and hydroxy fatty acids. Platelets that had been stored frozen at -40° still actively metabolized 20:4. More than 70% of the substrate was converted to metabolic products. The overall conversion was uniform within each group of subjects. Total conversion of 20:4 was similar in platelets from American and Italian subjects, and was almost 10% higher in platelets from Finnish subjects.

Conversion by platelets of 20:4 to thromboxanes did not differ among samples from the three areas. Conversion of 20:4 to products of lipoxygenase activity (mainly hydroxy fatty acids with 20 carbon atoms) was about 20% higher in platelets of Finnish than in those of American or Italian subjects.

The differences in function among platelets from the three groups were not explained by the equal production of thromboxanes. The high level of hydroxy fatty acids formed by the platelets from the Finnish subjects might, however, indicate an increase in lipoxygenase activity. A product of 20:4 oxidation in platelets depresses the enzyme involved in the conversion of the prostaglandin endoperoxide into the newly discovered (42-43) prostacyclin. Prostacyclin is the most potent inhibitor of platelet aggregation and release and appears to be produced by endothelial cells as well as by other tissues. If this is the case, it is possible that physiologically, a reduced production of prostacyclin might explain the high reactivity of the platelets from the Finnish subjects to aggregating agents.

SUMMARY

Some differences in the blood of farmers in Nurmijarvi, Finland, Canino, Italy, and Beltsville, Maryland in the United States apparently were associated with differences, among the areas, in the farmers' diets. Those associations suggested that diets that are high in saturated fats (Nurmijarvi) could predispose humans to develop intravascular disease. Such predisposition has been observed in experimental animals. Low levels of the parameters that are considered active in such predisposition apparently were associated with diets that were low in saturated fats (Canino) or with diets that were low in saturated and high in unsaturated fats (Beltsville). Within the limits of the experimental design, the data from the three population groups indicated that a more comprehensive study might establish a relation between diet and intravascular disease in humans.

ACKNOWLEDGMENTS

We wish to thank all of the subjects, their wives and families for their support of the dietary survey and for providing valuable data and blood samples. For the dietary survey we wish to acknowledge the expert work done by Ms. Maria Stanghellini in Canino, Italy; Ms. Riitta Peltonen assisted by Maarit Ahola, Seija Rantio, Leena Rajala and Marja Mutanen in Nurmijarvi, Finland; and Ms. Margaret McIntyre assisted by Karyn Lieberman, Natalie Hardison and Janet Sandberg in Beltsville, Maryland, USA. We wish to thank Drs. M. Capoccia and V. Barbagli, Canino, Italy; Dr. M. Heliovaara, Nurmijarvi, Finland; and Dr. J.J. Canary, Georgetown University Medical Center, Washington, D.C., USA, for carrying out the physical examinations and local town officials for providing assistance in locating subjects for the study. We also wish to thank Dr. T. Suomela, Nurmijarvi terveyskeskus, for providing space in the medical clinic at Nurmijarvi. We gratefully acknowledge laboratory assistants who provided support and included Mr. Edward Matusik, Mr. David West, Ms. Pauline Giannusi, Mr. Raymond Vaillancourt, Mr. Howard Kwong and Ms. Elizabeth Agradi. We wish to thank Mr. James Mowder and Mr. Robert Kling of the Data Systems Application Division at the National Agricultural Library at Beltsville, Md., USA, for their support in handling the dietary survey information. In addition, we want to acknowledge the help of Professors Martti Karvonen and Maija Pekkarinen of Helsinki, Finland, for providing us with the support to carry out the Finnish part of the study.

REFERENCES

1. Dietary Fats and Thrombosis (1974) (Renaud, S. and Nordøy, A., Eds.), Basel, Karger.

2. Thomas, W.A., and Hartroft, W.S. (1959) Circulation, 19, 65.

3. Hartroft, W.S., and O'Neal, R.N. (1962) Am. J. Cardiol. 9, 335.

4. Gresham, G.A., and Howard, A.N. (1960) Br. J. Exp. Path. 41, 395.

5. Nordøy, A., and Chandler, A.B. (1964) Scand. J. Haemat. 1, 202.

6. Renaud, S., and Allard, C. (1962) Circulation Res. 11, 388.

7. Renaud, S., and Lecompte, F. (1970) Circulation Res. 27, 1003.

8. Mustard, J.F., and Murphy, E.A. (1962) Br. Med. J. 1, 1651.

9. Mustard, J.F., Rowsell, H.C., Murphy, E.A., and Downie, H.G. (1963) J. Clin. Invest. 42, 1783.

10. Renaud, S., and Gautheron, P. (1974) Haemostasis, 2, 53.

11. Keys, A. (1975) Atheroscl. 22, 149.

12. Carnovale, E., and Miuccio, F.C. (1976) Tabelle di Composizione degli Alimenti, Istituto Nazionale della Nutrizione, Roma, Italia.

13. Seppanen, R., Hasunen, K., Pekkarinen, M., and Backstrom, L.A. (1976) Autoklinikan ravintotutkimuksen seuranta vuosina 1973-1975, Suunnitelma, toteutus ja menetelmat, Helsinki, Finland.

14. Watt, B.K., and Merrill, A.C. (1963) Composition of Foods, USDA Handbook No. 8.

15. Marr, J.W. (1971) World Rev. of Nutr. and Dietet. 13, 105.

16. Born, G.F.R. (1962) Nature (Lond.), 194, 927.

17. Jerushalmy, Z., and Zucker, M.B. (1966) Thromb. Diath. Haemorrh. 15, 413.

18. Lowry, O.H., Rosebrough, N.J., Farr, L., and Randall, R.J. (1951) J. Biol. Chem. 193, 265.

19. Block, W.D., Jarrett, J.R., and Levine, J.B. (1966) Clin. Chem. 12, 681.

20. Kessler, G., and Lederer, H. (1965) Automation in Analytical Chemistry (Skeggs, L.T., Ed.) New York, p. 341.

21. Rouser, G., Fleisher, S., and Yamomoto, A. (1970) Lipids, 5, 494.

22. Abell, L.L., Levy, B.B., Brodie, B.B., and Kendall, F.E. (1952) J. Biol. CHem. 195, 357.

23. Bartlett, G. (1959) J. Biol. Chem. 214, 466.

24. Mangold, H.K., and Malins, D.C. (1960) J.A.O.C.S. 37, 383.

25. Skipski, V.P., Peterson, R.F., and Barclay, M. (1964) Biochem. J. 90, 374.

26. Folch, J., Lees, M., and Sloane-Stanley, G.H. (1957) J. Biol. Chem. 226, 497.

27. Christie, W.W. (1972) _Analyst_, 97, 221.

28. Stoffel, W., Chu, F., and Ahrens, E.H., Jr. (1959) _Analyt. Chem._ 31, 307.

29. Hamberg, M., and Samuelsson, B. (1974) _Proc. Nat. Acad. Sci. USA_, 71, 3400.

30. Billimoria, J.D., Fahmy, M.F., Jepson, E.M., and MacLagan, N.F. (1971) _Atheroscl._ 14, 359.

31. Besterman, E.M.M., and Gillett, M.P.T. (1972) _Atheroscl._ 16, 89.

32. Durnin, J., and Womersley, J. (1974) _Br. J. Nutr._ 32, 77.

33. Gautheron, P., and Renaud, S. (1972) _Thromb. Res._ 1, 353.

34. Renaud, S., and Gautheron, P. (1975) _Atheroscl._ 21, 115.

35. Iacono, J.M., Zellner, D.C., Paoletti, R., Ishikawa, T., Frigeni, V., and Fumagalli, R. (1974) _Haemostasis_, 2, 141.

36. Carvalho, A.C.A., Coleman, R.W., and Lees, R.F. (1974) _N. Engl. J. Med._ 290, 434.

37. Bennett, J.S., Shattil, S.J., Cooper, R.A., and Coleman, R.W. (1974) _Blood_, 44, 918.

38. Iacono, J.M., Binder, R.A., Marshall, M.W., Schoene, N.W., Jencks, J.A., and Mackin, J.F. (1974) _Haemostasis_ 3, 306.

39. Ranud, S., Kuba, K., Goulet, C., Lemire, Y., and Allard, C. (1970) _Circ. Res._ 26, 553.

40. Goldenfarb, P.B., Cathey, M.H., Zucker, S., Wilbur, P., and Corrigan, J.J. (1971) _Circulation_ 43, 538.

41. Schoene, N.W., and Iacono, J.M. (1976) _Advances in Prostaglandin and Thromboxane Research_, Vol. 2, (Samuelsson, B. and Paoletti, R., Eds.), Raven Press, New York, p. 763.

42. Dusting, G.J., Moncada, S., and Vane, J.R. (1977) _Prostaglandins_ 13, 3.

43. Johnson, R.A., Morton, D.R., Kinner, J.H., Gorman, R.R., McGuire, J.R., Sun, F.F., Whittaker, M., Bunting, S., Salmon, J.A., Moncada, S., and Vane, J.R. (1976) _Prostaglandins_ 12, 915.

DISCUSSION FOLLOWING SECOND PLENARY SESSION:
RISK FACTORS FOR ATHEROSCLEROSIS AND THROMBOSIS

R.W. Wissler: Dr. McGill, I think we should reserve judgment regarding estrogens, particularly estradiol and its effect on atherosclerosis before we call it a deleterious factor.

The effects of estrogen present complex problems and it is, I believe, too early to dismiss it as a part of the remarkable protection of the female from severe coronary atherosclerosis which is so well documented in most populations that are relatively hypercholesterolemic. The International Atherosclerosis Project and many other studies have presented such data. We should keep in mind that estradiol has well documented effects in the right metabolic direction to be "protective" relative to atherogenesis by producing a relatively high level of HDL and phospholipids; inhibiting the proliferative response of arterial smooth muscle cells; and increasing or protecting endothelial integrity.

The fact that there are early deleterious effects of estrogen therapy is well documented both clinically and experimentally. That it increases the LDL disproportionately and increases the rate of atherogenesis in the early phases of clinical or experimental administration should not blind us to its overall protective effect against atherosclerosis in physiological quantities over long periods as found in both experimental animals and in several clinical studies.

C. Rhee: Dr. McGill, we have shown that estradiol suppresses surgically induced intimal hyperplasia in male rabbits (J. Lab. Clin. Med., July 1977). Also, we have preliminary findings that estradiol reduces balloon-induced intimal cell proliferation in male rabbit aorta and this hormone decreases cell proliferation of rabbit smooth muscle cells in vitro.

B.A. Kottke: In a study some years ago, Drs. K. Hannasa, J.L. Titus, and I compared the pathologic assessment of the degree of coronary and aortic atherosclerosis in three groups of patients: patients with prostatic cancer not receiving estrogens, those

receiving estrogen treatment and those dying of traumatic causes.
The degree of coronary and aortic atherosclerosis was the same
in all three groups.

J.A. Joist: Are there good data on the prevalence of unrecognized hyperlipidemia in patients with sudden death syndrome?

H.C. McGill, Jr.: Numerous epidemiological cohort studies
have shown that the profile of risk factors for sudden death is
similar to that for other forms of coronary heart disease. This
profile includes hyperlipidemia. In some studies, cigarette
smoking is a stronger risk factor for sudden death than for myocardial infarction or angina pectoris.

A.B. Chandler: Dr. Mitchell makes a plea for exactness in
distinguishing between atherosclerosis and thrombosis in the assessment of pathological studies in relation to risk markers. This is,
of course, an important point. Recently developed unincorporated
thrombi formed in association with plaques are obvious, but we must
also take into account those atherosclerotic plaques that contain
incorporated or buried thrombi as described yesterday by Dr. Woolf.
To make such a sharp distinction between atherosclerosis and thrombosis in atherothrombotic plaques might be misleading rather than
clarifying in regard to the role of thrombosis in the pathogenesis
of atherosclerosis.

J.R.A. Mitchell: Dr. Lees said that "the thrombotic complications of atherosclerosis are more common in Type II hyperlipidemia."
Can he substantiate that statement? I know that certain clinical
events are all too frequent in that 50% of Type II males will
develop myocardial infarction by the age of 50. Is that because
they have an excess amount of wall disease, an enhanced predilection to thrombosis, a propensity to both conditions, or is it due
to some other mechanism such as the myocardial response to ischemia?

A.B. Chandler: Dr. Lees, your observation that thromboembolic
events are five times more common in Type II than in Type IV hyperlipoproteinemia would seem crucial to the evaluation of in vitro
studies of platelet reactivity in these disorders. What kind of
thromboembolic events were they: arterial, venous, or both? How
were the events assessed: by autopsy or biopsy, or by other means?

R.S. Lees: Our data are to be considered very tentative, Dr.
Chandler, although they are published in Circulation. The events
we monitored were, as I recall, acute myocardial infarction, cerebral embolus, cerebral thrombosis, peripheral embolus, peripheral
arterial occlusion, thrombophlebitis and pulmonary embolism. The
end-points we used were electrocardiograph for myocardial infarction, clinical for thrombophlebitis, chest x-ray for pulmonary
embolus and, in general, angiography for the other diagnoses.

Dr. Mitchell, your point is well taken. Although I suspect
that patients with Type II hyperlipidemia have more arterial wall
disease than do those with Type IV, and can substantiate that
(Lancet 1, 928-930, 1976) for the coronary arteries, and also have
evidence which I presented today that they have a predilection to
thrombosis; I cannot tell you whether one or the other of these
abnormalities is the predisposing factor for their clinical events.
In partial answer to your first question, we do have evidence to
substantiate the fact that Type II patients have a higher incidence
of clinically recognizable thrombotic events than do Type IV
patients (Circulation 56, 114-118, 1977).

We are very uneasy about the extrapolation from in vitro platelet studies to clinical events, although our crude assessment of
the occurrence of thromboembolic events in two of our patient groups
is encouraging to us. What we find most exciting, however, is that
our data suggest that the two major and allegedly opposing theories
of atherogenesis are really related. In other words, hypercholesterolemia may predispose to atherogenesis not only by increasing
the entry of lipid into the arterial wall, but also by increasing
platelet activity. Since platelet interaction with the arterial
wall may increase arterial wall permeability and thus increase
lipoprotein entry, the filtration and the thrombogenic theories
of atherogenesis may really be but two sides of the same coin.

D.J. Hanahan: Dr. Lees, have you examined the fatty acid
composition of the platelets in patients with hypercholesteremia?
Are these platelets with high cholesterol and phospholipid representative of younger platelets? Have you examined the erythrocytes
from the same persons?

R.S. Lees: We are analyzing platelet fatty acid composition
now, Dr. Hanahan, and hope to have the results available within the
next year. Although we cannot conclusively prove that younger
platelets are not the cause of some of the compositional and functional changes that we see, platelet sizing suggests to us that
there are not sufficient differences in the age of platelets from
normal, Type II, and Type IV patients to explain the differences
which we have observed. We have examined the erythroctyes from
some of the same subjects and find similar changes in erythrocyte
lipids. We feel that this is further evidence that the differences
we see in the platelets are not due to platelet age or size.

M.R. Malinow: We have studied platelet behavior in cynomolgus
monkeys with dietary-induced hypercholesterolemia. We have found
that no changes were present in platelet aggregation that could be
related to the level of plasma cholesterol.

J.H. Joist: Dr. Mitchell, I have two comments. One probably
important point Dr. Mitchell did not raise in his sobering review
is the very difficult problem of separating the effect of an apparently established atherosclerosis risk factor such as hyperlipidemia on platelet function or platelet behavior from the effect of
the disease itself (atherosclerosis) on platelet behavior. There
is substantial evidence, of course, that patients with myocardial
infarction or stroke may have altered platelet behavior with respect
to in vitro tests and platelet survival measurements. Secondly,
for the record, Nordøy et al. did not observe increased platelet
aggregation in hypercholesterolemic patients as suggested by Dr.
Lees. Nordøy and Rodset in fact found increased platelet factor
3-availability in their patients, an observation which we were able
to confirm for both Type II and Type IV, hyperlipidemia patients.
Thus, although I do not quarrel with the concept that platelet behavior may be altered in hyperlipidemic patients, I question whether
platelet aggregometry is a method which is sensitive in detecting
this abnormality.

D.J. Hanahan: Dr. Iacono, did you assay your platelet lipids
for plasmalogen (vinyl ethers)? It could alter the pattern you
noted.

J.M. Iacono: The assay of plasmalogens in platelets, red cells
and plasma will be made by Dr. Fred Synder at Oakridge, Tennessee.
Although we do not know the function of this class of lipids, we
feel that these lipids should be carefully assessed.

S.G. Haynes: Dr. Mitchell, I have three questions. First,
you have quite clearly shown the major weaknesses in current clinical diagnoses for CHD and stroke. In designing epidemiological
studies, however, do we not have to rely on autopsy studies in order
to obtain the precision in diagnoses demanded by Dr. Mitchell? Epidemiologists are usually not satisfied with the response rates ob-
tainable in autopsy studies (at most 30-50%) and are uncertain
about their generalizability.

Second, if we were to collect some coagulation measures in a
large-scale epidemiologic study, like the Framingham heart study,
what should we measure? What is the reliability of current measures, like platelet aggregation, platelet survival, etc.?

Third, several studies have shown that women have higher
platelet aggregation than men, especially among women who are premenopausal and not on oral contraceptives. How might these studies
be interpreted vis-a-vis the lower rates of coronary heart disease
among women than men?

J.R.A. Mitchell: Low autopsy rates would obviously reduce the precision of the labels used in studies where death was an epidemiological end-point, and this was particularly true in studies on strokes. Only two solutions were possible: one, to improve the autopsy rate, which is unlikely to be practicable; two, to recognize the imprecision of the data and to avoid using falsely-precise words. Thus, the term athero-thrombotic brain infarction (ABI) used in the Framingham studies could only have been truthfully applied after necropsy, and conceals from the reader that what is meant is "stroke without blood in the CSF" which is a different ball game altogether.

There is no suitable test of platelet behavior which I would recommend for large-scale epidemiological use. Before contemplating such studies the questioner should read the reports from Dr. T.W. Meade and his colleagues at Northwick Park Hospital, England.

The uselessness of platelet aggregation as a clinical tool does not permit this question to be answered in a meaningful way.

SECOND WORKSHOP SESSION

LIPID-MEMBRANE INTERACTIONS OF PLATELETS, COAGULATION AND THE ARTERIAL WALL AT THE MOLECULAR LEVEL

Donald J. Hanahan, *Session Chairman*
Department of Biochemistry
University of Texas Health Science Center
San Antonio, Texas

WORKSHOP 2a: LIPID-MEMBRANE INTERACTIONS OF PLATELETS AND COAGULATION

Donald J. Hanahan, Moderator
Participants: P.G. Barton, L.C. Smith,
D.B. Zilversmit

WORKSHOP 2b: LIPID-MEMBRANE INTERACTIONS OF PLATELETS AND COAGULATION WITH THE ARTERIAL WALL

J. Bryan Smith, Moderator
Participants: J.M. Gerrard, G. Hornstra,
D.C.B. Mills, P.W. Ramwell, M.T.R. Subbiah

SUMMARY OF WORKSHOP 2a: LIPID-MEMBRANE INTERACTIONS

OF PLATELETS AND COAGULATION

Donald J. Hanahan

Department of Biochemistry
University of Texas Health Science Center
San Antonio, Texas

This workshop centered attention on approaches to an understanding of lipid interactions in biological systems. To this end, the topics for discussion focused on the behavior of phospholipids in the intrinsic coagulation process, the mechanism of exchange of cholesterol between vascular compartments and constituents, and the manner in which the lipid exchange proteins can be employed as membrane probes. In order to fully understand the complexities of lipid biochemistry in situ, one must know first about the behavior of purified cell components or comparable model substances in in vitro systems and then armed with this information to investigate their characteristics in the intact cell. Hence, it was the intent of this workshop to illustrate how the first part of this two pronged objective may be accomplished.

In his presentation, Dr. Peter G. Barton described the reactivity of mixtures of phospholipids in the reaction

$$\text{Prothrombin} \xrightarrow[\text{PL, Ca}^{2+}]{\text{factor Xa, factor V}} \text{Thrombin}$$

Phase diagrams of mixtures of dimyristoylphosphatidylglycerol (DMPG) and either dilauroyl-(DLPC), dimyristoyl-(DMPC) or dipalmitoylphosphatidylcholine (DPPC) in the presence and absence of Ca^{2+} were obtained by light scattering and differential thermal analysis. Prothrombin activation was measured at 30°C, 37°C and 44°C. Mixtures entirely in the gel phase were inert. Higher activity was manifested with the liquid-crystalline phase but optimal activity accrued from a biphasic lipid system (lateral lipid-lipid phase separation). Platelet membranes isolated after glycerol lysis or freeze-thawing were active in this model system and showed a phase separation induced by Ca^{2+}. Prothrombin activation may occur at the lateral interface between gel and liquid-crystalline lipid phases.

An equally fascinating topic, that of the mechanism of lipid transfer and exchange, was the subject considered by Dr. Louis C. Smith. Exchange and transfer of cholesterol and other lipids between plasma liporoteins and the various cell membranes of the vascular wall is an important determinant of normal lipoprotein and cellular metabolism and of pathological cellular lipid accumulation. To test whether the mechanism of transfer involves dissociation into the aqueous phase or formation of a collision complex, lipids containing the fluorescent moiety, pyrene, have been synthesized and characterized. The similarity of the fluorescent analog, 3-pyrenemethyl-23, 24-dinor-5-cholenic-22-acid-3β-ol (PMCA), and cholesterol was shown by efficient ester formation by lecithin cholesterol acyltransferase and by the suppression of HMG-CoA reductase by PMCA in cultured human fibroblasts. The fluorescence intensity of PMCA at two different wavelengths (393 nm and 470 nm) depends on the concentration of the probe in the lipoprotein. Transfer can be monitored continuously without isolating the donor and acceptor species by the change in fluorescence that accompanies a change in microscopic concentration. Lack of rate-dependence on the concentration of the reactants anf first order kinetics suggests that the rate-limiting step in the transfer of PMCA and cholesterol between lipoproteins is dissociation into the aqueous phase. Similar pehnomena were demonstrated for other pyrene containing lipids. Distribution of cholesterol and other lipids between the plasma lipoproteins and the cellular membranes of the vascular wall are determined, in part, by a simple physical process.

Dr. Donald B. Zilversmit addressed the provocative subject of phospholipid-exchange proteins as membrane probes. Phospholipid exchange proteins, first discovered in rat liver, have now been identified in a variety of animal and plant tissues. In rat liver one protein transfers phosphatidylcholine with a high degree of specificity. Another protein fraction is capable of transferring all major types of phospholipids as well as cholesterol. Beef heart is a good source of phospholipid exchange protein which transfers phosphatidylinositol and phosphatidylcholine. Studies with phospholipid exchange protein from beef heart, beef liver, and rat liver show that these proteins are useful for the study of membrane structure. When unilamellar vesicles of isotopically labeled phosphatidylcholine are incubated with nonlabeled mitochondria in the presence of phospholipid exchange protein only the outer portion of the phosphatidylcholine bilayer is exchangeable and translocation of lipids between inner and outer parts of the bilayer is exceedingly slow. Resealed red blood cell ghosts show an equilibration of phosphatidylcholine between the inner and outer portions of the bilayer with a tl/2 of 2 h. An even faster equilibration of various phospholipids in the micro-somal membrane appears to take place in rat liver microsomes.

REFERENCES

1. Barton, P.D. (1975) in Platelets, Drugs, Thromb., Proc. Symp. (Hirsh, J., Cade, J.F., Gallus, A.S. and Schonbaum, E., Eds.), Karger Publ., Basel, pp. 43-48.

2. Sterzing, P.R., and Barton, P.G. (1973) Chem. Phys. Lipids 10, 137-148.

3. Charlton, S.C., Olson, J.S., Hong, K-Y., Pownall, H.J., Louie, D.D., and Smith, L.C. (1976) J. Biol. Chem. 251, 7952-7955.

4. Kao, Y.J., Charlton, S.C. and Smith, L.C. (1977) Fed. Proc. 36, 936 (abstract).

5. Bloj, B., and Zilversmit, D.B. (1976) Biochemistry 15, 1277-1283.

6. Bloj, B., and Zilversmit, D.B. (1977) J. Biol. Chem. 252, 1613-1619.

DISCUSSION FOLLOWING WORKSHOP 2a: LIPID-MEMBRANE INTERACTIONS
OF PLATELETS AND COAGULATION

J.H. Joist: Dr. Barton, if the predominant phospholipid in
the outer layer of the platelet plasma membrane is phosphatidylcholine, as Dr. Schick's studies indicate, how and to what extent
is an increase in cholesterol in that membrane going to affect
the clot promoting activity (PF3) of the platelet?

Since hyperpyrexia, i.e., temperature elevation above 37°C,
occurs relatively frequently in man, would this have a likely
effect on platelet-related procoagulant activity (PF3) in view
of your observation on temperature-related lipid phase transition?

P.G. Barton: To answer this question one would need to have
more precise information about the locus of platelet factor 3
activity. Recent findings (Miletich, J.P., Jackson, C.M. and
Mayerus, P.W., P.N.A.S. 74) cast doubt on the idea that this
locus is the plasma membrane. Since we do not really know the
lipid composition and phase strucutre of platelet factor 3, it
would be impossible to predict the effects of altered cholesterol
content.

Since phase transitions in mammalian cell membranes take
place over a fairly broad temperature range, the elevation would
have to be very large to produce a significant effect on clotting
activity.

J.M. Iacono: Dr. Zilversmit, can you alter the phospholipids
and/or fatty acids in the microsome membrane system?

D.B. Zilversmit: It is possible to exchange phospholipids
within a given class, so that one can replace saturated phospha-
tidlycholine with a more unsaturated species. We are not yet
certain whether one can exchange once class of phospholipids for
another one with different polar head groups.

J.H. Joist: Dr. Zilversmit, are any of the phospholipid
exchange proteins normally present in circulating blood unassoci-
ated with formed elements?

341

D.B. Zilversmit: If there is any phospholipid exchange activity in lipoprotein-free plasma, it is of relatively low activity. It is true, of course, that the lipoproteins can serve as mediators for phospholipid exchange.

M.J. Karnovsky: Dr. Zilversmit, are any of these exchange proteins membrane-associated proteins?

D.B. Zilversmit: It is possible that in the intact cell exchange proteins are associated in part with membranes. However, the purified phospholipid exchange proteins have all been prepared from a standard sucrose medium homogenate, centrifuged at 100,000 g, i.e., the soluble fraction.

L.C. Smith: We have not tested any plasma lipoproteins as mutagens in the Ames test. In this context, Dr. Zilversmith has proposed that atherogenesis is related to lipoprotein lipase action on VLDL. This enzymic action may provide a link with the Benditt hypothesis in that reduction in particle size would increase the exchange rate of mutagens in the triglyceride-rich lipoproteins with the vascular membranes.

SUMMARY OF WORKSHOP 2b: LIPID-MEMBRANE INTERACTIONS OF

PLATELETS AND COAGULATION WITH THE ARTERIAL WALL

J. Bryan Smith

Cardeza Foundation
Department of Pharmacology
Thomas Jefferson University
Philadelphia, Pennsylvania

Both platelets and the arterial wall contain enzymes capable of converting arachidonic acid into the prostaglandin endoperoxides, PGG_2 and PGH_2. These endoperoxides are subsequently metabolized in platelets into thromboxane A_2 which causes platelet aggregation and is a potent vasoconstrictor. By contrast, the endoperoxides are converted in the arterial wall into prostacyclin, a potent inhibitor of platelet aggregation and vasodilator. In the presence of isomerases, the endoperoxides are converted into PGE_2 or PGD_2 .

Dr. Gerrard described the mechanism of platelet activation by prostaglandin endoperoxides and thromboxane A_2. Addition of PGG_2, PGH_2 or thromboxane A_2 to platelets produces an internal wave of contraction with centralization of the platelet granules as evidenced by electron microscopy. As the contractile process continues, secretion of the contents of platelet granules occur, the material being squeezed out of the platelet through the channels of the surface connected canalicular system. The synthesis of prostaglandin endoperoxides and thromboxane A_2 in platelets in response to thrombin or exposed constitutents of the vessel wall, occurs in the platelet dense tubular system, a smooth endoplasmic reiticulum membrane system which also stores the intracellular calcium. It appears that thromboxane A_2 probably acts by initiating a flux of calcium from the dense tubular system into the platelet cytoplasm thereby initiating the internal contraction. The effect of thromboxane A_2 does not appear to be mediated by changes in cyclic AMP or cyclic GMP in platelets. The structure of thromboxane A_2 suggests that it might act as an ionophore which directly transports calcium and experiments showing that thromboxane A_2 can transport calcium into an organic phase (diethyl ether) support this hypothesis.

343

Activation of phospholipase A_2 is required to release arachidonic acid from platelet membranes for thromboxane A_2 synthesis. This appears to be stimulated by an early localized flux of calcium. An attractive hypothesis is that the calcium flux required to activate the phospholipase A_2 is linked in series by thromboxane A_2 with the calcium flux required to initiate contraction. Since the initial processes appear to be localized in the dense tubular system, the thromboxane A_2 may act to transport calcium to the secondary contractile processes occurring in the platelet cytoplasm.

Dr. Mills described how several prostaglandins, which may be released from cells other than platelets, act on platelets to inhibit platelet aggregation. Prostaglandins E_1, E_2, D_1, D_2 and prostacyclin (PGI_2) all elevate cyclic AMP in platelets by stimulating adenylate cyclase in the platelet plasma membrane. The cyclic AMP apparently in turn stimulates a protein kinase which causes protein phosphorylation leading to inhibition of aggregation. This effect may be mediated by a calcium flux out of the platelet cytoplasm into the dense tubular system. The aggregating agent ADP inhibits the stimulation of adenylate cyclase by the prostaglandins. This effect of ADP appears to involve sulfhydryl groups at the platelet membrane, since it can be selectively blocked by a non-penetrating sulfhydryl group reagent (PcMBS). Several pieces of evidence indicate that the adenylate cyclase in platelets has several receptors at the platelet surface including two which recognize prostaglandins. One prostaglandin receptor recognizes PGE_1, PGE_2 and PGI_2 and is present on the surface of platelets from animals as well as man. A second receptor recognizes PGD_1 and PGD_2 and is present predominantly in human platelets. There is no evidence that more than one adenylate cyclase exists in platelets.

Dr. Ramwell demonstrated a marked sex difference in thrombotic tendency in mice and rats. Males were much more susceptible to thrombosis than females. This sex difference was present in in vivo models of thrombosis using either arachidonate administration or a loop cannula in the abdominal aorta. Testosterone dramatically promoted the thrombotic process while the sex difference was markedly reduced by either the anti-androgen Flutamide or by aspirin pretreatment.

In contrast to the results obtained with mice and rats, studies of aggregation in human platelet-rich plasma indicate that platelets obtained from females are aggregated more readily than platelets obtained from males. It appears that these results may be an artifact of in vitro experiments and may not be indicative of a thrombotic tendency. In fact, it has been observed that men have a shorter bleeding time than women, and that they have a higher incidence of thrombosis in hemodialysis shunts.

Sex differences are also present in blood pressure changes in response to vasocative agents. A greater pressor response is produced by norephinephrine in male dogs or rats than in female animals. The pressor response is promoted by testosterone treatment. By contrast, the relaxation of vessels induced by arachidonic acid (an effect probably mediated by prostacyclin) is reduced by testosterone but not by estradiol.

As a result of their greater contractility, male vessels may be subjected to greater shear stress than female vessels. These findings implicate testosterone as a factor in the development of atherosclerosis and suggest that it is a risk factor in arterial thrombosis.

Dr. Ravi Subbiah described his investigations of the biosynthesis of PGE_2 in the aorta of spontaneously atherosclerosis-susceptible White Carneau pigeons and in the aorta of atherosclerosis-resitant Show Racer pigeons. About 80% of the PGE_2 synthetase activity is located in the microsomal fraction of homogenates of aorta. The conversion of $1-^{14}C$-arachidonic acid into PGE_2 is linear up to one hour and shows an optimum pH of 7.4. The formation of PGE_2 by microsomes prepared from the aorta of young white Carneau pigeons is significantly higher than the formation of PGE_2 by microsomes of aortas of age-matched Show Racer pigeons. Prostaglandin E_2 strongly inhibits the cholesteryl ester hydrolase activity present in the supernatant fraction of homogenates of the aorta of atherosclerosis-susceptible pigeons. Its effect on specific enzymes controlling cholesteryl ester concentration in the aorta strongly suggest that PGE_2 and possibly other prostaglandins play a significant role in atherogenesis.

Dr. Hornstra described the results of experiments performed in rats fed a diet without linoleic acid. These essential fatty acid-(EFA)-deficient rats have a reduced content of both linoleic acid and arachidonic acid in the phospholipids of platelets and other tissues, with an associated increase of 20:3, n-9 fatty acid which very actively competes with arachidonic acid to prevent prostaglandin formation. Aggregation of platelets obtained from EFA-deficient rats in response to thrombin or collagen does not differ markedly from the aggregation of platelets obtained from control rats. Moreover, serotonin release does not differ between EFA-deficient platelets and controls although the formation of prostaglandins is essentially abolished. These results show that an additional release mechanism has to exist which is independent of thromboxane A_2 formation.

The ability of the aorta from EFA-deficient or control rats to produce prostacyclin was investigated by testing the capacity of material released from the aorta to inhibit ADP-induced aggregation. Prostacyclin production is very much lower in the aorta of

EFA-deficient rats. Moreover, incubation of aortas from EFA-deficient animals with platelets from EFA-deficient animals causes
more platelet aggregation than is seen when the same test is performed with normal rat platelets and tissue. This would suggest
that EFA-deficient rats would have an increased thrombotic tendency in vivo. However, when the thrombotic tendency of EFA-deficient rats was tested in vivo using the aorta-loop technique it
was found that EFA-deficient rats have a decreased thrombotic
tendency. These findings show that there must be mechanisms other
than those involving thromboxane and prostacyclin formation which
can lead to thrombosis formation in vivo.

RECOMMENDATIONS

Platelets possess the capacity to produce large amounts of
the highly unstable lipid, thromboxane A_2 and it seems probable
that this potent vasoconstrictor performs some function in vivo,
although what this function is has not been clearly defined. Perhaps thromboxane A_2 acts solely within the platelets to mobilize
calcium as discussed by Dr. Gerrard and permit the platelets to
secrete granule-bound substances such as the smooth muscle mitogenic factor. However, thromboxane A_2 might also act on the vessel wall to change the vascular permeability or restrict blood flow.
Methods for measuring the levels of thromboxane B_2 in vivo should
be encouraged as well as in vivo experiments involving the use of
selective thromboxane synthetase inhibitors. The speculation by
Dr. Gerrard that thromboxane A_2 acts as a calcium ionophore to
facilitate contraction is worthy of further experimentation especially since it may shed light on the mechanisms of cellular contraction in general. Progress in this area will obviously require
the chemical synthesis of stable analogs of thromboxane A_2.

The discovery of the lipid prostacyclin which potently inhibits
platelet aggregation and stimulates adenylate cyclase has resolved
the, until now, paradoxical existence of the cyclic AMP system in
platelets. It is important to learn more about which cells in the
vessel wall can produce prostacyclin and which stimuli enhance or
inhibit prostacyclin formation. As shown by Dr. Mills, human platelets also possess receptors for D-type prostaglandins. It is important to learn which cells produce prostaglandin D_2 and which
stimuli enhance the synthesis of this prostaglandin in vivo.

The synthesis of both thromboxane A_2 and prostacyclin is
dependent on the biosynthesis and metabolism of arachidonic acid,
and on the enzymes which control its turnover in phospholipids
and other ester forms. In particular, a great deal more needs to
be learned about the phospholipase A_2 activities that make arachidonic acid available for prostaglandin biosynthesis. The influence

of steriods on the availability and effect of arachidonic acid require further investigation. It is quite clear from Dr. Ramwell's
presentation that a systematic assessment is warranted of testosterone as a risk factor in the thrombosis and atherosclerosis models
discussed in this conference.

The studies of Dr. Subbiah point to the fact that prostaglandin
synthesis is increased in atherosclerotic lesions. It is important
to learn whether prostaglandins influence low density lipoprotein
receptors on smooth muscle cells or the transport of fat into the
atherosclerotic lesion. The effect of prostaglandins on the synthesis of glycosaminoglycans associated with the atherosclerotic plaque
is worthy of investigation.

Finally, it is apparent from the work of Dr. Hornstra that
mechanisms exist for the development of thrombosis and probably is
consistent with in vitro studies showing that platelets can undergo
platelet aggregation and secretion independently of the formation
of thromboxane A$_2$. Furthermore, the work of Dr. Hornstra suggests
that the synthesis of prostacyclin by the vessel wall may also only
play a modulatory role in vivo. These findings by no means indicate that prostaglands do not play a signification role in the development of atherosclerosis or thrombosis, but do indicate that
research efforts should be kept in perspective. We must continue
to examine all the potential mechanisms that may lead to thrombosis
and atherosclerosis. Without doubt these mechanisms will become
better understood as basic research advances our knowledge of lipid-
membranes.

REFERENCES

Dr. Gerrard

Gerrard, J.M., Townsend, D., Stoddard, S. Witkop, C.J., and
White, J.G. (1977) Am. J. Pathol. 86, 99-116.

Gerrard, J.M., White, J.G., Rao, G.H.R., and Townsend, D.
(1976) Am. J. Pathol. 83, 283-298.

Glass, D.B., Gerrard, J.M., Townsend, D., Carr, D.W., White,
J.G., and Goldberg, N.D. (1977) J. Cyclic Nucl. Res. 3, 37-94.

Gerrard, J.H., White J.G., and Peterson, D.A. Thrombosis and
Hemostasis. In press.

Dr. Mills

    Mills, D.C.B., and Smith, J.B. (1971) <u>Biochem. J</u>. 121,185-188.

    Mills, D.C.B., and Smith, J.B. (1972) <u>Ann. N.Y. Acad. Sci. USA</u> 201, 391-396.

    Mills, D.C.B., and Macfarlane, D.E. (1974) <u>Throm. Res</u>. 5, 401-408.

    Mills, D.C.B., Macfarlane, D.E., and Nicolaou, K. (1977) <u>Blood</u> 50, Suppl. 247, Abstract No. 517.

Dr. Ramwell

    Uzunova, A.D., Ramey, E.R., and Ramwell, P.W. (1977) <u>Prosta-glandins</u> 13, 995-1002.

    Uzunova, A. Ramey, E., and Ramwell, P.W. (1976) <u>Nature</u> 261, 712-713.

    Johnson, M., Ramey, E., and Ramwell, P.W. (1975) <u>Nature</u> 253, 355-357.

    Uzunova, A.D., Ramey, E.R., and Ramwell, P.W. <u>Gonadal Hor-mones and Pathogenesis of Occlusive Arterial Thrombosis</u>. In press.

Dr. Subbiah

    Subbiah, M.T., and Dicke, B.A. (1977) <u>Atherosclerosis</u> 27, 107-111.

    Subbiah, M.T. (1977) <u>Sixth Int. Symp. on Drugs Affecting Lipid Metabolism</u>, Aug. 29-Sept. 1, 1977, Philadelphia, Pa. In press.

Dr. Hornstra

    Hornstra, G., and Haddeman, E. (1977) <u>Thromb. Haem</u>. 38, 19.

    Hornstra, G. (1977) <u>Thromb. Haem</u>. 38, 256.

    Hornstra, G., Haddeman, E., and Don, J.A. (1977) <u>Thromb. Res</u>. In press.

DISCUSSION FOLLOWING WORKSHOP 2b:

LIPID-MEMBRANE INTERACTIONS OF PLATELETS
AND COAGULATION WITH THE ARTERIAL WALL

F.A. Pitlick: Dr. Ramwell, have you looked at the effect of
progesterone, which might be expected to be similar to testosterone,
or hydrocortisone, which has effects on membrane stability similar
to estradiol?

P.W. Ramwell: We have found that progesterone treatment like
testosterone also enhances the pressor response to norepinephrine
in anesthetized dogs. (See Waldman et al., Fed. Proc. 1976).

F.A. Pitlick: Dr. Subbiah, have you any kinetic data (Km, Vmax
for arachidonic acid) for differences in PGE₂ synthesis in the
two types of pigeon aortas you have tested?

M.T.R. Subbiah: No, we do not.

A. Nordøy: Endothelial cell monolayers have been prepared
as primary cultures from human umbilical cords. During the last
24 hours of growth, the calf serum of the medium is replaced with
lipoprotein-free human serum. At the time of the experiment, the
dishes are washed and incubated with purified lipoprotein fractions (LP) (LDL, VLDL and HDL, and combinations of these) diluted
in lipoprotein-free plasma. After 2 hours incubation at 37°C,
the LP are aspirated off the dishes, washed three times, and then
incubated with citrated PRP (300,000/1) for 30 minutes at 37°C.
The reactivity of this PRP to ADP (10 μM) and to collagen (70 μg/ml)
are tested with regard to platelet aggregation and MDA production.

Increasing concentrations of LDL up to 1600 μg protein/ml
have an inhibitory effect on the platelet inhibitory behavior of
the endothelial cells. HDL and VLDL are largely without effect
and HDL partly counteracts the effect of LDL.

THE THROMBOTIC PROCESS AND ATHEROGENESIS IN SPECIFIC ARTERIAL INJURY

Carl G. Becker, *Session Chairman*
Department of Pathology
Cornell University Medical College
New York, New York

WORKSHOP 3a: HEMODYNAMIC INJURY

Donald L. Fry, Moderator

Participants: S. Chien, R.J. Forstrom, J.F. Mustard, R.M. Nerem

WORKSHOP 3b: IMMUNOLOGIC INJURY

Carl G. Becker, Moderator
Participants: P.M. Henson, C.R. Minick, F. B. Taylor

SUMMARY OF WORKSHOP 3a: HEMODYNAMIC INJURY

Donald L. Fry

Laboratory of Experimental Atherosclerosis
National Heart, Lung, and Blood Institute
Bethesda, Maryland

The workshop began with five-minute presentations from each
of the participants who were asked to give a brief panoramic view
of the present state of knowledge regarding intravascular fluid
mechanics as a factor in thromboatherogenesis. This served as a
review for those in related fields and as a point of departure
for subsequent discussion. Dr. Nerem began with a review of basic
fluid mechanics. Hemodynamic stress was defined and shown to be
resolved into two components: a pressure and a shear stress.
Types of flow fields that can occur in a variety of conduit geome-
tries were also reviewed (1). The extraordinary complexities that
can occur in these fields were emphasized. Although flow tends
to be streamlined in the vascular system, a branching conduit
such as the arterial tree can manifest significant variation of
shear stress from point to point and is particularly vulnerable
to localized areas of disturbed flow patterns and flow separation.
It was noted that the maintenance of a stable flow pattern in any
conduit configuration depends on subtle geometric considerations
and that, given a stable flow conduit system, subtle distortions
of this geometry will destroy its streamlined properties. For example, the overdistended and distorted arterial tree associated
with hypertension might be particularly predisposed to unstable
flow patterns. The endothelial surface was found to be sensitive
to adjacent hemodynamic events. Endothelial permeability was
shown to increase monotonically with acute exposure to increasing
levels of shear stress.

Dr. Chien (2) reviewed current knowledge regarding the role
of the endothelial vesicular system as a mechanism for transendothelial transport of plasma substances and discussed how this

353

mechanism might be related to the fluid mechanical events in the zone of adjacent flow. It was noted that vesicular transport depends on the random Brownian motion of the vesicles across the endothelial cell; therefore, the net flux of material that is transported will depend not only on the concentration difference across the cell but also on the average velocity of this vesicular shuttle system. It was noted that this vesicular traffic appears to be greatest in the "fluid" regions of the cell interior away from the more structured organelles.

The fluid mechanical convection of platelets by the blood stream in stable and unstable flow situations was reviewed. Data was presented to show that the "dwell-time" of a platelet in the vicinity of an endothelial surface is a function of the local blood velocity gradient. Areas of low shear and areas of flow separation have particularly long dwell times as compared to regions of high shear suggesting that if platelet-endothelial interaction is to occur, it will be much more likely in the low shear areas.

Dr. Forstrom then extended this discussion based on the results of mathematical and experimental work performed by him and others (3). He noted that particles flowing in a suspension are normally repelled from impervious surfaces by various forces and contact the wall only infrequently. With permeable surfaces, however, radial convection drags the particles closer to the surface and if repulsion is overcome, significant particle deposition is expected. If the surface is nonadhesive, the particle concentration at the surface may still be enormously high, if the convection of cells to the surface by the increased wall permeability exceeds the capability of the particle to escape by diffusion or downstream convection. He presented a number of ingenious studies demonstrating this phenomenon in physical models, but noted that the relevance of this phenomenon to atherogenesis must await comparable measurements in the in vivo situation.

Dr. Mustard reviewed evidence showing that various substances extracted from platelets are potent agents in increasing the permeability of the microcirculation of the subcutaneous tissues in a rat model. The role of these substances in altering arterial endothelial permeability remains to be shown. He then presented data on the deposition of blood cellular elements on the luminal surface of a scaled model of a porcine thoracic aorta which was placed in an extracorporeal shunt of a pig (4). The pattern of platelet and fibrin deposition on the luminal surface in the region of the intercostal orifices was of particular interest. The deposition formed a striated pattern radiating from the lateral lips of the intercostal orifices onto the postero-lateral aspects of the aortic surface. The overall pattern resembled a

butterfly wing stretching laterally from the circular orifice
(body). Comparison of this butterfly pattern to the pattern of
sudanophilic staining from actual porcine aortas demonstrated an
extraordinary similarity.

Dr. Fry (5) reviewed work from his group showing the congruence of the patterns of increased permeability as measured by the
parenteral Evans blue technique in normal animals with the patterns
of sudanophilic staining that occur along the arterial tree of the
same species that have been on an atherogenic regimen. Examples
of impressive congruence were shown for the Erythrocebus patas
monkey, the Sinclair minipig, and the dog. Ultrastructural differences between the highly permeable (blue) and the impermeable
(white) regions were described. As compared to white regions,
blue regions were characterized by subtle subendothelial edematous
changes, a greater incidence of degenerating and eroded endothelial
cells, and a more disordered cell alignment when viewed enface with
scanning electron microscopy. The topographic distribution of
these "lesion-susceptible" blue regions cannot be clearly identified with either high or low shear stress exposure. It was suggested that the blue areas might correlate better with areas frequently exposed to disturbed flow, e.g., flow separation, or to
relatively stable flow patterns that change direction and magnitude periodically throughout the day with the varying metabolic
and blood flow demands.

Many aspects of the foregoing presentations were pursued in
depth during the subsequent portions of the workshop, much of which
is reported in detail below. If one were to attempt to summarize
the conclusion to be drawn from this workshop, it would be that
evidence linking hemodynamics with thromboatherogenesis must still
be considered only presumptive.

With the exception of hypertension, most evidence relating
hemodynamic events with atherogenesis is highly indirect. In certain special animal preparations, such as the surgically constructed arteriovenous shunt preparation, it is possible to show
that induced hemodynamic changes appear to correlate with increased
atherogenesis. As noted above, it has been shown that in normal
animals the topographic distribution of regions of increased endothelial permeability and "injury" along the vascular tree tends to
correlate with the patterns of sudanophilia that develop in the
same kind of animal on an atherogenic regimen. These observations
might be interpreted in light of the known relationship between
hemodynamic forces and endothelial permeability, noted earlier,
to suggest a causative role for hemodynamic forces. However, convincing direct evidence is lacking.

There are a number of reasons for lack of progress in evaluating the role of hemodynamics in atherogenesis. One is related to

the extraordinary difficulty in making the discrete hemodynamic
measurements in the highly restricted regions in which atherosclerotic lesions occur. Another is the unavailability of the requisite
methodology for obtaining discrete topographic information regarding the normal patterns of this disease process in man and in the
experimental animal. Neither of these problems are trivial, and
until we can develop the necessary technology to map discrete
hemodynamic measurements at sites that are lesion-susceptible and
sites that are lesion-resistant in the vascular tree during the
evolution of this disease process; our knowledge regarding the
role of hemodynamic events in atherogenesis will remain purely
inferential.

REFERENCES

1.   Nerem, R.M., Rumberger, J.A., Jr., Gross, D.R., Muir, W.W.,
     and Geiger, G.L. (1976) J. Cardiovasc. Res. 10(3), 301-313.

2.   Chien, S. (1976) Ann. N.Y. Acad. Sci. 275, 10-27.

3.   Forstrom, R.J., Bartelt, K., Blackshear, P.L., and Wood, T.
     (1975) Trans. Am. Soc. Artif. Int. Organs 21, 602-607.

4.   Murphy, E.A., Rowsell, H.C., Downie, H.G., Robinson, G.A.,
     and Mustard, J.F. (1962) Can. Med. Assoc. J. 87, 259-274.

5.   Fry, D.L. (1976) Cerebrovascular Diseases (Scheinberg, P.,
     Ed.), Raven, New York, pp. 77-95.

DISCUSSION FOLLOWING WORKSHOP 3a: HEMODYNAMIC INJURY

H.C. McGill, Jr: Two important considerations for those
studying the role of hemodynamic factors in atherogenesis are the
relevance of these factors to 1) the localization of the majority
of human atherosclerotic lesions and 2) the modulation of human
lesions among individuals and among populations.

1) Localization -- By far the majority of human lesions occur
in relatively straight, cylindrical, and non-branching segments of
the aorta, coronary arteries, and peripheral arteries. In fact, in
the thoracic aorta, most fatty streaks and fibrous plaques tend to
spare the orifices of the intercostal vessels and involve the intervening intima. The abdominal aorta below the renal artery orifices
and above the bifurcation is the most severely involved aortic
segment; this segment has very few branches. Also, in the coronary
arteries, the topography of most fatty streaks, fibrous plaques,
and advanced occlusive and complicated lesions does not seem related
to major branches but rather seems to involve mainly the straight
segments.

Most of the emphasis in describing hemodynamic effects is
usually placed upon what occurs at or very near branches, and therefore the relationship of those conditions to the bulk of human
atherosclerotic lesions is obscured. If hemodynamic factors are
involved in atherogenesis (and I have no doubt that they are, in
some way), they should be tested for association with direct quantitative topographic descriptors of human atherosclerosis rather
than by association with isolated anecdotal cases. If existing
topographic description is not adequate, such information should
be accumulated. The 23,000 sets of arteries collected in the International Atherosclerosis Project could be made available for
this purpose.

2) Modulation -- Do variations in hemodynamic characteristics
"explain" any of the variance that we see among individuals (other
known "risk factors" being equal) or among populations with widely
varying levels of "risk factors"? Do they "explain" any of the
residual 50% of variance that is not "explained" by the established
risk factors? I have heard much speculation about heart rate,

357

pulse pressure, etc., but if hemodynamic effects are real and if
they vary between individuals and populations, there must be some
way to test for these hypothesized relationships. Until such an
association can be demonstrated, we are limited only to considering hemodynamics as localizing factors (as discussed above) and
not as modulating factors among individuals or populations. Investigators in this field can perhaps suggest to epidemiologists
techniques by which such characteristics can be measured, and
thereby tested for association with disease.

D.L. Fry: Localization -- For reasons discussed elsewhere
(1), I would speculate that regions of the arterial tree that are
exposed to unstable hemodynamic stress patterns will become more
permeable and, if certain other conditions are met, be more susceptible to disease. Although orifice regions are susceptible to
unstable flow patterns, so are vessel bends (e.g., in the coronary
tree of the beating heart, leg arteries near joints, etc.) and
vessels (e.g., lower abdominal aorta) downstream from effluent
systems, the flow of which must vary throughout the day with changing metabolic demands (e.g., the celiac, superior mesenteric, and
renal orifices). Thus, I would expect the influence of hemodynamic
forces to be felt not only at vessel branches but also in regions
that are nominally straight (particularly when dissected and
pinned out at necropsy) and in regions away from orifices. The
hemodynamocist is well aware of the predominance of "non-orifice"
disease.

There are two reasons for the emphasis on the orifice lesions
by hemodynamocists. 1) We have some remote possibility of defining
the associated detailed fluid mechanical behavior of these areas
(2), and 2) orifices form a relatively unambiguous coordinate
system in which to define the requisite detailed topography of the
disease for correlation with the above hemodynamic measurements.
Until we have succeeded with these simpler problems, we have little hope of solving the far more difficult set of measurements and
associated topography posed by the beating coronary tree or lower
abdominal aorta. Obviously, new technology must be developed.

Modulation -- If one believes that certain local hemodynamic
events are adversely affecting the endothelial surface to promote
atherogenesis at that particular site (localization effect), then
it is reasonable to assume that accentuation of this local hemodynamic "injury" would accent the probability of disease as well
as its severity at that site. In this sense "aberrant" hemodynamics could be considered an added risk factor and might "explain"
at least part of the residual 50% variance referred to in Dr.
McGill's comment. Until we have better evidence and deeper insight into hypothesized relationships between hemodynamic stress
and disease, the hemodynamocist should be conservative in making

recommendations for collection of hemodynamic data by the clini-
cians, pathologists, and epidemiologists. Careful standardized
documentation of relevant observations such as heart rate, blood
pressure, and necropsy material is of obvious importance. However, if we are to gain the depth of insight necessary to evaluate
this important area of "risk factor" less ambiguously, it will be
necessary to enlist other basic disciplines to develop new nonin-
vasive technology for detailed flow measurements, continuous blood
pressure sensing, etc., that can be applied to appropriately
selected samples of the population.

1.   Fry, D.L. (1976) Cerebrovascular Diseases (Scheinberg, P.,
     Ed.) Raven, New York, pp. 77-95.

2.   Lutz, R.J., Cannon, J.N., Bischoff, K.B., Dedrick, R.L.,
     Stiles, R.K., and Fry, D.L. (1977) Circ. Res. 41(3), 391-399.

J.R.A. Mitchell: Flow has been implicated in thrombus formation even since Virchow's postulates. If the stimulus for thrombus
formation is a chemical message from diseased vessel wall, the presumably slow flow would allow this chemical message to reach a high
level of activity. If on the other hand thrombosis depends on the
arrival of particulate building units such as platelets, then a
fast delivery system and a fast flow is necessary for rapid thrombus growth. Finally, how quickly can arriving cells respond to
whatever the local thrombotic message is? If the response time is
slow, and flow is fast, then the cells will only become modified
when they have passed by the site. Could the panel tell us whether
slow, fast flow, or disturbed flow is the prerequisite for thrombus
formation and whether this differs in the arterial and venous sides
of the circulation?

D.L. Fry: Dr. Mitchell has posed an interesting and very
important question. A satisfactory answer would presume a depth
of knowledge and a highly complicated and sophisticated analysis
of the relevant chemical, diffusive, convective, and fluid mechanical events in this ensemble of processes that we simply do not
have. The relatively structured, low-profile, streamlined-form of
many arterial thrombi as contrasted to the venous counterpart
strongly implicate flow factors as a significant modulating influence on the associated cascade of processes in thrombosis.

J.F. Mustard: Would Dr. Fry and his colleagues try to explain
the butterfly pattern of endothelial changes around the orifice
of right angled branches and the butterfly pattern of formed element deposition around equivalent orifices in extracorporeal
shunts?

D.L. Fry: By "explain" I shall assume you mean suggest possible mechanical events that might be related to the pattern.

Flow from the aorta into the orifice of a right angled branch
such as you describe will be accompanied by an extremely complicated system of secondary flows and vortices. Let us begin by
looking at Fig. 1 representing the situation when flow through
the orifice is zero. Panel A shows the system in the longitudinal
plane and panel B in a cut-away perspective shows the aortic
luminal surface in the region of the orifice corresponding to
the views that Dr. Mustard showed. Flow is from left to right.
A pressure (p) and a velocity (v) will exist at each point in
the system as indicated at the solid circles on the segments of
the two representative streamlines (dashed lines) shown in panel
A. Since the flow moves in straight parallel lines, no pressure
gradients will exist in the cross-sectional plane. Thus, in
panel B the pressures on the streamlines (p_1 and p_2) and at the
wall (p_3) are all equal. Similarly, the shear stresses (τ_3 and
τ_4) shown as open arrows at points 3 and 4 on the wall lumen will
be equal and in the direction of the longitudinal mainstream of
the flow.

Consider now Fig. 2A which represents a situation in which the
side branch is now open. The lower streamline now bends into the
side branch. The associated fluid velocity vectors (represented
by v_2) must be accelerated, perhaps to different magnitudes but
certainly to a new direction that is approximately 90° from the
original (as represented by v_2 in Fig. 1A). A pressure difference
(δp_{accel}) must exist across the stream between points 1 and 2 to
produce the acceleration of the intervening flow to this new direction as indicated by the light arrow pointing downward from p_1
toward the orifice as shown in both panels of Fig. 2. Since velocities and acceleration toward the lateral walls (from point 1 to
point 3) are relatively small or negligible, the pressures across
the horizontal diameter of this system are virtually equal; thus
$p_1 \approx p_3$. It follows, therefore, that p_3 is also greater than p_2.
This means that a pressure difference (δp_τ), which approximates
δp_{accel}, will act circumferentially between points 3 and 2 in the
boundary layer flow (the thin sleeve of slowly moving "viscous"
flow between the wall and the more rapidly moving mainstream).
Since boundary layer flow is governed principally by its viscous
properties, this pressure difference will create a direction of
flow in the boundary layer that is different from that of the mainstream which is governed principally by its inertial properties.
This "secondary" flow in the boundary layer is in the circumferential direction toward the orifice. An associated circumferential
shearing stress (τ_4) will be created on the wall surface by this
secondary flow as indicated by the lower open arrow in panel B at
point 4. Somewhat farther away, up on the lateral aspect of the
wall at point 3, the shear stress is still essentially in a longitudinal direction or the direction of the mainstream.

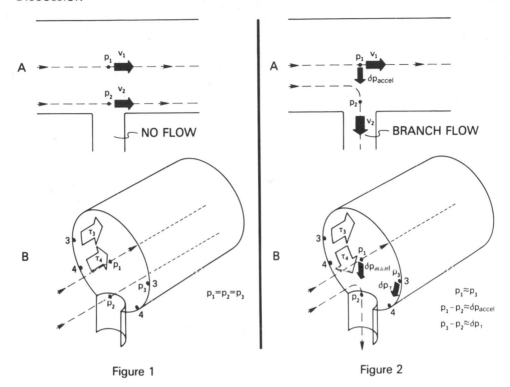

Figure 1   Figure 2

The direction and magnitude of τ will vary between point 3
and the orifice rim depending on a number of variables including
the instantaneous values of the velocities in the mainstream and
in the branch. In a very simplified model it can be shown that δp_τ
is approximately equal to ρv_2 where ρ is the fluid density and
v is the average magnitude of the fluid velocity in the mainstream.
Thus, the strength of the circumferential secondary flow can vary
greatly in magnitude throughout the cardiac cycle as well as
throughout the day and accordingly the distribution of both the
magnitude and the direction of the shear stress on the endothelial
surface in regions lateral to the orifice will also vary throughout the cardiac cycle and with the distal metabolic demands for
flow.

Although for simplicity the pressure gradient δp_τ has been
shown as a single arrow in the illustration, it is actually a
field of pressure gradient which may be visualized as a pattern
of δp_τ arrows, the heads of which will point toward the orifice
and the tails of which will fan out in a pattern that could resemble the butterfly pattern of cellular debris shown earlier on the
wall of the extracorporeal model. Accordingly, the associated
field of flow in the boundary layer will have a similar shape and
pattern of directions that converge on the orifice rim.

It should be noted also that in any flow system in which two streams of differing velocities interface (in the present case the mostly circumferential boundary flow and the mostly longitudinal mainstream) complicated systems of vortices commonly form in the interfacial region between these streams thus adding to the unstable nature of the stress exposure in this butterfly region.

The relationship of the butterfly-shaped region of lipid deposition in the pig to the strikingly similar area of postulated disturbed flow in the model could be explained on the assumption that endothelial surfaces which are exposed to unstable shear stress patterns suffer some, as yet undefined, latent injury that predisposes them to cellular deposition in a manner exactly analogous to the deposition on the foreign surface of the model. On the other hand, the endothelial surface may be entirely normal and simply exercising a normal physiologic response to changing or unstable stress patterns by increasing its permeability in a manner described in greater detail elsewhere (1). If endothelial surfaces that are exposed to unstable stress patterns are more permeable, then the increased lipid accumulation in the butterfly region of the pig may simply reflect an increased intimal accumulation of lipid-bearing plasma substances. While the foregoing does not necessarily "explain" the pathogenesis of the butterfly pattern of the lesions in the pig, it does suggest a plausible sequence of mechano-chemical mechanisms for further study.

1.   Fry, D.L. (1976) Cerebrovascular Diseases (Scheinberg, P., Ed.), Raven, New York, pp. 77-95.

A. Nordøy: According to explanations given by Dr. Fry on the hemodynamic forces acting at bifurcations, one might wonder what this situation may be in muscular arteries during acute episodes of physical exercise particularly where associated with hyperlipoproteinemia. It is known that the flow will increase significantly to the muscular areas, and one could easily imagine that the acute changes in the hemodynamic forces would favor the process of deposition and probably damage the endothelial cells. Have the panel or Dr. Fry any thoughts about the relevance of such a situation?

D.L. Fry: The role of exercise in altering the physiologic state of the endothelial surface of arteries supplying the cardiac and skeletal muscle masses is probably quite different in the two types of exercise regimens, i.e., acute episodic as opposed to chronic programmed exercise, and in the two lipemic states, normal as opposed to hyperlipemic. The shear stress on the endothelial surface due to the drag of the associated blood flow will vary monotonically with the flow. Thus, acute episodic exercise will expose the surfaces of the relevant arteries to acute increases in shear stress which are probably associated with acute increases in endothelial permeability (1). These will be associated with an increased intimal influx of plasma substances and diffusive efflux of wall substances. Depending on the chemical composition and relative magnitude of these two fluxes, this event could lessen or aggravate atherogenesis. In the situation where the endothelial surface may have been unfavorably altered by some prior immunologic or chemical event, e.g., hypercholesterolemia, one might not only expect an exaggeration of the foregoing flux changes in response to acutely increased shear stress exposure, but also an increased incidence of structural failure, i.e., endothelial cell erosion. As noted in earlier discussions, this event will be associated with platelet adhesion followed by intimal proliferation responses which clearly would be undesirable.

Events might be quite different in a planned program of progressively increased exercise over a suitably long period of time. We have studied chronic, surgically-prepared, arterial-venous shunts in the carotid and iliofemoral systems of normolipemic dogs. To the extent that the arteries that supply the shunted side may be considered the extreme case of an artery supplying a chronically exercised muscular bed, the observations indicate that although permeability increases acutely in response to the creation of the shunt, the endothelial surface responds to this increased unidirectional shear stress exposure within approximately a week to decrease its permeability back toward levels comparable to the normal contralateral control artery. Thus, the endothelial surface appears programmed to respond to an increased unidirectional shear stress load by returning the transendothelial flux of plasma substances to normal. Although this is not initially associated with obvious structural changes in the endothelial surface, within a matter of weeks the endothelial cells are seen to have developed a very strong longitudinal orientation in the direction of the flow and by scanning electron microscopy present a highly ordered structural appearance. We might speculate that the chronically exercised muscular beds in normolipemic subjects might also have analogous arterial changes such that the endothelial surface becomes less permeable and may even be mechanically stronger, (perhaps in a manner analogous to callous formation in epidermis that is exposed to chronic friction). If so, the arterial tree supplying exercised muscular beds might become conditioned to be more impermeable and to be more resistant to injury and atherosclerosis, at least over portions of the conduit system in which relatively stable flow patterns can be maintained such that a reasonably unidirectional stress is created.

In hyperlipemic dogs the incidence of atherosclerosis is higher in the arterial segment supplying a shunt. This would suggest caution in applying the above speculation to the hyperlipemic state (2).

1.   Fry, D.L. (1976) Cerebrovascular Diseases (Scheinberg, P.,
      Ed.), Raven, New York, pp. 77-95.

2.   Flaherty, J.T., Ferrans, V.J., Pierce, J.E., Carew, T.E.,
      and Fry, D.L. (1972) Atherosclerosis and Coronary Heart
      Disease, Chapter 6, (Likoff, W. et al., Eds.), Grune and
      Stratton, New York, pp. 40-83.

R.S. Lees: In discussing the effects of shear on the arterial wall and on the entry of macromolecules, I think it's important not to forget that shear may affect the concentration of
lipoproteins at the wall, where filtration is occurring. Like
Dr. Forstrom, we have performed some studies with synthetic semi-
permeable membranes (J. Clin. Invest. 51, 2472-2481, 1972). The
behavior of macromolecules at the membrane surface was complex
and determined by molecular size, rate of fluid flux through the
membrane and shear rate. Furthermore, the presence of one macromolecule strongly affected the concentration, at the membrane
surface, of other macromolecules. LDL, for instance, achieved
high concentration in the fluid layer at the surface when shear
was low: high shear kept the surface concentration much lower.
When VLDL was present, it formed a highly concentrated layer on
the membrane and actually kept LDL away from the surface.

My point is that the effects of shear may be complex and the
entry of lipoproteins may be determined by changes in local lipoprotein concentration at the wall, as long as some fluid flux is
going on. This may be of particular importance, for instance, in
the ballooned animal model. Since trans-arterial fluid flux is
normally very slow, it should be of little significance where
damage to the vessel wall has not occurred. On the other hand,
spontaneous damage to the arterial wall may occur, and if it does
occur in areas of low shear, local lipoprotein concentration may
become much greater than the average plasma level.

M.D. Ezekowitz: Dr. Nerem, the rate of egress of material
from the arterial wall into the plasma has not been emphasized in
the preceding discussion. What roles do hemodynamic factors play
in controlling egress of material? Secondly, do you think these
egress-influencing factors within the walls are important in determining the accumulation of material?

R.M. Nerem: Although studies of transendothelial macromolecule transport have invariably addressed the problem of the uptake
of material by the arterial wall, it is clear that there can also
be egress of material from the wall. The former has been demonstrated to have a shear dependence, and it would not be surprising,
in fact, it is tacitly assumed by many, that the rate of egress
of material is also shear dependent. Whether it is the uptake of
material or the egress of material from the arterial wall that is

important in the atherogenic process is literally not known, and this uncertainty only adds to our present lack of knowledge about hemodynamics as a factor in atherogenesis.

S. Chien: I agree with Dr. Nerem that sometimes it is difficult to define whether a given shear stress level is high or low. For example, when a shear stress of 400 dyn/cm² is applied for a long time, Dr. Fry found this was sufficient to cause endothelial damage. If a shear stress of several thousand dyn/cm² is applied only for a very short period (e.g., a few milliseconds), however, there may be no resultant injury. I also would like to comment on the effect of exercise and high shear stress. An increase in shear stress causes an increase in endothelial permeability to macromolecules probably in both directions; thus efflux as well as influx may be enhanced. Therefore, if there is any accumulation of lipoproteins in the sub-endothelial layer, exercise and the resulting high shear stress may help to reduce the intramural concentration.

R.G. Gerrity: I have several comments with respect to areas of Evans blue uptake. First, our ferritin uptake data which Dr. Chien referred to do not indicate an increased rate of vesicular movement. They do show an enhanced activation of vesicles in the uptake process. That is, although blue and white areas contain the same number of vesicles per unit area of endothelium cut in cross-section, and the same average number of ferritin particles per vesicle, there are two to three times as many vesicles carrying ferritin in blue areas as compared to white areas. Moreover, this ferritin does accumulate in the intima at a greater rate in blue areas, and undergoes phagocytosis by intimal cells at a greater rate and in greater numbers in blue than in white areas. I would agree with Dr. Karnovsky that a larger number of particles per vesicle is not necessarily indicative of enhanced or more rapid transport. In fact, what we have shown here is that there is not an increase in this parameter, but an increased number of labeled vesicles, and that the ferritin does accumulate in the intima.

We have also demonstrated that the endothelium in blue areas is much less polarized, and is more cuboidal in shape, with less complex junctions than in white areas. The endothelial glycocalyx in blue areas is some three times thinner in blue areas than in white areas, and this layer is decreased in thickness within two weeks of the initiation of cholesterol feeding.

C.G. Becker: Is vesicle motion purely random or is it directed, perhaps by contractile events in the endothelial cell?

S. Chien: The current understanding of vesicle diffusion in the endothelial cell is that this is due to thermal Brownian motion without any polarity. The work of the Simionescus and Palade have shown that macromolecular markers introduced into the sub-endothelial space in the capillary are transported by vesicle motion toward the blood front. Therefore, vesicle motion in the endothelial cell can result in macromolecular efflux as well as influx.

C.G. Becker: Do local changes in blood flow such as those which may be induced by mediators of inflammation effect vesicle transport?

S. Chien: Hemodynamic factors may induce intracellular fluid motion thus causing enhanced vesicle transport. The asymmetry of the endothelial cell near the junction area and the visoelastic nature of the cell may contribute to this enhancement.

J.H. Joist: Dr. Chien, if these vesicles are involved in transcellular transport of macromolecules, how do you explain their apparently selective localization close to the plasma membrane? Why are they not seen throughout the cell?

S. Chien: Vesicles are excluded from the nuclear and organelle regions of the endothelial cell, probably because of the inability of the vesicle to diffuse through these regions. Therefore, the distribution of vesicles in the endothelial cell is not uniform.

J.H. Joist: I am not totally satisfied with your answer. Are you suggesting that the vesicles move along the inside layer of the cell plasma membrane?

S. Chien: The vesicle moves between the luminal and the abluminal membranes in the peripheral zone of the endothelial cell.

M.J. Karnovsky: To amplify on Dr. Chien's answer to Dr. Joist: the assymmetric distribution of vesicles in the cell may reflect a slow loading phase at the membrane and rapid transit. Thus, the number of free vesicles in the cytoplasm at any point of time -- point of fixation -- would be only a proportion of those at the periphery.

J.C. Lewis: Dr. Gerrity's comment, which points out the subtle morphologic differences found by SEM and TEM when aortic endothelial cells in the Evans blue areas are compared to the non-blue areas, are most interesting. These observations are significant in that our attention is again focused on the endothelial layer as the primary site of alteration which ultimately leads to the more complex disease. When considering the luminal aspect of endothelial cells, it seems reasonable to suggest that alterations in the glycoprotein surface coat (glycocalyx or endo-endothelium as described by Dr. Majno) are instrumental in deter-mining the susceptibility of endothelial cells to injury. Along these lines, Dr. Marion Barnhart's group has recently demonstrated that in vitro enzymatic alteration of umbilical vein endothelial cell surface coats leads to extensive irregularities in the mor-phology of the endothelium. Subsequent to neuraminidase treat-ment, Chien and Barnhart found that, although the altered endothe-lial cells were no more thrombogenic than controls, there had occurred endothelial cell swelling, junctional separation and focal loss of cells exposing the fibrous subendothelial network. Platelets did adhere to the exposed subendothelium. These results by Chien and Barnhart suggest a role for the cell surface coat in maintaining endothelial integrity. Such a protective role for the cell surface coat is significant with respect to hemodynamic injury. Latta has shown for kidney that the appearance of endothelial cell surface coats can be altered by simply modifying the conditions under which the tissue is processed. This emphasizes the suscep-tibility of cell coat integrity to environmental fluctuation. It is conceivable therefore that hemodynamic forces directed at focal points on the vessel wall can alter endothelial cell surface coats, and by so doing render endothelial cells susceptible to more exten-sive injury.

J.F. Mustard: I would like to ask Dr. Lewis a question in respect to his comments and then make a comment. In the experi-ments of Dr. Barnhart, was the neuraminidase purified so that it did not contain contaminating enzymes? If red blood cells or platelets are treated with neuraminidase their surface sialic acid is removed and they are recognized as foreign and rapidly removed from the circulation. Neuraminidase-treated platelets adhere to normally intact endothelium and to the subendothelium and have a normal or slightly enhanced response to aggregating and release-inducing agents. Thus, removal of sialic acid from platelets does not have a major effect on their adherence or aggregation. How-ever, it does cause the rapid clearance of the platelets from the circulation. The mechanism responsible for this rapid clearance is not known, but the speculation is that gamma globulin may be bound to the surface when the membrane sialic acid is removed and this results in the uptake of platelets by the phagocytic cells. If this is true, it could mean that the surface of endothelial cells treated with neuraminidase may take up gamma globulin and that this alters the properties of the endothelium.

J.C. Lewis: I cannot answer with certainty; however, I assume the neuraminidase was purified to remove other proteases. Enzymes from several sources were used in the studies.

Your suggestion that neuraminidase treatment may alter endothelial cells leading to gamma globulin uptake is important. It
is essential to keep in mind that the result of neuraminidase
treatment is not restricted to sialic acid removal with concomitant charge alteration. Changes in membrane electrochemical configuration have ramifications with respect to membrane recognition, receptor site function, membrane fluidity, and as you have
pointed out, interaction with circulating molecules.

S. Chien: I would like to follow up Dr. Mustard's answer to
Dr. Lewis' question. First, studies on neuraminidase-treated red
blood cells indicate that they have the same deformability as normal cells with the sialic acid present. Second, the range of
electrostatic force due to cell surface charge is at most 100 Å
in physiological environments. Therefore the removal of surface
charge should not alter the probability of interactions between
cell surfaces, unless they have been brought together to very
close range by some other force.

G. Majno: As regards the interpretation of Dr. Gerrity's
results, I would like to emphasize that "more ferritin in the
vesicles" does not necessarily mean "more active vesicular transport." It could just as well mean a traffic jam in vesicular
transport. Also, there is a paper by G. Weber suggesting that
(in one model of experimental atherosclerosis) the carbohydrate
coating of the endothelium is reduced. From other sources, there
is evidence that this coating can slow down the penetration of
particles into the caveolae. So, "more ferritin in the vesicles"
could also be interpreted as "decreased coating of the endothelium."

C.J. Schwartz: I was delighted to see Dr. Donald Fry's convincing evidence that sites of in vivo arterial Evans blue accumulation
correspond very closely with sites developing atheromatous lesions
in the hypercholesterolemic pig. These findings are consistent
with our observation that such pre-lesion sites preferentially
accumulate cholesterol and cholesterol esters before any lesions
have become apparent.

Additionally, it is of interest to note that such sites of
dye accumulation which represent areas of enhanced permeability
to proteins and ferritin and which exhibit an increased endothelial
cell turnover, are sites which are more prone to injury from other
causes, such as endotoxin and hypercholesterolemia. In other
words, these areas are prone to recurring injury, a process possibly of great importance in terms of atherogenesis, and the insults
inflicted during aging.

M.J. Karnovsky: I do not think that transport by vesicles
should be regarded as a filtration process; it is rather quantal
in nature. Therefore, I do not see how the proposed increased

vesicular transport could relate to the proposed deposition of platelets by increased filtration flux.

The comments of Drs. Schwartz and Gerrity do not convince me of increased labeling. Furthermore, the data with ferritin do not relate directly to the Evans-blue-albumin data, in my opinion.

SUMMARY OF WORKSHOP 3b: IMMUNOLOGIC INJURY

Carl G. Becker

Department of Pathology
Cornell University Medical College
New York, New York

The purpose of this workshop was to consider how immunologic mechanisms might injure blood vessel walls, initiate thrombosis, or both, and ultimately contribute to the development of athero-arteriosclerosis and its complications.

Attention was also focused on the increasing number of known inter-relationships that exist between immunologic systems involving antibody and the complement system, leukocytes, platelets, and proteins of the hemostatic system, and how these various components often act synergistically in both physiologic and pathologic processes.

Dr. Peter Henson reviewed current knowledge of mechanisms responsible for the deposition of circulating immune complexes in blood vessel walls and ensuing injury, with special emphasis on IgE mediated reactions between basophils and platelets.

In earlier studies of experimental serum sickness Kniker and Cochrane (1) demonstrated in rabbits that immune complex deposition in vessel walls could be prevented by antagonists of histamine or serotonin, or by depleting the rabbits of platelets.

Earlier observations of Barbaro and Zvaifler indicated that platelets and leukocytes could cooperate in producing allergic reactions mediated by homocytophilic antibody (2). Further analysis of this phenomenon in the rabbit revealed that when antigen reacts with specific IgE on the surface of basophils; histamine is released from basophils, and both histamine and serotonin are released from the dense granules of platelets (3). This noncytotoxic

371

release of vasoactive amines by platelets is induced by a soluble, phospholipid also released by the sensitized, challenged basophils. This phospholipid has been named platelet-activating factor or PAF (4). PAF can also be released when a basophil attempts to ingest an immune complex containing IgE. PAF induces transient aggregation of platelets and the transient disappearance from the circulating blood of both neutrophils and platelets (5). PAF-induced platelet aggregation occurs at a lower concentration than that required to induce release of vasoactive amines (6). The latter appears to be accomplished by a secretory mechanism similar to secretory mechanisms in other cells, but also requiring activation of a specific serine protease (7).

PAF appears to be a specific mediator of platelet aggregation in that PAF-induced aggregation is resistant to agents which destroy ADP and occurs with platelets made unresponsive to ADP. On the other hand, platelets which have returned from the circulation after anaphylactic challenge in rabbits are refractory to stimulation by PAF, but are responsive to collagen, thrombin, epinephrine and $C3_b$ (5). According to comments contributed by Dr. Hanahan, who is studying PAF with Drs. Henson and Pinckard; PAF is neither a prostaglandin nor a thromboxane, indicating that it is a unique, phospholipid mediator of inflammation. PAF has been demonstrated in rats, rabbits, and man, and future research is aimed at its characterization.

Dr. Henson also reviewed briefly the ways in which immune complexes, complement and leukocytes can induce injury to blood vessels. Deposition of immune complexes in arterial walls and activation of the complement cascade leads to generation of chemotactic factors ($C5_a$, C567) which attract polymorphonuclear neutrophils and, in turn, to severe arteritis (8). The severity of the injury is, in part, due to the fact that when polymorphonuclear neutrophils attempt to phagocytize immune complexes on nonphagocytizable surfaces, exocytosis of granules occur along the stimulated membrane of the cell. The released enzymes then injure vascular membranes. This release is much less when complexes are not on nonphagocytizable surfaces (9). Immune complex deposition in renal glomeruli can induce proteinuria in the absence of complement, although the latter is necessary for attraction of leukocytes (8).

The question arises as to how IgE-mediated release of PAF and the effects of the latter on platelets might be related to the pathogenesis of atherosclerosis and/or its complications. IgE-mediated release of PAF and the subsequent release of vasoactive amines from platelets can enhance immune complex deposition in vessel walls, probably by enhancing permeability, and thus set in motion processes that lead to vessel injury as described above (8). It must be pointed out that, at present, the mechanism(s) by which

release of PAF and/or vasoactive amines promotes immune complex
deposition in blood vessel walls is obscure. IgE mediated release
of PAF can apparently also cause accumulation of platelets at sites
of immune complex deposition (10).

A unique feature of this system is that a reaction involving
a small quantity of antigen and specific IgE antibody is translated
into an augmented, nonimmunologic, pharmacologic stimulus. This
might favor the deposition of any circulating immune complexes in
vessel walls, even those unrelated to the specific antigen-IgE-
antibody reaction that triggered the event. It might also enhance
permeability to other macromolecules such as lipoproteins.

IgE mediated release of vasoactive amines can also affect myocardial function, and cardiac anaphylaxis can be demonstrated
experimentally (11). It is intriguing to think that IgE-mediated
release of vasoactive amines and/or platelet aggregation occurring
in myocardial vessels might also contribute to sudden cardiac
death, independent of their possible role in the pathogenesis of
athero-arteriosclerosis.

Dr. Fletcher Taylor focused on interactions between complement, proteins of the coagulation cascade and blood platelets and
developed the concept of the platelet membrane as a surface for
catalysis on which other processes are focused and augmented.

Studies presented here grew out of experiments directed at the
question of whether and how coagulation and fibrinolytic activity
were coupled. The assay system used involved observation of clotting, clot retraction, erythrocyte shedding, and lysis of clots
formed when whole human blood was diluted in phosphate buffer,
clotted at 4°C by addition of thrombin, and subsequently incubated
at 37°C. Removal of platelets, IgM, C_3, C_4, C_5 or plasminogen inhibited clot retraction and lysis. Platelet fusion is necessary
for clot retraction and lysis. Deactivation or removal of thrombin
IgM, C_3, C_4 or C_5 inhibited platelet fusion and reconstitution of
these components reactivated it. It was further shown in these
studies that factor Xa, thrombin, C_3 and C_5 were bound to platelet
membranes during this reaction (12, 13).

Further evidence for the role of the complement cascade in
coagulation came from the observation that agents which promoted
coagulation of rabbit blood by complement-dependent mechanisms did
so by activating the alternate pathway (14). More recently it has
been demonstrated that ultrastructural lesions identical to those
that develop on erythrocytes following activation of the alternate
complement pathway, occur in normal human platelet membranes during
coagulation in vitro. The development of these lesions requires
both thrombin and C_3 (15).

On the other hand, it has been reported that the platelet release reaction, as measured by serotonin release, occurs after C_3 fixation to platelets of patients with paroxysmal nocturnal hematuria (PNH), but not to normal human platelets (16). This observation would appear to be in keeping with the often stated conclusion that normal human platelets have no C_{3b} receptors, and suggests that PNH patients are more likely to suffer thrombosis because of a unique capacity to react with C_3.

However, in experiments presented here by Dr. Taylor it was observed that when purified factors II, V, Xa, radiolabeled C_3, and human platelets were mixed, C_3 bound to platelets, before peak thrombin generation occurred, potentiated the release of serotonin from platelets. The presence of C_3 did not affect the amount of thrombin generated. These experiments indicate that normal and PNH platelets differ more in the degree to which they bind C_3, and raise the question of whether C_3 binds to platelet membranes via a different kind of receptor than the C_{3b} receptor.

Since platelet membranes and endothelial cell membranes have many features in common, the obvious question is whether they also react similarly with components of the complement cascade and whether endothelial cell surfaces, too, can potentiate certain aspects of coagulation. With respect to hemostasis it would appear highly adaptive for them to do so; but the cost may be related to the pathogenesis of atherosclerosis and thrombosis. On the other hand, in experiments presented by Dr. Taylor, C_3 appears to modify platelet membranes to amplify reactions that would proceed in the absence of C_3. It is intriguing to think that reduction of this amplification step, particularly if it did not interfere with the immunologic functions of C_3 would be an effective means of preventing thrombosis without sacrificing hemostasis.

Dr. Becker presented data suggesting that constitutents of tobacco might be related to cardiovascular disease through IgE mediated mechanisms, through activation of the clotting cascade, and/or the synergistic action of both.

In these experiments, a glycoprotein of approximately 18,000 daltons was purified from flue-cured Virginia Bright tobacco leaves and from cigarette smoke condensate. Approximately one-third of human volunteers exhibited immediate cutaneous hypersensitivity when inoculated intracutaneously with tobacco glycoprotein (TGP), whether or not they were smokers. The high incidence of hypersensitivity among both groups may be due to either a) the presence of TGP in cigarette smoke and sensitization of smokers and, vicariously, of nonsmokers, and/or b) the presence of cross reacting antigen in commonly eaten members of the family Solanaceae to which tobacco belongs. These include tomatoes, eggplant, green peppers, and potatoes (17).

Neonatal sensitization and subsequent boostering of rabbits with TGP resulted in the selective production of heat labile homo-cytophilic (hence IgE) antibodies to TGP that could mediate pas-sive cutaneous anaphylaxis reactions when challenged with TGP derived from either cured tobacco leaves or cigarette smoke con-densate (18).

In further experiments TGP was demonstrated to contain rutin, which closely resembles quercetin, a substance known to activate factor XII. The capacity of TGP to activate factor XII was measured and it was observed that addition of TGP to normal human plasma shortened the partial thromboplastin time, activated fibrinolysis, and stimulated generation of bradykinin. These effects were not demonstrable in factor XII deficient plasma (19).

These experiments taken together suggest that constituents of tobacco can initiate an inflammatory response through either IgE-mediated mechanisms reviewed by Dr. Henson, or through activation of factor XII-dependent pathways, and thereby injure blood vessels in both the pulmonary and systemic circulation. The capacity of TGP to activate the intrinsic pathway of coagulation might also contribute to both the growth of arteriosclerotic plaques and to the lethal complications of arteriosclerosis by initiating thrombus formation. In this connection, Dr. Nossel commented that large quantities of fibrinopeptide A were found in the blood of human subjects who had been challenged with allergens (20).

Finally, the question arises as to whether TGP is a model for many other commonly ingested substances that contain plant polyphe-nols and whether these as yet unidentified substances might also contribute to the pathogenesis of atherosclerosis and/or thrombosis.

The last presentation in this section was by Dr. C. Richard Minick who focused and summarized our discussion of immunologic injury and athero-arteriosclerosis by presenting several experimen-tal models in which immunologic injury of different kinds was shown to act synergistically with dietarily-induced hyperlipidemia to initiate athero-arteriosclerosis.

In the first sets of experiments rabbits were divided into three groups. Groups I and III were fed cholesterol-supplemented diets and groups II and III were, in addition, repeatedly injected with foreign serum. Rabbits of group III developed fatty-prolif-erative lesions of large, medium, and small coronary arteries that closely resemble some stages of human atherosclerosis. In contrast, control rabbits of group I developed predominantly fatty lesions which occurred primarily in small coronary arteries and bore little resemblance to human atherosclerosis. Rabbits of group II devel-oped fibromuscular intimal thickening in large, medium, and small

coronary arteries. Rabbits in groups I and III exhibited atherosclerotic change in the aorta, though it was significantly greater
in rabbits of group III (21).

When this basic experiment was modified so that a cholesterol-
poor, lipid-rich diet was fed instead of a cholesterol-supplemented
diet, essentially the same results were obtained even though the
mean serum cholesterol level was between 200-250 mg% (22).

In subsequent experiments rabbits were repeatedly injected
intravenously with horse serum and the resultant arterial lesions
allowed to heal for 40-80 days. One group of these rabbits was then
fed a cholesterol-supplemented diet. Fatty-proliferative lesions
were found in large, medium, and small arteries of these rabbits,
whereas musculoelastic intimal thickening was found at the same
sites in rabbits that had serum sickness, but were not subsequently
fed a cholesterol-supplemented diet (23). The results of these
experiments support the hypothesis that, in man, sites of fibromuscular intimal thickening that result from one or several instances
of immunologic injury may continue to have increased avidity for
lipid for weeks, months, or perhaps even years after the initial
injury.

Athero-arteriosclerosis may also be mediated by cellular immune mechanisms. Unexpectedly severe and rapidly developing atherosclerotic changes in coronary arteries have been found to occur
in some human cardiac homografts and an experimental model was
developed to test the hypothesis that the synergy of immunologic
injury to coronary arteries due to graft rejection and dietarily-
induced hypercholesterolemia could initiate and accelerate atherosclerosis. Heterotopic cardiac homotransplants were performed in
the necks of 60 rabbits. Addition of cholesterol to the diet
intensified and accelerated the development of atherosclerosis in
the segment of aorta attached to the transplanted heart and in
the coronary and myocardial arteries of the transplanted heart.
Often very advanced atherosclerosis was observed in these arteries
within a few weeks after transplantation. Fatty-proliferative
lesions were also found, but in lesser number, in arteries from
hearts transplanted to rabbits which did not receive cholesterol
supplements. Aortas, coronary and myocardial arteries of recipient
rabbits were found to be normal indicating that neither receiving
foreign tissue antigens nor dietary cholesterol supplement alone
were capable of inducing atherosclerotic change (24). These experiments also indicate that, if the intensity of injury is severe
enough, lipid deposition can occur in vessel walls in the absence
of hyperlipidemia.

Dr. Minick also described experiments performed in collaboration with Dr. Julius and Catherine Fabricant in which specific,
pathogen-free chickens were infected with Marek's disease herpes

virus. Infected chickens develop extensive arteriosclerosis and
addition of cholesterol to their diet accelerates the development
of atherosclerosis. However, the intensity of injury is such that
some chickens develop atherosclerotic lesions even when cholesterol
is not added to the diet and their serum cholesterol level is 135
mg% (25). At this time it is not known whether the arterial injury
is due to cytopathic effects of the virus or to cellular or humoral
immunologic reactions to the virus, or some combination thereof.
Viral antigen can be demonstrated in the lesions.

The experimental models described above clearly demonstrate
that immunologically-mediated injury and dietarily-induced hyperlipidemia act synergistically to induce atherosclerosis closely
resembling that in man. There is increasing evidence that preco-
cious coronary artery disease occurs in systemic lupus erythematosus: it may occur in patients who develop arteritis associated
with hepatitis virus B and circulating antibodies to it, and it
has been described in some patients with rheumatic heart disease.
Furthermore, we are familiar with the effects of syphilis on blood
vessels. The question arises as to whether these disease states
are unique in this respect, or whether they represent an extreme
expression of a common phenomenon. The latter hypothesis tends to
be supported by the fact that 50% of patients with heart attacks
cannot be classified into any known risk group, suggesting the
existence of as yet unidentified risk factors. Further, the experiments with Marek's disease herpes virus, cited above, are very
important in this connection since herpes type viruses are ubiqui-
tous in the human population and severe hyperlipidemia is not.

REFERENCES

1. Kniker, W.T., and Cochrane, C.G. (1968) J. Exp. Med. 127, 119-
    136.

2. Barbaro, J.F., and Zvaifler, N.J. (1966) Proc. Soc. Exp. Biol.
    Med. 122, 1245-1247.

3. Henson, P.M., and Benveniste, J. (1971) in Biochemistry of
    Acute Allergic Reactions (Austen, K.F. and Becker, E., Eds.),
    Blackwell Scientific Publications, Oxford, pp. 111-126.

4. Benveniste, J., Henson, P.M., and Cochrane, C.G. (1972) J. Exp.
    Med. 136, 1356-1377.

5. Henson, P.M., and Pinckard, R.N. J. Immunol. In press.

6. Henson, P.M. (1977) J. Clin. Invest. 60, 481-490.

7. Henson, P.M., and Oades, Z.G. (1976) J. Exp. Med. 143, 953-968.

8. Henson, P.M. (1977) in Bayer Symposium VI, Experimental Models
    of Chronic Inflammatory Diseases, Springer-Verlag, 94-106.

9. Henson, P.M., and Oades, Z.G. (1975) J. Clin. Invest. 56, 1053-
    1061.

10. Kravis, T.C., and Henson, P.M. (1977) J. Immunol. 118, 1569-
    1573.

11. Capurro, B., and Levi, R. (1975) Circ. Research 36, 520-528.

12. Taylor, F.B., Jr., and Muller-Eberhard, H.J. (1970) J. Clin.
    Invest. 49, 2068-2085.

13. Taylor, F.B., Jr., et al., (1973) Ser. Haemat. VI, 527-548.

14. Zimmerman, T.S., and Muller-Eberhard, H.J. (1971) J. Exp. Med.
    134, 1601-1606.

15. Polley, M.J., and Nachman, R.L. (1975) J. Exp. Med. 141, 1261-
    1268.

16. Dixon, R.H., and Rosse, W.F. (1977) J. Clin. Invest. 59, 360-
    368.

17. Becker, C.G., Dubin, T., and Wiedemann, H.P. (1976) Proc. Natl.
    Acad. Sci. USA 73, 1712-1716.

18. Becker, C.G., Levi, R., and Zavecz, J. (1977) Circulation 55-56.

19. Becker, C.G., and Dubin, T. (1977) J. Exp. Med. 146, 457-467.

20. Theorell, H., Blomback, M., and Kockum, C. (1976) Thrombos.
    Haemostas. 36, 593-604.

21. Minick, C.R., Cambell, W.G., Jr., and Murphy, G.E. (1966) J.
    Exp. Med. 124, 635-652.

22. Minick, C.R., and Murphy, G.E. (1973) Am. J. Pathol. 73, 265-
    292.

23. Hardin, N.J., Minick, C.R., and Murphy, G.E. (1973) Am. J.
    Pathol. 73, 301-322.

24. Alonso, D., Starek, P., and Minick, C.R. (1977) Am. J. Pathol.
    87, 415-422.

25. Fabricant, C.G., Fabricant, J., Litrenta, M.M., and Minick,
    C.R. (1977) Circulation 55-56, Suppl. III, 144.

DISCUSSION FOLLOWING WORKSHOP 3b:
IMMUNOLOGIC INJURY

J.H. Joist: First, I would like to repeat a comment made by
Dr. Nemerson at a recent Gordon Conference in which he pointed out
with respect to some of the recently discovered complex interactions
of activated coagulation factors that we seem to know a lot about
what can happen in vitro but relatively little about what actually
happens in vivo. Concerning the interaction of platelets, immune
complexes, basophils and the vessel wall, how crucial is the presence of platelets, and do they serve predominantly as a localizing
factor for the deposition of immune complexes on the vessel wall or
can immune complexes attach to the vessel wall without the platelets
Second, what is so peculiar about the kidney, which makes it attractive for immune complex deposition?

P.M. Henson: I agree totally that it is imperative to extend
in vitro observations to the whole animal. In the case of PAF, we
have gone to considerable lengths, as outlined in my presentation,
to show that PAF does act in vivo and has acted on platelets during
the course of the anaphylaxis and the immune complex deposition.
Similarly, the abrogation of anaphylaxis and immune complex deposition following platelet depletion argues strongly for their role in
these processes in these experimental models.

It is not completely understood what makes the kidney a predilection site for immune complex deposition, but presumably its
unique blood flow characteristics are in some way involved.

D.J. Hanahan: Dr. Taylor, how was Factor X_a binding monitored?
Was this done with human or bovine material? Could you tell whether
the bound Factor X_a is still active towards prothrombin? And how
do you correlate this possibility of Factor X_a binding in vivo with
the large amount of antithrombin III present in plasma?

F.B. Taylor: Factor X_a binding to platelets was monitored by
harvesting platelets from a Factor II, V, platelet reaction system,
centrifuging against a silicone oil gradient, and counting the
radioactivity of the platelets. Studies were done with X_a. Studies

to measure bound Factor X_a activity towards prothrombin were not
done. Since the experiments presented were performed in buffer,
not plasma, the possibility of Factor X_a binding to antithrombin
III was not a practical problem. However, theoretically the studies
of Yin and Wessler suggest that, if the reactions in which Factor
X is activated in the presence of both platelets and AT III, the
reaction will go to completion, whereas in the absence of platelets
the X_a will be inhibited by AT III. This suggests that reactions
occurring on or near the surface of the platelets are not as easily
inhibited as those which occur in monophasic solutions.

M. Tiell: Many of our distinguished speakers have suggested
that inflammatory responses may play an integral role in atherogenesis. We have examined this phenomenon in our balloon-injured hypophysectomized rats, animals which consistently fail to develop
intimal smooth muscle cell plaques for periods up to two weeks following balloon injury.

Five days prior to ballooning, we injected subcutaneously
into the dorsal flank of our hypophysectomized rats a mixture of
turpentine and oil. Other hypophysectomized rats, serving as controls, received only oil subcutaneously. Both groups were sacri-
ficed one week after ballooning. Hypophysectomized rats, which
received turpentine in oil, developed intimal lesions, comparable
to the lesions obtained in one week, post-ballooned pituitary
intact rats. One week post-ballooned hypophysectomized rats,
receiving only oil subcutaneously, remained lesion-free.

The mechanism by which the inflammatory response, due to the
turpentine abscess, achieved its effect in overcoming the inhibitory effects of hypophysectomy on smooth muscle cell proliferation
is by no means fully understood. However, the results obtained
with our model concerning non-specific inflammatory reactions
warrants further investigation.

G. Majno: I was amused to hear that turpentine is still being used in 1977. It has been with us ever since the beginnings
of experimental pathology. In this case the results are fascinating, - but I want you to realize the rationale for the use of turpentine. The rationale is a tradition of some 5,000 years. Turpentine was originally the resin of a bush quite common in the
Mediterranean world; it was used by the Greeks and probably also
by the Sumerians, presumably because it smells good and gives a
warm feeling on the skin. Then it stayed on as one of the most
popular "drugs" of Western medicine. It was the standard means
for producing inflammation 100 years ago. But we still have no
idea of what it does.

C.J. Schwartz: Severely atheromatous arteries in man are frequently (80% of blocks) associated with a significant and rela-

tively homogeneous lymphocytic infiltration of the adventitial coat. This was reported in detail by Dr. J.R.A. Mitchell and myself some years ago. Such a cellular response would on general pathologic principles be regarded as cellular evidence for a chronic inflammatory process; the nature of the cellular infiltrate would additionally suggest an immune or auto-immune basis for this inflammation. For a given degree of plaque severity, it is of interest that in the presence of recent thrombus, the degree of the adventitial lymphocytosis is more extensive than would have been anticipated, suggesting either that thrombosis might cause this cellular response, or alternatively, that an underlying "immune" inflammatory process might in some manner contribute to thrombogenesis. I would appreciate the comments of the panel.

J.R.A. Mitchell: Colin Schwartz has commented on the focal lymphocyte collections in the adventitia of atherosclerotic vessels. If these were in the thyroid gland, they would be labeled as "auto-immune."

We have looked at age-matched subjects with severe peripheral vascular disease and normal subjects and find very significant elevations of IgG and IgM levels, although there is no difference in C'3, IgA, IgE, and lymphocyte transformation.

G. Majno: Regarding the possibility of an auto-immune component of atherosclerosis: this is precisely how we interpret the observations that we presented Sunday (mononuclear cells in the intima of the "normal" rat). The lymphocytes that stick to the endothelium and penetrate into the intima appear to choose areas where smooth muscle antigens are extruded across the endothelium.

H.L. Nossel: Elevated fibrionopeptide A levels have been reported in a number of immunological disorders - transient extremely high levels in acute food allergy and elevated levels in systemic lupus erythematosus and rejection of renal transplant.

T.A. Pearson: Dr. Minick, the photomicrographs and gross photographs of the disease in chickens you presented seemed to be examples of diffuse, end-stage disease. I would like to ask Dr. Minick if, at early stages, the disease is focal and if evidence of active inflammation is present? Secondly, do ultrastructural studies provide evidence for the presence of virus or evidence for the presence of cell transformation?

C.R. Minick: In the short time available for this part of the presentation we chose to illustrate end stage disease to document the severity of the process and emphasize the striking similarity to chronic human atherosclerosis. What we would interpret

to be early lesions are often exceedingly focal, often involving
only a small portion of the arterial wall. We have been able to
find Marek's disease antigen in arterial lesions by immunofluorescence microscopy. Ultrastructural studies are in progress.

S. Moore: Dr. Minick's work on virus is very exciting in providing a more biologically realistic model than many of those we
have been using in the study of arterial injury. I would like to
ask Dr. Minick if the Marek virus intimal lesions occur in the
aorta? I can think of an analogous model in human disease, that
of polyarteritis nodosa associated with hepatitis virus antigen
where lesions occur classically - lesions in vessels the size of
mesenteric arteries and coronary arteries.

C.R. Minick: We are also intrigued by the potential biological significance of this model of injury, because we believe it
offers an opportunity to test the validity of many of the hypotheses we have evolved in other model systems. Lesions do occur
in the aorta, but generally they are not as impressive as those
in the coronary and mesenteric arteries.

ANIMAL MODELS OF ATHEROSCLEROSIS INVOLVING THE THROMBOTIC PROCESS

K.M. Brinkhous, *Session Chairman*
Department of Pathology
School of Medicine
University of North Carolina

WORKSHOP 4a: THROMBOTIC MODELS

K.M. Brinkhous, Moderator
Participants: M.J. Karnovsky, R.L. Kinlough Rathbone,
B.A. Kottke, K.T. Lee, R.W. Mahley, M.R. Malinow,
R.H. More

WORKSHOP 4b: ATHEROSCLEROSIS IN HEMORRHAGIC DISORDERS

E.J.W. Bowie, Moderator
Participants: D.N. Fass, R.J. Friedman, T.R. Griggs

SUMMARY OF WORKSHOPS 4a & 4b:

ANIMAL MODELS OF ATHEROSCLEROSIS INVOLVING THE THROMBOTIC PROCESS

K.M. Brinkhous and E.J.W. Bowie

Department of Pathology, University of North Carolina, Chapel Hill, NC and Hematology Research, Mayo Clinic, Rochester, Minnesota

This section of the Workshop on Thromboatherosclerosis dealt with the present "state of the art" of producing experimental atherosclerosis in different animals, in which the thrombotic process is part of the development sequence in the pathogenesis and histogenesis of the lesion. The consideration of this topic was under two headings: (a) The use of normal animals of various species in which thromboatherosclerotic lesions are induced by diverse procedures; and (b) The use of animals with either induced or genetic impairment of the hemostatic mechanism, in which either naturally occurring or induced atherosclerosis is examined.

THROMBOATHEROSCLEROSIS IN DIFFERENT SPECIES

Experience in producing thrombosis/atherosclerosis in several different species was reviewed in seven separate presentations dealing with six species, pigeon, dog, rat, rabbit, pig, and non-human primates. Well characterized, experimentally-produced thromboatherosclerotic lesions have been described in all of these species.

Pigeon as a Model

The pigeon as a model for studying the thrombotic process in atherogenesis was described by Bruce A. Kottke, Mayo Clinic, Rochester, Minnesota. The potential of this model for the study of atherogenesis was first identified by Clarkson and associates in 1959 (1). They described the occurrence of a nearly 100% incidence of aortic atherosclerosis in White Carneau pigeons over three years

of age. A control breed, the Show Racer, had a less than 5% incidence under identical environmental conditions, including a
cholesterol-free diet. The aortic lesions occur in a constant
location and progress with age. In addition, the White Carneau
pigeons develop coronary atherosclerosis with an incidence of 70%
by age seven to eight years (2).

By conducting biochemical and morphologic studies of age-
matched groups of White Carneau and Show Racer breeds from newborn
to five years of age, an attempt has been made to elucidate the
sequence of critical changes that are associated with the pathogenesis of atherosclerosis (3). The earliest change is the occurrence of spontaneous endothelial damage with adherence of thrombocytes in the lesion-prone area of the susceptible breed at two to
three months of age (4). This is rapidly followed by the appearance of microscopic fat. Between 6 to 12 months of age the smooth
muscle cells in this area proliferate and by 12 months a chemically
detectable increase in aortic cholesteryl oleate is found. This
accumulation is preceded by a decrease in the activity of microsomal cholesteryl ester hydrolase and an increase in the cholesteryl
ester synthetase enzymes (5). After 12 months of age large quantities of microscopically detectable mucopolysaccharides accumulate.
By studying the mechanisms that control these critical events in
susceptible and resistant breeds, the molecular and cellular aspects
of the pathogenesis of atherosclerosis can be studied.

Dog as a Model

The dog as a model for studying the thrombotic process in
atherogenesis was described by Robert W. Mahley and Russell W.
Jaffe, National Institutes of Health, Bethesda, Maryland. They
pointed out that there is much to recommend the dog as a model for
studies of experimental atherosclerosis, including ease of handling, availability, and large size which provides sufficient blood
and arterial tissue for analysis. In addition, the dog does not
develop spontaneous atherosclerosis so that any arterial lesions
observed are the result of the experimental protocol. However, the
dogs are resistant to the development of hypercholesterolemia and
atherosclerosis and require maneuvers beyond simply feeding a high
cholesterol diet. Two different protocols have been shown to be
successful. One utilizes the hypothyroid dog (foxhounds) fed a
diet containing fat, cholesterol, and bile salts (6). The other
protocol requires the feeding of a semisynthetic diet which contains coconut oil as the only fat in the diet plus cholesterol
(7). It was found that the type of fat in the diet (saturated
vs. unsaturated) has profound influence on the severity of the
disease and on the complications associated with the atherosclerosis. When the dietary fat fed in association with cholesterol

is primarily saturated (beef tallow or lard in hypothyroid dogs
or coconut oil with the semisynthetic diet), the atherosclerosis
is more severe and is often associated with thrombosis. The sites
at which thrombosis is observed include the terminal abdominal
aorta, coronary arteries, and the internal carotid, iliofemoral
and basilar arteries (6). On the other hand, when the fat is
primarily unsaturated (cottonseed or corn oil), the atherosclerosis is less complicated, and no thrombosis has been observed.

Two parameters of platelet function, platelet aggregation and
platelet survival, were measured in dogs on the saturated fat-
cholesterol diets. Platelet aggregation studies were performed
with special attention paid to adaptation of the animals to the
environment and handlers; unrestrained phlebotomy by the two-syringe
technique, free-flow technique; pH control of the platelet-rich
plasma; and definite titratable endpoints for both ADP and collagen.
The minimum concentration of aggregating agent required to achieve
the largest and most rapid change in optical density is the end-
point. Dogs fed tallow and cholesterol for 7 to 12 days become
hypercholesterolemic (mean = 1756 mg/dl) and hypertriglyceridemic
(856 mg/dl). These animals show a mean 19.5-fold increase in sensitivity to ADP when the on-diet concentration of ADP is compared
to the pre-diet concentration required for maximal aggregation.
In response to bovine type I fibrillar collagen, sensitivity increases 4.3-fold. In animals fed the unsaturated cottonseed oil-
cholesterol diets, comparable hyperlipidemia occurs (cholesterol =
1852 mg/dl; triglyceride = 420 mg/dl), yet the platelet sensitivity
is not significantly changed from pre-diet values. For ADP, the
mean on-diet to pre-diet ratio is 1:2 and for collagen the ratio
is 1:1. Similar sensitivity of the platelets in dogs on the saturated fat diets and lack of responsiveness of the platelets in
the dogs on unsaturated fat are also observed after 20 weeks on
diet. Platelet survival was measured with ^{51}Cr-tagged platelets
before initiation of the diet and after 21 weeks on diet. The
diet-induced changes in the survival times are expressed as a
ratio of the on-diet survival to the pre-diet value. For animals
fed tallow and cholesterol, the mean ratio of on-diet to pre-diet
survival of the platelets is 0.68 as compared to 0.80 for the
cottonseed oil and cholesterol-fed dogs. The decrease in survival
time is significant for the dogs on the saturated fat.

In summary, there appears to be a definite association between
saturated fat and cholesterol and the occurrence of thromboatherosclerosis. In addition, there are marked alterations in platelet
function, including increased sensitivity to platelet aggregation
and a decreased survival time in the animals with the thrombotic
tendency.

Rat as a Model

The rat as a model for studying the thrombotic process in atherogenesis was described by Morris J. Karnovsky, Harvard Medical School, Boston, Massachusetts. A new model was developed (8) to study the reaction of components of the arterial wall following endothelial injury. Complete endothelial denudation was produced in a precisely defined unbranched segment of the rat common carotid artery, 1.5 cm long, by briefly drying the isolated segment with a gentle stream of dry air (50 ml/min for 3-5 min), blown along the arterial lumen. Upon restoration of blood flow, the endothelial cells begin to fall away within 10 min and denudation is complete within 12 hours. Platelets rapidly attach to the denuded surface. Endothelial regeneration occurs from each end of the denuded segment, and is complete by 10 days. Myointimal proliferation occurs in the central region of the segment to a predictable and defined degree which can be quantitated by morphometry. In this model, the clear demarcation and completeness of endothelial denudation allows for study of the kinetics of endothelial replacement, avoiding the complications imposed by residual islands of non-denuded endothelium or contributions from branch vessels. The method of inducing denudation does not cause detectable damage to the underlying media, and thus the model offers the opportunity of studying the relationships between relatively specific endothelial injury and changes in components of the arterial wall, such as the kinetics and extent of myointimal proliferation. The effects of stress, manipulation of the diet (9, 10) and the administration of drugs can readily be assessed (11, 12).

Rabbit as a Model

The rabbit as a model for studying the thrombotic process in atherogenesis was described by Robert H. More and Bernard I. Weigensberg, McGill University, Montreal, Canada, and R.L. Kinlough-Rathbone, H. Groves, J.-P. Cazenave, S. Moore, and J.F. Mustard, McMaster University, Hamilton, Ontario, respectively, in two separate presentations as follows: In the model reported by More and Weigensberg, a polyethylene catheter is placed in the aorta of the rabbit by way of the femoral artery. On the catheter, massive amounts of platelet thrombus material accumulate that can be studied at sequential time intervals for as long as a year. In the normolipidemic rabbit this thrombus progresses, in a period of six months, to a rather classic atherosclerotic plaque with a core of intracellular and extracellular lipid overlayed with a connective tissue cap. The thrombus material is of sufficient amount to permit the study of parallel morphologic and chemical profiles over short and long periods of time. These studies can

be conducted under varying experimental conditions such as with
various levels of lipidemia and/or with various drugs and diets
that affect the rate and quality of cell proliferation and rate
and quality of connective tissue production. A number of observations made on this model have been reported (13-19).

Kinlough-Rathbone et al. reported that rabbits are not ideal
for studying the effects of diet-induced hypercholesterolemia on
the development of atherosclerosis and relating it to the process
in man (20). However, they do appear useful for studying the
effects of endothelial injury on the development of atherosclerosis
and thrombosis. Cannula-injury to the umbilical vessel of neonates
(21) produces a spectrum of intimal lesions similar to those produced in the aortae of rabbits by indwelling cannulae (22). Thus,
in young animals or humans the response of the arterial wall to
endothelial injury is similar. With rabbits parallel results can
be obtained from in vitro and in vivo studies of platelet interactions with subendothelial structures. Repeated endothelial
injury in rabbits changes the properties of the subendothelium
and it becomes more thrombogenic (23). As a result of a single
injury to the rabbit aorta induced by a balloon catheter, a monolayer of platelets is deposited on the exposed subendothelium and
there is relatively little turnover of this initial platelet layer
(24). In contrast to results obtained with monkeys (25), platelet
survival is unchanged by a single injury to the endothelium (24).
Within 30 minutes of the initial injury and for at least 7 days
after injury, the damaged surface is relatively non-reactive to
circulating platelets (unpublished observations). Thus, the initial platelet interaction with the damaged vessel wall is probably
crucial for the smooth muscle cell response to injury. It was
shown in rabbits that dipyridamole reduces platelet adherence to
subendothelial structures in vitro but does not block release from
platelets adherent to collagen. In contrast, anti-inflammatory
drugs such as aspirin or sulphinpyrazone do not block platelet
adherence to collagen or to exposed subendothelial structures in
vitro or in vivo, nor the release reaction of platelets adherent
to collagen (26, 27). This is consistent with the observation
that aspirin and sulphinpyrazone have little effect on smooth muscle cell proliferation secondary to endothelial injury (11, 28,
unpublished observations).

Pig as a Model

K.T. Lee and W.M. Lee, Albany, New York, reported on their
experience in producing advanced coronary atherosclerosis in swine
by a combination of balloon-denudation procedure and high cholesterol diet (29-36). Advanced atherosclerotic lesions were produced
in coronary arteries in cholesterol-fed swine within a short period

of time by inserting a balloon-catheter via the right carotid artery into the coronary artery, inflating it so as to distend the lumen, and pulling it back quickly, which resulted in extensive denudation of the endothelium of coronary arteries. Atherosclerotic lesions developed at the site with eventual narrowing of the lumen leading to myocardial ischemia, myocardial infarction, and occasional sudden death, thus resembling in many aspects human coronary disease. Among 22 swine studied, 10 had severe atherosclerosis with virtual occlusion of the proximal portion of either or both coronary arteries and developed myocardial infarction within 2-3 months. Seven of these swine died suddenly, probably due to arrhythmia. The evidence of thromboembolism was found in half of the swine studied. This model should be appropriate for studies where advanced coronary atherosclerosis with its complications is needed.

Non-Human Primate Models

M.R. Malinow, W.P. McNulty and S.H. Goodnight, Jr., Oregon Regional Primate research Center and University of Oregon, Portland, Oregon, raised the question if the thrombotic process is involved in diet-induced atherosclerosis in non-human primates (37-48). A survey of the literature indicated that diet-induced atherosclerosis has been reported in several thousand non-human primates, but these reports have, for the most part, failed to disclose evidence of thrombosis. That incidence of arterial thrombosis seems much higher in atherosclerotic vessels of human beings than in those of non-human primates could be due to several factors, including (1) inadequate animal studies and/or (b) differences in the pathogenesis of arterial lesions and/or in the thrombotic process. However, it seems unlikely that possibility (a) would explain the absence of thrombosis in the numerous reports from different experienced investigators. The observations of Malinow et al. on several hundred monkeys agree with the above. A survey of possibility (b) indicates obvious differences between diet-induced atherosclerosis in monkeys and human atherosclerosis. In addition, differences may also occur in the thrombotic process; for instance, Malinow et al. have documented that platelets in several species of monkeys react less well to aggregating agents than do platelets in human beings. A non-human primate model is needed in which to predictably induce arterial thrombosis superimposed on experimental atherosclerosis. At present, though, there are limitations in the use of monkeys as a model for the study of the thrombotic process superimposed on atherosclerotic vessels.

Comparative Levels of Clotting Factors in Different Species

Another aspect of selection of a suitable animal species for inducing experimental thromboatherosclerosis was presented by one

of us (K.M.B.). It was pointed out that a considerable body of
data exists regarding comparative levels of clotting factors and
platelet function in normal animals of various species (49-52).
Since both fibrin clotting and platelet activation represent basic
biological mechanisms underlying thrombosis, knowledge of species
differences in the various components of these mechanisms can be
helpful in species selection. On the one hand, one may wish to
select an animal in which fibrin clotting and hemostatic plug formation are comparable to those observed in man. Or one may select
species in which certain factors are qualitatively or quantita-
tively greatly different from those in man, so that an assessment
of the influence of a given biological mechanism on the thromboatherosclerotic process can be made. Two examples were cited.
One example is the natural deficiency observed in birds in the
contact activation system of the intrinsic clotting pathway. Also,
birds have nucleated thrombocytes rather than platelets. The
other example related to species variation in the plasma levels
of platelet aggregating factor/von Willebrand factor (PAΓ/vWF).
This aggregating factor is part of the factor VIII macromolecular
complex which provides a bridge between the intrinsic pathway of
clotting and platelet function. In a recent study (53) it was
found that certain species, pig and two non-human primates, rhesus
monkey and chimpanzee, had PAF/vWF levels in the same range as
human plasma. On the other hand, all of the ruminants tested,
cow, sheep and goat, had very high levels of this platelet aggregating factor. There is still a need to characterize more fully
the various species of animals used in thromboatherosclerotic
studies as to the relative thrombus-promoting and thrombus-retard-
ing activities of their blood.

ATHEROGENESIS IN HEMORRHAGIC DISORDERS

The interaction of platelets, smooth muscle cells and endothelium seems to be of major importance to an understanding of atherosclerosis. This has led several workers to look at the applicability
of animal models of hemorrhagic diseases to this research. The two
main animal models that have been developed so far are (a) the von
Willebrand pig, and (b) the thrombocytopenic rabbit. Preliminary
data is also being obtained in other animal models.

Pig with von Willebrand's Disease as a Model

The pig as a model for atherosclerosis in hemorrhagic disorders was described by V. Fuster, E.J.W. Bowie and D.N. Fass, Mayo
Clinic, Rochester, Minnesota and T.R. Griggs, University of North
Carolina, Chapel Hill, North Carolina, in three separate presentations. Fuster and Bowie reported that normal pigs have an ar-

terial system closely resembling man's. They both develop spontaneous atherosclerosis early in life, and the lesions are similar
in distribution and development (54-56). Because of their size,
the lesions are easy to quantitate macroscopically and structurally
Furthermore, porcine atherosclerosis may be induced by a high
cholesterol diet in less than 6 months (57-59). The development
of atherosclerosis was studied in the aortas of 11 pigs (age 1-3
years) with homozygous von Willebrand's disease (vWD) (60) and in
11 normal pigs of the same ages. Multiple atherosclerotic plaques
with intimal thickening of 63 to 130 μm was found in 6 of the controls. None of the vWD pigs, in contrast, had multiple plaques
and only 1 had a lesion with a diameter of more than 2 mm. Subsequently, a 2% cholesterol diet for up to 6 months was given to
3-month-old pigs (11 controls and 7 with vWD). Aortic atherosclerotic plaques developed in all of the controls, in 9 of which at
least 12% of the aortic surface was involved. Intimal thickness
ranged to 390 m. On the other hand, no lesions developed in 4
of the vWD pigs and 2 developed lesions affecting only 6% and 7%
of the aortic surface. One vWD pig had 13% of the aortic surface
involved. Most of the vWD pigs, however, developed fatty infiltration of the intima (flat fatty lesions), whereas this was rarely
seen in the normal pig. Two vWD pigs were injected with Evans
blue dye antemortem, and there was blue staining of the flat fatty
lesions. Severe endothelial damage was found in the stained areas
by electron microscopy, but there was no intimal proliferation.
All of these findings may be related to impaired platelet arterial
wall interaction in vWD and confirm the importance of the pig
model for atherosclerosis research (61, 62).

    D.N. Fass described platelet responses to von Willebrand fac-
tor. Two lines of evidence indicate that, in the porcine model,
platelet endothelial interaction is dependent upon the presence
of Willebrand factor in the vessel wall. In studies conducted in
collaboration with Drs. Didisheim, Grabowski, and Lewis it was
seen that in flowing whole blood, platelet adhesion to kidney
dialysis membrane was possible only if Willebrand factor containing blood components were first adsorbed to the membrane surface
(63). This adhesion was abolished by treatment of the coated
membranes with anti-Willebrand factor antibodies.

    Investigations carried out with Drs. Booyse, Lewis, and Bowie,
utilizing cultured porcine aortic endothelium, in part corroborate
these findings (64). The endothelial cells of normal pigs contain
immunoreactive fibers detectable by both indirect immunofluorescence and peroxidase linked second-antibody. While scanning electron microscopy reveals filaments in the von Willebrand porcine
cultures, these are immunologically unreactive when stained with
antiporcine Willebrand factor. Platelets adhere to damaged normal
cultures but not to similarly treated von Willebrand endothelial

cultures. This platelet adhesion is also abolished by pretreatment of the culture with antibody to porcine Willebrand factor.

T.R. Griggs described the induction of atherogenesis in pigs.
Studies comparing normal pigs with swine from an inbred colony with
homozygous von Willebrand's disease have shown that the abnormal
swine, even at an advanced age and in spite of exposure to an
atherogenic diet, tend to develop fewer lesions than do normal pigs.
This phenomenon may result from a decreased response of platelets
to endothelial injury in the abnormal animals. Studies are in
progress on the response to endothelial injury caused by balloon
denudation and carbon monoxide inhalation in normal swine and in
swine with von Willebrand's disease. In preliminary studies it
was shown that coronary atherosclerosis with myocardial infarction
and death can be induced in animals heterozygous for the von Willebrand trait. Homozygous animals have been prepared and are being
studied also. These experiments are designed to examine the
effects not only of the von Willebrand factor on atherogenesis,
but also to provide a model for studying the relationship of carbon monoxide, a major component of cigarette smoke and an atmos-
pheric pollutant, to the development of these lesions.

Thrombocytopenic Rabbit as a Model

R.J. Friedman, Albert Einstein College of Medicine, Bronx,
New York, described studies on rabbits as models for experimental
atherosclerosis. A knowledge of the interaction of platelets,
smooth muscle cells, and endothelium is of importance to a better
understanding of the pathobiology of atherosclerosis. Endothelial
injury evokes a smooth muscle cell proliferative response (65,
66). The resulting neointimal smooth muscle cell lesion is considered to be a precursor of the more complicated lesions of
atherosclerosis (67, 68). Ross et al. have observed that a platelet-derived constituent in serum is required for growth of cultured arterial smooth muscle cells (38). This constituent, known
as "platelet growth factor" may be involved in initiating and/or
maintaining the smooth muscle proliferative response in vivo.
Removal of platelets from the general circulation with a crude
antiplatelet serum markedly inhibits experimentally induced atherosclerotic lesions in rabbits (69). The present study was designed to investigate the role of the platelet in the migration
and proliferation of smooth muscle cells (SMC) following selective
de-endothelialization by the intra-arterial balloon catheter in
rabbits made thrombocytopenic with a specific anti-platelet serum
(70). Thrombocytopenia (mean platelet count of 5,300/cu.mm) was
induced and maintained for up to 1 month. Control animals (mean
platelet count of 360,000/cu.mm) received identically treated
normal sheep serum on the same schedule as their experimental
pair-mates. The purpose of the present study (70) included inves-

tigation of (a) the role of thrombocytopenia on SMC migration and proliferation following the endothelial removal; (b) the effect(s) of the various sera themselves on the SMC proliferation; (c) the effect of thrombocytopenia and the various sera on the re-endothelialization process, and (d) the effect of thrombocytopenia and the sera on the white blood count. Evidence for re-endothelialization was obtained by administering IV Evans blue dye one half hour before sacrifice. Evaluation of SMC proliferation was determined by a count of cell layers in semi-thin sections. The results of the study show that SMC intimal thickening in thrombocytopenic rabbits was strikingly suppressed when contrasted with that occurring in animals with normal platelet count. These results indicate that the proliferation of SMC which is characteristic of arteriosclerotic lesions is markedly inhibited by reduction of platelets.

In a second series of experiments (unpublished observations) designed to answer the question what the platelet's role is in the initiation of the SMC proliferative response following endothelial injury, rabbits were given antiplatelet serum (APS) 1 hr, 3 hr, and 1 day post- de-endothelialization. At the time of balloon injury, these rabbits had normal platelet counts (range 320,000-410,000 cu.mm). Following administration of APS, platelet counts fell to less than 7,000/cu.mm and were maintained at those levels for 7 and 14 days. Control groups included animals given APS 3 days prior to ballooning and maintained thrombocytopenic until sacrifice. These animals had platelet counts at the time of ballooning of about 5,000/cu.mm. Additional control groups included non-treated ballooned animals and animals given normal sheep serum and ballooned. The results indicate that animals which were thrombocytopenic at the time of ballooning had marked inhibition in the SMC response. In contrast were non-treated control animals, animals given normal sheep serum and animals made thrombocytopenic 1 hr, 3 hr, and 1 day following balloon de-endothelialization. These animals had the normal proliferative response to balloon de-endothelialization with a mean SMC proliferation of 6.9 SMC at 14 days post-injury. These data indicate that the platelet seems to be important in the initiation of the SMC proliferative response. Its role in the maintenance of this response is as yet unclear.

In an effort to determine a role of lipids, if any, in the SMC proliferative response following balloon de-endothelialization, a series of experiments was done with thrombocytopenic rabbits fed a normal rabbit chow diet and those fed a high lipid diet (unpublished observations). Appropriate normal sheep serum and nontreated controls were run. In addition, a group of animals fed the high lipid diet alone and not ballooned were included. The animals were fed the egg-supplemented diet for 6 weeks prior to ballooning. All lipid supplemented animals had mean serum cholesterol levels of approximately 260 mg% prior to balloon de-endothelialization. Animals fed the non-supplemented diet had mean

serum cholesterol levels of about 55 mg%. The results indicated
marked inhibition of the SMC proliferative response in the non-
diet supplemented thrombocytopenic animals as has been previously
reported (70). In marked contrast, however, were the hypercholesterolemic, thrombocytopenic animals who developed the SMC proliferative response equivalent to control animals. These findings
implicate a possible important role of lipids in the SMC response
which may be independent of the platelet related response.

In summary, the data presented indicate the following: (a)
the SMC proliferative response following balloon de-endothelialization is markedly inhibited if animals are severely thrombocytopenic at the time of endothelial injury; (b) the platelet appears
to play a role in the initiation of the SMC response; (c) lipids
play an important, as yet undefined, role in the SMC response
which may be independent of the platelet's role.

CONCLUDING COMMENTS

In summary, animal models are powerful tools in the experimental pathological study of thromboatherosclerosis. Morphologic, biochemical, and physiological effects can all be studied to advantage.
Recent methods for production of accelerated atherosclerosis in
animal models have provided much evidence for the importance of the
thrombogenic process in the initiation and progression of atherosclerosis. Any of a number of animals have been successfully used
for development of the thromboatherosclerotic lesions. Different
species may serve both a common and a specific purpose. The qualitative and quantitative aspects of various biologic mechanisms which
on activation contribute to thrombogenesis can be selected and
manipulated to determine the importance of selected factors in
atherogenesis (52). This may be done by (a) taking advantage of
natural species differences, well exemplified by the relative deficiency in contact activation in birds or the very high levels of
the von Willebrand factor in ruminants, (b) by utilizing mutant
strains, such as pigs with von Willebrand's disease and dogs with
hemophilia or other bleeder states, or (c) by inducing changes by
drugs, such as with coumarin or platelet-anti-aggregating drugs.

REFERENCES

1. Clarkson, T.B., Prichard, R.W., Netsky, M.G., and Lofland,
    H.B. (1959) Arch. Pathol. 68, 143-147.

2. Prichard, R.W., Clarkson, T.B., Goodman, H.O., and Lofland,
    H.B. (1966) Arch. Pathol. 81, 292-301.

3. Subbiah, M.T.R., Unni, K.K., Kottke, B.A., Carlo, I.A., and Dinh, D.M. (1976) Exp. Mol. Pathol. 24, 287-301.

4. Lewis, J.C., and Kottke, B.A. (1977) Science 196, 1007-1009.

5. Subbiah, M.T.R., and Dicke, B.A. (1977) Arterosclerosis 27, 107-111.

6. Mahley, R.W., Nelson, A.W., Ferrans, V.J., and Fry, D.L. (1976) Science 192, 1139-1141.

7. Mahley, R.W., Innerarity, T.L., Weisgraber, K.H., and Fry, D.L. (1977) Am. J. Pathol. 87, 205-226.

8. Fishman, J.A., Ryan, G.B., and Karnovsky, M.J. (1976) Lab. Invest. 32, 339-351.

9. Clowes, A.W., Ryan, G.B., Breslow, J.L., and Karnovsky, M.J. (1976) Lab. Invest. 35, 6-17.

10. Clowes, A.W., Breslow, J.L., and Karnovsky, M.J. (1977) Lab. Invest. 36, 73-81.

11. Clowes, A.W., and Karnovsky, M.J. (1977) Lab. Invest. 36, 452-464.

12. Clowes, A.W., and Karnovsky, M.J. (1977) Nature 265, 625-626.

13. Sumiyoshi, A., More, R.H., and Weigensberg, B.I. (1973) Atherosclerosis 18, 43-57.

14. Weigensberg, B.I., More, R.H., Sumiyoshi, A., and Mullen, B. (1974) Exp. Mol. Pathol. 20, 154-167.

15. Weigensberg, B.I., More, R.H., and Sumiyoshi, A. (1975) Lab. Invest. 33, 43-50.

16. Weigensberg, B.I., and More, R.H. (1975) in International Workshop Conference on Atherosclerosis (Haust, M.D. and Manning, Eds.), Plenum, New York.

17. Gotlieb, A., More, R.H., and Weigensberg, B.I. (1977) Am. J. Pathol. 86, 52a-53a.

18. Rabinovitch, J., Weigensberg, B.I., More, R.H., and Gotlieb, A. (1977) Thromb. Haemost. 38, 154.

19. Weigensberg, B.I., Gotlieb, A.I., Lough, J., and More, R.H. (1977) Fed. Proc. 36, 1161.

20. Wissler, R.W., and Vesselinovitch, D. (1974) in Atherosclerosis III (Schettler, G. and Weizel, A., Eds.), Springer, Berlin-Heidelberg-New York, pp. 253-267.

21. Tyson, J.E., de Sa, D.J., and Moore, S. (1976) Arch. Dis. Child. 51, 744-754.

22. Moore, S. (1973) Lab. Invest. 29, 478-487.

23. Stemerman, M.B. (1973) Am. J. Pathol. 73, 7-26.

24. Groves, H.M., Kinlough-Rathbone, R.L., Richardson, M., and Mustard, J.F. Blood. In press.

25. Ross, R., and Harker, L.A. (1976) Science 193, 1094-1100.

26. Cazenave, J.P., Packham, M.A., Kinlough-Rathbone, R.L., and Mustard, J.F. (1977) in Brook Lodge Workshop on Models for Thrombosis Research. In press.

27. Cazenave, J.P., Kinlough-Rathbone, R.L., Packham, M.A., and Mustard, J.F. Blood. In press.

28. Baumgartner, H.R., and Studer, A. in Workshop on Thrombosis and Atherosclerosis, IV International Symposium on Atherosclerosis. In press.

29. Lee, W.M., and Lee, K.T. (1975) Exp. Mol. Pathol. 23, 491-499.

30. Nam, S.C., Lee, W.M., Jarmolych, J., Lee, K.T., and Thomas, W.A. (1973) Exp. Mol. Pathol. 18, 369-379.

31. Lee, K.T., Lee, W.M., Han, J., Jamolych, J., Bishop, M.B., and Goel, B.G. (1973) Am. J. Cardiol. 32, 62-73.

32. Scott, R.F., and Briggs, T.S. (1972) Am. J. Cardiol. 29, 782-787.

33. Stemerman, M.B., and Spaet, T.H. (1972) Bull. N.Y. Acad. Med. 48, 289-301.

34. Baumgartner, H.R., and Spaet, T.H. (1970) Fed. Proc. 29, 710 Abstract.

35. Bjorkerud, S. (1969) Virchows Arch. A. 347, 197-210.

36. Thomas, W.A., Florentin, R.A., Nam, S.C., Kim, D.N., Jones, R.M., and Lee, K.T. (1968) Arch. Pathol. 86, 621-643.

37. Weber, G., Fabrini, P., Resi, L., Jones, R., Vesselinovitch, D., and Wissler, R.W. (1977) Atherosclerosis 26, 535-547.

38. Ross, R., Glomset, J.S., Kariya, B., and Harker, L.A. (1974) Proc. Natl. Acad. Sci. USA 71, 1207-1210.

39. Stemerman, M.B., and Ross, R. (1972) J. Exp. Med. 136, 769-789.

40. Wu, K.K., Armstrong, M.L., Hoak, J.S., and Megan, M.B. (1975) Thromb. Res. 7, 917-924.

41. Taylor, C.B., Manalo-Estrella, P., and Cox, G.E. (1963) Arch. Pathol. 76, 239-249.

42. Scott, R.F., Morrison, E.S., Jarmolych, J., Nam, S.C., Kroms, M., and Coultson, F. (1967) Exp. Mol. Pathol. 7, 11-33.

43. Scott, R.F., Jones, R., Daoud, A.S., Zumbo, O., Coultson, F., and Thomas, W.A. (1976) Exp. Mol. Pathol. 7, 34-57.

44. Chakravarti, R.N., Kumar, M., Singh, S.P., and Das, K.C. (1974) Atherosclerosis 21, 349-359.

45. Prathap, K. (1972) J. Pathol. 110, 203-212.

46. Harker, L.A., Slichter, S.J., Scott, C.R., and Ross, R. (1974) N. Engl. J. Med. 291, 537-543.

47. Barnett, H.J.M. (1977) Adv. Neurol. 16, 45-70.

48. Mason, R.G., Sharp, D.E., Chuang, H.Y.K., and Mohammad, S.R. (1977) Arch. Pathol. Lab. Med. 101, 61-64.

49. Hawkey, C.M. (1974) Thromb. Diath. Haemorrh. 31, 103-118.

50. Mason, R.G., and Read, M.S. (1967) Exp. Mol. Pathol. 6, 370-381.

51. Mason, R.G., and Read, M.S. (1971) J. Biomed. Mat. Res. 5, 121-128.

52. Brinkhous, K.M. (1978) in Thrombosis: Animal and Human Models (Day, H.J., Molony, B.A., Nishizawa, E.E. and Rynbrandt, R., Eds.), Plenum Press, New York. In press.

53. Brinkhous, K.M., Thomas, B.D., Ibrahim, S.A., and Read, M.S. (1977) Thromb. Res. 11, 345-355.

54. French, J.E., Jennings, M.S., and Florey, H.W. (1965) Ann. N.Y. Acad. Sci. 127, 780-799.

55. Getty, R. (1965) in Comparative Atherosclerosis: The Morphology of Spontaneous and Induced Atherosclerotic Lesions in Animals and Its Relation to Human Disease (Roberts, J.D. and Straus, R., Eds.), Harper and Row, New York, pp. 11-20.

56. Ratcliffe, H.L., Luginbuhl, H., and Pivnik, L. (1970) Bull. W.H.O. 42, 225-234.

57. Imai, H., and Thomas, W.A. (1968) Exp. Mol. Pathol. 8, 330-357.

58. Florentin, R.A., and Nam, S.C. (1968) Exp. Mol. Pathol. 8, 263-301.

59. Hill, E.G., Lundberg, W.D., and Titus, J.L. (1971) Mayo Clin. Proc. 46, 621-625.

60. Bowie, E.J.W., Owen, C.A., Zollman, P.E., Thompson, J.H., and Fass, D.N. (1973) Am. J. Vet. Res. 34, 1405-1407.

61. Fuster, V., Bowie, E.J.W., and Brown, A.L. (1977) Adv. Exp. Med. Biol. 82, 315-317.

62. Fuster, V., Bowie, E.J.W., Lewis, J.C., Fass, D.N., Owen, C.A., and Brown, A.L. (1978) J. Clin. Invest. In press.

63. Fass, D.N., Didisheim, P., Lewis, J.C., and Grabowski, E.F. (1976) Circulation 53-54, Suppl. II, Abstract 454.

64. Booyse, F.M., Quarfoot, A.J., Bell, S., Fass, D.N., Lewis, J.C., Mann, D.C., and Bowie, E.J.W. (1977) Proc. Natl. Acad. Sci. USA. In press.

65. Spaet, T.H., Stemerman, M.B., Veith, F.J., Lejnieks, I. (1975) Circ. Res. 36, 58-70.

66. Ross, R., and Glomset, J.S. (1973) Science 180, 1332-1339.

67. Arteriosclerosis, Report by National Heart and Lung Institute. Task Force Arteriosclerosis (1972) DHEW Publ. No. 72-219, 13.

68. Geer, J.C., and Haust, M.D. (1972) Monograph on Arteriosclerosis, Karger, Basel.

69. Moore, S., Friedman, R.J., Singal, D.P., Gauldie, J., Blajchman, M.A., and Roberts, R.S. (1976) Thromb. Haemost. 35, 70-81.

70. Friedman, R.J., Stemerman, M.B., Wenz, B., Moore, S., Gauldie,
     J., Gent, M., Tiell, M.L., Spaet, T.H. (1977) J. Clin. Invest.
     60, 1191-1201.

71. Brinkhous, K.M., Davis, P.D., Graham, J.B., and Dodds, W.J.
     (1973) Blood 41, 577-585.

DISCUSSION FOLLOWING WORKSHOPS 4a & 4b:

ANIMAL MODELS INVOLVING THE THROMBOTIC PROCESS

K.M. Brinkhous, the Chairman, asked the audience, on the
basis of what had been presented at the Workshop, which animals
they would use for models of thromboatherosclerosis in their own
studies. Of those interested in using animal models, the largest
number favored the pig, with the rabbit second, non-human primates
third, and the dog fourth. Other animals were favored by only a
few investigators. Most of the Workshop participants indicated
that for their own work they favored studies on human subjects.
The Chairman then noted that there appeared to be a potential increase in the use of the dog in the light of the recent studies
presented by Mahley. This should be an advantage since the dog,
of the various animals, has been best characterized in relation
to normal clotting and platelet functions. Likewise, in the dog,
there are many more well studied genetic strains with deficiencies
of one or more factors which contribute to thrombogenesis. At the
University of North Carolina there is an inter-strain breeding
program in progress in dogs with different genetic deficiencies
of the hemostatic mechanism. The separate deficient strains are
hemophilia A dogs (coagulant factor VIII deficiency), hemophilia
B dogs (Factor IX deficiency) and von Willebrand's disease (PAF/
vWF and related factor VIII complex deficiency). Of the possible
crosses among three strains, 3^3, or 27, 15 have been obtained
(see ref. 52, 71 above). In this way a combination of deficiency
states can be studied in relation to atherogenesis, in addition to
a single deficiency state.

G. Hornstra: Dr. Mahley, did you find in your EFA-deficient
fed dogs any sign of EFA-deficiency, such as an increase in the
triene-tetraene ratio of the plasma or tissue lipids?

R.W. Mahley: Dogs fed the essential fatty acid deficient diet
(hydrogenated coconut oil plus cholesterol) were 9 to 12 months of
age before they were started on the diet and did not develop physical signs of EFA-deficiency. We have not determined the triene-
tetraene ratio. However, this question has been extensively
studied by investigators at the Cleveland Clinic, and the role of

EFA-deficiency is discussed in a recent paper (McCullagh, K.G., Ehrhart, L.A., and Butkus, A. (1976) Lab. Invest. 34, 371-405).

A. Nordøy: I also have a question to Dr. Mahley. You have used two protocols to produce hypercholesterolemia in dogs, one including hypothyroid drug. In humans, it has been shown that hypothyroidism may be associated with impaired platelet function not unlike the findings in patients with von Willebrand's disease. I wonder if you observed any differences in platelet function or thrombotic lesions in the hypercholesterolemia dogs from the two groups.

R.W. Mahley: We have found that the type of atherosclerosis which develops in the hypothyroid, saturated fat-cholesterol-fed dogs is very similar to the atherosclerosis which developed in the euthyroid coconut oil cholesterol-fed dogs on the semisynthetic diet. Both of these protocols have led to the production of thrombosis. Hypothyroidism is not required when the semisynthetic diet contains cholesterol and coconut oil as the only fat.

N. Woolf: There are cogent advantages in the choice of the pig as a model for the production of experimental thromboatherosclerosis. It has an artery wall closely resembling that of the young human; if left alone for long enough time, it will develop spontaneous atherosclerosis. Perhaps most important of all, the pig is omnivorous and does not require the use of grossly unphysiological maneuvers to produce plasma lipid levels in the human range.

I should also like to make a plea that we should characterize the models we use accurately. I have been struck by the fact that in all the single injury balloon catheter models we have had described to us, on no occasion has what a practicing histopathologist would call a thrombus resulted. Instead we see a "carpet" of platelets adhering to the abraded surface with no buildup of aggregated platelets and no fibrin formation. In my own experience, focal abrasion of the aortic intima under direct vision is followed by the formation of large thrombi and the natural history of these lesions inevitably differs somewhat from what we have seen in the balloon catheter model. One system is not necessarily either more or less useful than another but they are different and the differences should be appreciated.

H.J. Weiss: In fact, I am somewhat surprised by Dr. Griggs' findings as I would have expected some inhibition of the atherosclerotic process in the ballooned vessels of von Willebrand swine. As you know, we have shown impaired adhesion of human von Willebrand platelets to rabbit subendothelium and that this is correctable by factor VIII. We have recently shown that their defect can be demonstrated in native (non-anticoagulated) blood and is highly shear-rate dependent. What Dr. Griggs has shown is that severe von Willebrand's disease does not confer absolute protection against atherogenesis in the ballooned von Willebrand vessels. One wonders, however, whether the process is slowed in any way. Perhaps this could be answered by studying the rate of atherogenesis in these animals. I would also like to raise one other point. Dr. Bowie indicated that the basic defect in von Willebrand's disease is impaired adhesion to endothelium, whereas we have postulated that impaired adhesion to subendothelium accounts for the hemostatic defect and possibly the atherogenic-sparing effect in von Willebrand swine. That is, we would suggest that platelets adhere to areas of the vessel wall where the endothelium has been removed and subsequently release mitogenic factor into the vessel. Your theory would suggest that platelets attach to endothelium, and, perhaps, release mitogenic factor at this site.

T.R. Griggs: In response to the question of Dr. Weiss, it may indeed be possible that severe von Willebrand's disease in our swine does slow the rate of development of atherogenesis following balloon denudation and feeding of an atherogenic diet. We fear, however, that the use of the balloon denudation itself may introduce an uncontrollable variable making detection of rate differences impossible. Therefore, we presently are developing a model for study of this question which utilizes a more subtle endothelial injury.

E.J.W. Bowie: I was not really surprised by Dr. Griggs' findings, because I suspect that von Willebrand platelets can, indeed, adhere to collagen which would be exposed by balloon denudation of the subendothelial tissues. You mention Baumgartner's rabbit aorta work; and as a matter of fact, I carefully reviewed the data and find that significant numbers of von Willebrand platelets did, indeed, adhere to the subendothelial tissues - quite enough, I think, to induce a mitogenic response in the smooth muscle.

In my view balloon denudation is rather a severe insult to the blood vessel, and I suspect that the initiating lesion of atherosclerosis is something much more subtle. I would suggest that the initial lesion is damage to the endothelium (which can be produced in a number of ways) and that this exposes the fibrils of von Willebrand factor to which the platelets adhere. Obviously, the situation is more complicated than this and the thromboxane-prostacyclin data must also be taken into account. In any case, for the reasons I have outlined, I do not find it surprising that balloon denudation and exposure of the subendothelial tissues would result in atherosclerosis in von Willebrand pigs.

H. Stormorken: In conjunction with the reports on the findings in von Willebrand swine, I would like to report briefly on our

results of assaying F. VIII Ag (von Willebrand factor) and antithrombin III (AT-III) in a prospective study of men aged 40-50.
Of 2014 presumably healthy men, 115 had strong clinical evidence
of coronary heart disease, never diagnosed nor suspected prior to
the study. Coronary angiography was performed in 105 of these
cases. In 80 of these 105, of whom 57 were angiopositive and 23
angionegative, AT-III and F. VIII Ag were assayed, together with 35
normals. The results showed: 1) AT-III was significantly lower
in angiopositive than in normals. 2) Subdivision into those with
and those without angina pectoris revealed significantly lower
AT-III values in the former. 3) Within angiopositive individuals,
those with blood group A had significantly lower AT-III. 4) Blood
group O had significantly lower F. VIII Ag than all other groups,
which has not been previously reported.

It cannot be excluded that these results might be secondary,
but on the other hand, when they are compared with previously published results on differences between blood groups, it is a fair
chance that they are of primary concern, in that changes in coagulation and platelet function can influence the development of coronary atherosclerotic disease.

As shown in the table, blood group O has a "bleeder profile."
Clinical observations have shown that group O has lower arterial
and venous thrombosis, but more intestinal bleeding than the other
groups. As our angiopositive individuals showed a "clotter profile,"
in line with the more thrombosis-prone groups, it is not unlikely
that our findings support the notion that coagulation and platelet
function is of causal importance for the development of atherosclerosis.

BLOOD GROUP O vs. OTHER GROUPS

Lower F. VIII Activity

Lower F. VIII Antigen

Lower F. II, VII and X Levels

Higher AT-III Levels

The blood group O cases have a lower frequency of venous and arterial thrombosis
and increased intestinal bleeding.

J.C. Lewis: Dr. Friedman, if you stop treatment with anti-
platelet serum, how long will the rabbits remain thrombocytopenic?
And have you done experiments where the thrombocytopenic rabbits
were maintained in a platelet-deficient state for a limited time

subsequent to balloon injury, but were allowed to return to normal platelet levels before termination of the experiment?

R.J. Friedman: The duration of action of the antiplatelet serum varies from animal to animal. The mean duration of action was about 18 hours with a range of 8-30 hours. Thereafter, the platelet count rose slowly. Animals which were thrombocytopenic for three days prior to, and three-four days post-balloon injury and then allowed to return to normal platelet levels for several days before being made thrombocytopenic again, were found to develop neointimal smooth muscle cell proliferation about 20-30% greater than corresponding control groups. We postulate that the smooth muscle cells are somehow "turned on" following intimal injury but are not stimulated to migrate and proliferate. In essence they are "running in place." When the appropriate stimulus is received (? platelet growth factor), they may proliferate for a longer period of time than cells which are exposed to the mitogenic stimuli at the time of intimal injury. I must stress that this is totally speculation and we are currently studying the processes involved.

B.A. Kottke: If, as some investigators believe, the platelet obtains its mitogen factor from some other source such as the pituitary, could it be that you are depleting the available mitogen until new platelets containing newly acquired mitogen become available? Have you any evidence for this hypothesis?

R.J. Friedman: This is quite possible. However, the animals were made thrombocytopenic and maintained as such by daily injections of anti-platelet serum. Thus, very few platelets were made available to the circulation because of their continuous antibody-mediated destruction. However, one hypothesis which is under consideration is that some source, possibly the pituitary, may supply the mitogen and, if platelets were allowed to return to the circulation in sufficient numbers, they would be available to deliver the mitogen to areas of vessel wall injury. This has been shown to be true in animals whose platelet counts have been allowed to return to normal after ballooning at a time when they were thrombocytopenic. Normal or enhanced lesion development occurred. Thus, it is conceivable that new platelets may be carrying a pituitary-derived mitogen which they can deliver at sites of endothelial injury.

H.L. Nossel: In comment on Robert Friedman's paper, Charles Scher reported at a workshop chaired by me at the International Society on Thrombosis and Hemostasis meeting in June 1977, that in the tissue culture system the platelet-derived growth factor acted as a commitment factor and had done its work within one hour. Thereafter, one or more serum factors were required as maintenance factors - low density lipoproteins are necessary but it was not known if they are a sufficient factor. These data appear to support Dr. Friedman's interpretation of his data.

R.J. Friedman: I thank Dr. Nossel for presenting supporting evidence for our hypothesis which indicates that the platelet-derived growth factor acts as an initiator of the smooth muscle cell proliferative response. As yet, we have no in vivo evidence for the role of platelet mitogenic factors in the maintenance of the smooth muscle proliferative response.

R.W. Wissler: I would like to comment briefly on Dr. Fried-man's interesting results and questions that have been raised. There is now evidence that smooth muscle cells can be stimulated to grow without platelet factor. I believe that if Russell Ross were here he would agree with this statement. Furthermore, until we know more about the mitogenic effects of LDL from hyperlipidemic serum, we should keep an open mind about the results that indicate that hypercholesterolemic serum can produce a proliferative and lipid-filled lesion. We need an intensive study of the mechanisms involved.

R.J. Friedman: I appreciate Dr. Wissler's comments regarding the results of our work. Dr. Sean Moore has mentioned some con-cern with the interpretation of our findings that hyperlipemia (hypercholesterolemia) seems to be a sufficient stimulus for smooth muscle cell proliferation following endothelial injury even in the absence of platelets. His comments centered upon the fact that "some platelets" (about 7,000/cu.mm) were present in our thrombo-cytopenic, hyperlipemia animals and that it is possible that these platelets, in conjunction with hyperlipemia, may be sufficient to stimulate the smooth muscle cell response to intimal injury. While this is possible, it should be stressed that in non-lipid supple-mented thrombocytopenic animals with platelet counts similar to those of lipid-supplemented rabbits, the smooth muscle cell response did not occur. Dr. Wissler and others have shown that hyperlipemic serum, LDL, etc., can and does stimulate smooth muscle cells to grow in the absence of platelet-derived growth factors. Thus, al-though platelets seem to be an important part of the smooth muscle cell proliferative response following intimal injury, it seems that other factors, such as hypercholesterolemia, LDL, etc., play at least a supplemental and perhaps a more dominant role in the response of the vessel wall to injury. I completely agree with Dr. Wissler that an intensive and comprehensive study of the mechanisms involved be undertaken.

Dr. Bowie inadvertently omitted the fact that lipids seem to play a significant role in the smooth muscle cell proliferative response following intimal injury. Our data suggests that the role of lipids may be independent of the platelet's role. This is ob-viously an important point which warrants further study.

A.B. Chandler: Certainly, the myointimal or smooth muscle cell
is important in the production of atherosclerotic lesions. However,
another cell that should not be overlooked, particularly in relation
to lesions with a thrombotic component, is the blood monocyte.
Thrombi usually contain plentiful monocytes which can undergo transformation to macrophages and participate along with granulocytes and
plasma fibrinolytic activity in the resolution of thrombi. Moreover,
macrophages that engulf lipid-rich platelets of thrombi may undergo
transformation to foam cells and thus along with the plasma lipids
contained in thrombi contribute to the fat content of thromboatherosclerotic plaques.

G. Hornstra: It has been stated that location as well as composition of the atherosclerotic lesion in rabbits is different from
that in man. This is definitely true when the animals are fed additional cholesterol which is mostly done in order to speed up the
atherogenic process. However, if we are somewhat less impatient,
lesions can be produced in the rabbit which are so similar to the
human lesion that essentially all pathologists visiting our laboratory are unable to discriminate between both. The trick is, to feed
the animals a semi-synthetic diet enriched with vegetable saturated
fats, such as coconut fat or palm oil. Lesions develop after a
period of about one year. This model is now being used by us for
over ten years and appeared very useful in the assessment of the
dietary fat effect in atherogenesis. Recently, Kloeze, from our
laboratory, showed that the presence of insulin is a prerequisite
for the development of the atherosclerotic lesion in rabbits, since
it did not develop in animals made insulin-deficient by alloxan
injection. The implication of this finding for the mechanism of
atherogenesis is presently being investigated.

ATHEROTHROMBOLOGY

Stanford Wessler

Department of Medicine
New York University School of Medicine
New York, New York

The lipid and thrombotic views of the genesis of atherosclerosis have, until recently, gone their separate ways despite linkages reaching back many generations. One of the goals of this workshop has been an attempt to bring these two schools of thought together.

It is perhaps permissible to coin a word to move an important idea clearly into focus. Walter Kaufmann, the Princeton philosopher noted that humility and ambition are widely considered antithetical. Although he had no brief for either so long as they appeared separately, he found their fusion into the word humbition a cardinal virtue (1). It was on this basis that I have entitled my remarks to you as Atherothrombology. Even at this I restrained myself; at one time I thought up, but quickly discarded, the title Atherolipothrombology.

The field of atherothrombology has been plagued and perhaps retarded by schools of thought and theories. Accordingly, some brief remarks on both these topics may be appropriate.

Those who belong to a school of thought are usually more interested in their small differences with fellow members, than they are in what they have in common. These differences can be defined without much trouble, and, in their publications, those who write, develop differences of this sort. What one has in common with those with whom one differs, is much harder to specify. Distance is required to behold such family resemblances and those inside the family lack this distance. But they rarely find it difficult to say who does not belong (1).

Supported by NHLBI Grant #2 RO1 HL18333, NIH, DHEW.

Can one say what the members of a school have in common without even specifying the school? They tend to deal with a few clusters of problems, not with others and they tend to deal with them in the same way. They share a way of thinking, a style and a tradition that they see in much the same perspective (1). A few investigators, and unfortunately I am not among them, may be key figures in more than one tradition, but different schools still see these Leonardos differently.

How might one best go about destroying another man's theory? If one spent one's time attempting to disprove it, he merely demonstrates his subservience to it. The way to fully refute a man is to ignore him for the most part, and the only way to do this is to substitute new fundamental categories of his own, so that one is simply pursuing a different path (2). I hope some of the discussions at the workshop have led in this direction.

In point of fact, however, most reactions to members of a rival school is simply lack of interest. Rival schools are not so much tolerated as they are ignored. For it is easier to be rational about what one takes to be false results, than it is to deal deliberately with a radically different approach that calls into question one's whole style of thinking (1).

Theories, like schools, also have their problems. Darwin's theory of evolution by natural selection was propounded long before he or anyone else had any clear idea about the true mechanism of heredity. By the early twentieth century, the Darwinian theory of evolution had acquired such an all-encompassing explanatory glibness that natural historians had become quite uneasy about it. Nowadays we should probably attribute this uneasiness to the realization that a theory that explains everything explains nothing, and indeed, today we can see a general parallel between the explanatory facility of the older forms of Darwinism, the doctrines of psychoanalysis and the Marxian interpretation of history. Nevertheless, Darwinism is a theory of evolution that prevails today, entirely refounded though it has been on the basis of Mendelian genetics and the concepts of population dynamics (3).

If it is indeed a truism that a theory that explains everything explains nothing, then the data in support of the lipid theory and experiments supporting the thrombotic concept of atherosclerosis must accommodate each other.

Perhaps, after this workshop, such an achievement will not prove any more difficult than the manner in which Medawar resolved the theories about the viability of viruses. Some properties of viruses (extractability, infectiousness, mutability) tempt us to think of them as minute organisms smaller even than bacteria. But

other properties, especially their ability to subvert the synthetic
machinery of a living cell in such a way that they will produce
more copies, make us think of them as no more than neat packages
of genetic information. So instead of arguing whether or not viruses are alive, Medawar said, why not think of a virus simply as
a piece of bad news wrapped up in a protein (3)!

Having expressed myself on schools and theories, I should like
to turn now to some of our own work that may, in the future, relate
to the problems under consideration at this workshop. I do this
with more humbition than you may appreciate, since my past contributions to the genesis of either atherosclerosis or arterial thrombosis have been marginal. My own investigative bent has been directed toward venous thromboembolism -- a much easier field with
which to engage.

As a tool to study thrombosis we have utilized, for over two
decades, an animal model for the production of fibrin thrombi in
isolated veins, arteries and the microcirculation that has contributed to our understanding of venous thromboembolism, but not
materially abetted our understanding of the genesis of the typical
platelet lesion of arterial thrombosis (4, 5). Although embolization of limb thrombi to the lung bear some morphologic resemblance
to atheromatous plaques deposited on normal pulmonary arteries (6),
this observation is of no originality whatsoever.

If it were only to demonstrate that this model has grown in
the breadth of its potential usefulness concerning the mechanisms
involved in the initiation, growth or retardation of thrombosis, I
would not mention it this evening. I present it now because data
has surfaced recently that may have some relevance to atherothrombology.

Animal models never provide final answers, but offer only
approximations: for no single animal model can ever duplicate a
disease in man. Thus, animal models should not be expected to be
ideal, not to be universally suited to all foreseeable uses. On
the other hand, for a model to be a good one, it must provide a
new insight, have relevance to a particular problem and respond
predictably (7).

Granted these constraints, let me briefly describe the method.
A rabbit jugular vein is freed from its surrounding structures. If
one injects, into the contralateral ear vein, a thrombogenic substance, such as a clotting protease, and then isolates by ligation
the freed jugular vein segment; there forms a thrombotic cast of
the isolated venous segment. This cast resembles a typical red
thrombus, an impression confirmed by light and scanning electronmicroscopy where one sees mostly erythrocytes enmeshed in a network

of fibrin with only an occasional platelet visualized. That a
fibrin gel can occur in the base of a valve cusp of a peripheral
vein capped by a platelet nidus had, in fact, been observed in
human autopsy material (8).

Various sizes of thrombi can be produced in this model. If
one injects lesser amounts of protease than the quantity necessary
to induce the thrombus that forms a cast of the isolated lumen (a
score 4 thrombus) one can obtain score 3, 2 or 1 thrombi as read by
an independent observer, and, if the quantity of the infusate is
sufficiently reduced, no thrombus will form. Despite its apparent
crudity, quantitative relationships can be derived from the model.
A linear plot of the log of infused thrombin concentration against
the resulting average thrombotic score indicates that a 100% increase in the amount of thrombin infused is required to raise a
score 1 to a score 2 thrombus. To raise a score 2 thrombus to
score 3, an additional 40% increase in thrombin is necessary.

Various infusates affect in at least five ways the response in
the stasis assay. A substance may be immediately thrombogenic as
with clotting proteases (9), trypsin (10), endotoxin (11), long-
chain saturated and unsaturated fatty acids (12), ellagic acid (13),
and tobacco glycoprotein. It can induce delayed thrombogenicity
as with small doses of 6-azauridine. The substance can be itself
non-thrombogenic, but if the clotting cascade has been initiated,
it can facilitate and augment thrombosis. This response can be
immediate as with certain phospholipid mixtures (14), or it can be
delayed as with estrogen-containing oral contraceptives which have
been shown in our laboratory to be related to a retarded reaction
rate between anti-thrombin III and activated Factor X (15). The
model also responds to anti-thrombotic drugs (9), as well as to
thrombolytic agents (16).

The versatility of the system can be further enhanced by examining histopathological sections of vessels from within and without
the occluded arteries and veins in treated and control animals.
The response to a given substance is dependent on dose, duration
and route of administration.

Thus, the model can provide potential information on the thrombogenicity of a proposed drug early on in the course of toxicity
studies -- in a sense perhaps analogous to the Ames test for carcin-
ogenicity (17). For example, the stasis assay correctly predicted
that some factor IX concentrates used in the treatment of hemophil-
iacs would be thrombogenic in man, if the concentrates were contaminated with trace amounts of Xa or IXa (18). In fact, infusions of
as little as 0.04 nanomols of Xa or 2 picomols of IXa are thrombogenic in rabbits (9).

Because of the possible relation to the topic of this workshop,
I should like to spend my remaining few minutes on one drug (6-
azauridine) and one compound (tobacco glycoprotein) both of which
we have begun to investigate in the stasis model. The experiments
with 6-azauridine have been carried out with Drs. Sanford Gitel,
Anthony Grieco and Selma Snyderman of NYU; those with tobacco protein with Dr. Gitel and with Drs. Carl Becker and Theodore Dubin of
Cornell.

The drug, 6-azauridine-triacetate, is a potent inhibitor of
pyrimidine biosynthesis (19). The site of the blockade is believed
to be the enzyme that decarboxylates orotidine-5'-phosphate (19).
Its administration results in man and animals in unique serum elevations of homocystine, β-alanine, β-aminoisobutyric acid, γ-amino-
butyric acid, cystathione, methionine and other amino acids (20, 21).
Some of these amino acids appear in three different inborn metabolic
diseases in man: β-alaninemia, cystathioninuria and homocystinuria.
Aside from trials of the drug in certain viral diseases and mycosis
fungoides, it has been most widely used in psoriasis (22). The
drug was recently removed from the market because of what appeared
to be a remarkable incidence of arterial thrombosis including cases
with acute myocardial infarction as well as venous thromboembolism
in psoriatric patients. To our knowledge, it is the first drug
identified as causing, by itself, arterial thrombosis in man. Of
considerable relevance is the finding that 6-azauridine induces
homocystinemia. Homocystinuria is associated in children with
arterial and venous thromboembolic phenomena as a cause of death;
and Harker and associates have reported data relating homocystinemia
to chronic endothelial cell desquamation, arterial thrombosis and
atherosclerosis (23). In addition, Ratnoff has shown in vitro that
homocystine activates Hageman Factor (240.

It was with this background that we administered 6-azauridine
to rabbits. Preliminary data show that the compound does not cause
thrombosis immediately after intravenous injection of less than
10 mg/kg; while doses of 50 mg/kg or greater do initiate immediate
thrombosis. However, when given orally for three weeks (at low
doses ranging from 2.5-5 mg/kg/day as well as at high doses of
50-500 mg/kg/day, or for three days (at 1,000 mg/kg/day), over 80%
of the rabbits developed score 1 or 2 thrombi irrespective of regimen, whereas saline treated controls did not develop thrombi. In
this regard, the dose in man has varied between 125-250 mg/kg/day.
Thrombosis in rabbits occurs spontaneously in arteries and veins
without injection of an additional thrombogenic stimulus. From
the experiments completed to date, the extent of thrombosis (unlike
protease injections) appears not to be dose-related over a 200-fold
range for a period of three weeks. Although the mechanism of the
thrombogenic stimulus is obscure, the picture, as we presently see
it, is one of persistent low-grade thrombogenicity, possibly by

activation of Hageman Factor and consistent with a compound that
induces damage of the vascular endothelium or stimulates chronic
infiltration of leukocytes into the endothelium. Alternatively,
upon long-term ingestion, the compound may simply build up to thrombogenic levels. We are presently attempting to resolve these possibilities in part by electronmicroscopy. More importantly, 6-
azauridine may provide another potential tool to explore the genesis
of atherothrombology.

And finally, in regard to cigarette tobacco, Becker and Dubin
have isolated from cured tobacco leaves a glycoprotein with the
capacity to activate Hageman Factor. A requirement for the in
vitro effect on Hageman Factor is the presence of rutin (25), a
substance chemically related to quercetin and ellagic acid which
Ratnoff had shown to be activators of Hageman Factor (13).

Tobacco glycoprotein appears at first glance to be a classic
thrombogenic agent. Its thrombogenic effect, as one might expect
from its activation of Hageman Factor, is evident immediately after
intravenous injection. The material, however, has several unique
properties. First, heating the purified tobacco protein at 65°C
for 15 minutes has no effect on its thrombogenicity. Second, although decreasing by 50% the amount of protein infused resulted in
a decrease in the average thrombotic score; doubling the amount of
glycoprotein injected did not increase the average thrombotic score
as occurs with the clotting proteases. This latter observation is
consistent with in vitro data showing that the tobacco protein exhibits a biphasic curve in changing the partial thromboplastin time
(25). In the rabbit, the amount of tobacco protein injected (0.5
mg/kg -- from two different lots) was initially chosen to obtain a
plasma concentration approximately equal to the concentration of
the protein that optimally activated the partial thromboplastin
time in vitro. Thus, no additional increase in thrombosis would
be expected with an increase in tobacco glycoprotein administration.
Tar may, of course, be more meaningful than leaf. More recently,
glycoprotein from tobacco tar has been found to be as thrombogenic
as that from tobacco leaf.

Of further interest is Gitel's preliminary finding that, if
he infuses tobacco protein into female rabbits on oral contraceptives, he doubles the average thrombotic score over comparable
rabbits infused with tobacco protein who were not receiving oral
contraceptives. As a further control, he showed that female rabbits
on oral contraceptives, injected with saline, never develop thrombosis.

This increase might have been anticipated: for while tobacco
protein is activating Hageman Factor and thus initiating intravascular coagulation; estrogen-containing oral contraceptives are inducing a hypercoagulable state by decreasing the reactivity of

antithrombin III, thereby facilitating the thrombotic process.
This effect of estrogen, incidentally, may explain why the femini-
zation of men led to their observed increased risk of coronary
artery thrombosis.

If one examines some of the epidemiological data on cigarette
smoking in man, one finds that atherosclerosis is augmented (26,
27) and that sudden cardiovascular deaths are increased by tobacco
(28). It has been suggested that vasoactive substances such as
nicotine (29) and catechol amines, normally found in cigarette
smoke, may be, in part, responsible for the increase in sudden cardiac deaths. May we now consider acute arterial thrombosis as a
possible additional factor causing this phenomenon? It has also
been suggested that the carbon monoxide present in cigarette smoke
may be related to the development of atherosclerosis (30). Is it
possible that the low-grade thrombogenicity induced by tobacco
protein may also be involved in the increased atherosclerosis seen
among long-term cigarette smokers? Finally, epidemiological data,
incomplete as they are, suggest that cigarette smoking, particularly among older premenopausal women, increases their risk of
acute myocardial infarction, if they are taking oral contraceptives
(31). Our rabbit studies would support such a synergism between
tobacco and estrogen.

Let me say, in closing, that it is not the promise of
easy victories, but rather the existence of an intellectual challenge that is the most effective means of stimulating research.
Although it sounds sententious, this generalization can be illustrated over and over again in the history of biology: one thinks,
for example, of the recruitment of biologists into embryological
research in the 1930's, into ethology in the 40's, and into molecular biology today (3).

Who knows but that this normo-cholesterolemic, normo-lipemic,
non-ballooned rabbit may in the 1980's shed some light on atherothrombology -- if we can teach him to smoke cigarettes, her to take
oral contraceptives and both sexes to use 6-azauridine, even if
they do not have psoriasis.

REFERENCES

1. Kaufmann, W. (1973) Without Guilt and Justice. In Decidopho-
    bia to Autonomy, Peter H. Wyder, New York, p. 274.

2. Hartz, L. (1955) The Liberal Tradition in America. An Inter-
    pretation of American Political Thought Since the Revolution,
    Harcourt Brace and World, New York, p. 329.

3. Medawar, P.B., and Medawar, J.S. (1977) The Life Science.
   Current Ideas of Biology, Harper and Row, New York, p. 196.

4. Wessler, S., Reiner, L., Freiman, D.G., Reimer, S.M., and
   Lertzman, M. (1959) Circulation 20, 846-874.

5. Wessler, S., Reimer, S.M., and Sheps, M.D. (1960) J. Appl.
   Physiol. 14, 943-946.

6. Wessler, S., Freiman, D.G., Ballon, J.D., Katz, J.H., Wolff,
   R., and Wolf, E. (1961) Am. J. Pathol. 38, 89-101.

7. Frenkel, J.K. (1969) Fed. Proc. 28, 160-161.

8. Chandler, A.B., personal communication.

9. Gitel, S.N., Stephenson, R.C., and Wessler, S. (1977) Proc.
   Natl. Acad. Sci. USA 74, 3028-3032.

10. Wessler, S., Reimer, S.M., Freiman, D.G., and Thomas, D.P.
    (1961) in Anticoagulants and Fibrinolysins, MacMillan, Toronto,
    pp. 108-116.

11. Thomas, D.P., and Wessler, S. (1964) Circ. Res. 14, 486-493.

12. Connor, W.E., Hoak, J.C., and Warner, E.D. (1963) J. Clin.
    Invest. 42, 860-866.

13. Botti, R.F., and Ratnoff, O.D. (1964) J. Lab. Clin. Med. 64,
    385-398.

14. Barton, P.G., Yin, E.T., and Wessler, S. (1970) J. Lipid Res.
    11, 87-95.

15. Gitel, S.N., Stephenson, R.C., and Wessler, S. Haemostasis.
    In press.

16. Freiman, A.H., Bang, N.U., Grossi, C.E., and Clifton, E.E.
    (1960) Am. J. Cardiol. 6, 426-431.

17. Ames, B.N. (1976) Science 191, 241-244.

18. Kingdon, H.S., Lundblad, R.L., Veltkamp, J.J., and Aronson,
    D. (1975) Thromb. Diath. Haemorrh. 33, 617-631.

19. Handschumacher, R.E., Calabresi, P., Welch, A.D., Bono, V.,
    Fallon, H.J., and Frei, E. (1962) Cancer Chemother. Rep. 21,
    1-18.

20. Slavik, M., Hyanek, Elis, J., and Homolka, J. (1969) Biochem. Pharm. 18, 1782-1784.

21. Slavik, M., Keiser, H.R., Lowenberg, W., and Sjoerdsma, A. (1971) Life Sciences 10 (Part II), 1293-1295.

22. Milstein, H.G., Cornell, R.C., and Stoughton, R.B. (1973) Arch. Dermatol. 108, 43-47.

23. Harker, L.A., Slichter, S.J., Scott, C.R., and Ross, R. (1974) N. Engl. J. Med. 291, 537-543.

24. Ratnoff, O.D. (1968) Science 162, 1007-1009.

25. Becker, C.G., and Dubin, T. (1977) J. Exper. Med. 146, 457-567.

26. Auerbach, O., Hammond, E.C., and Garfinkel, L. (1965) N. Engl. J. Med. 273, 775-779.

27. Strong, J.P., Richards, M.D., McGill, J.C., Jr., Eggen, D.A., McMurry, M.T. (1969) J. Atheroscler. Res. 10, 303-317.

28. Feinleib, M., and Williams, R.R. in Proceedings - Third World Conference on Smoking and Health (Wynder, E.L., Hoffman, D. and Gori, G.B., Eds.), DHEW Publication No. (NIH) 76-1221, U.S. Government Printing Office, pp. 243-256.

29. Hill, P. In Proceedings - Third World Conference on Smoking and Health (Wynder, E.L., Hoffman, D. and Gori, G.B., Eds.), DHEW Publication No. (NIH) 76-1221, U.S. Government Printing Office, pp. 313-319.

30. Astrup, P., Kjeldsen, K., and Wonstrup, J. (1967) J. Atheroscler. Res. 7, 343-   .

31. Ory, H.W. (1977) JAMA 237, 2619-2622.

CLINICAL ASSESSMENT OF THE THROMBOTIC PROCESS IN RELATION TO ATHEROSCLEROSIS

Hymie L. Nossel, *Session Chairman*
Department of Medicine
College of Physicians and Surgeons of Columbia University
New York, New York

PLATELET FUNCTION IN THROMBOSIS AND ATHEROSCLEROSIS

Robert W. Colman

Coagulation Unit, Hematology-Oncology Section,
Department of Medicine
University of Pennsylvania Medical School
Philadelphia, Pennsylvania

Thrombosis, frequently the final event in coronary or cerebral arterial occlusion, is a result of the interplay of abnormalities of the arterial intima, hemodynamic stresses, plasma coagulant proteins and platelets. Platelets initiate a series of intricate reactions by adhering to the injured arterial lining, aggregating to form a platelet plug (1) and releasing vasoactive metabolites and hydrolytic enzymes that might in turn alter both the function and structure of the vessel. Heightened platelet function thus might not only participate in the formation of thrombi but may also play a role in the development of progression of some forms of atherosclerosis. Two blood components which may be implicated in atherosclerosis are plasma lipoproteins and platelets. Epidemiologic evidence points to hyperbetalipoproteinemia as an important risk factor in coronary and cerebral arterial occlusion (2). Over the past five years, our laboratory has been gathering clinical and experimental evidence that the plasma lipoprotein composition may influence platelet reactivity by altering either the lipid composition directly or being associated with critical changes in the cholesterol/phospholipid ratio. Membrane protein function may change in an altered lipid environment. Investigations also suggest that lipid soluble drugs such as clofibrate and halofenate can reverse the increased platelet sensitivity probably through altering membrane lipid structure by inducing a phase separation.

Individuals with type IIa hyperlipoproteinemia have elevated plasma levels of low density lipoproteins (LDL) and cholesterol. Other reported causes of increased platelet aggregation such as diabetes, angina and symptomatic peripheral occlusive atherosclerosis were excluded. Two separate studies of the effect of epinephrine on platelet function are shown in Fig. 1. Platelet sen-

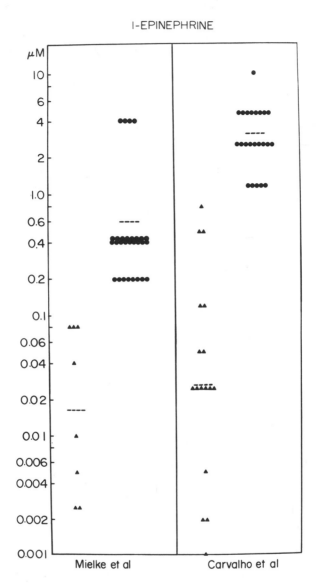

Fig. 1. Platelet sensitivity to epinephrine in normal individuals and patients with hyperbetalipoproteinemia. Normal individuals = ●; Type IIa hyperlipoproteinemia = ▲; Geometric mean = ---.

sitivity is defined as the lowest concentration of aggregating
agent capable of evoking a complete second wave aggregation response
in platelet-rich plasma as monitored in an aggregometer. Platelets from 17 patients with type IIa hyperlipoproteinemia were
140-fold more sensitive to epinephrine than normal (3) and 200-fold
more sensitive in 8 patients studied by Mielke (personal communication). In addition, platelets from IIa patients were significantly more sensitive to ADP and collagen. Furthermore, Type IIa
platelets released increased amounts of nucleotides and serotonin
in response to the aggregating agents ADP, epinephrine and collagen.

The defining feature of the type IIa hyperlipoproteinemia is
the elevation of LDL but we were concerned that there might be a
qualitative abnormality as well. When 19 patients were compared
with 23 controls a striking elevation of the cholesterol to phospholipid ratio was found in the isolated LDL (Fig. 2).

Platelets cannot synthesize cholesterol de novo. Evidence
from red cell studies (4) suggest that in the presence of elevated
cholesterol in serum, an increase of the cholesterol to phospholipid
ratio occurs in the cell membranes. Therefore, the lipid composition of the platelet subcellular fractions of normal and Type IIa
(5) was examined. The ratio of cholesterol to phospholipid in whole
platelets is increased 8% over normal. Most of the increase can
be accounted for by changes in the platelet membrane concentration.
The cholesterol to phospholipid ratio (C/PL) is increased 20% over
normal in the membrane (Fig. 2), while no significant change is
found in the granule fraction. Moreover, a reasonable correlation
exists between the C/PL in LDL and in platelets suggesting that
cholesterol may be transferred in vivo. Alternatively, the elevated
ratio of cholesterol to phospholipid may simply reflect the same
genetic defect expressed in the liver which synthesized LDL and the
megakarocyte from which platelets are derived.

To support further the hypothesis that the mechanism of platelet hypersensitivity in IIa relates to the platelet lipid composition and the lipid composition of the plasma environment an in vitro
model was developed (6). Normal platelets were incubated for 5
hours at 37°C in plasma, the free cholesterol to phospholipid molar
ratio (C/PL) of which had been increased by the addition of sonicated free cholesterol-dipalmitoyl lecithin dispersions rich in
cholesterol. These dispersions transferred cholesterol selectively
to the platelet membrane resulting in an increase of 39% in the
platelet C/PL ratio. This was associated with a 35-fold increase
in sensitivity to epinephrine-induced aggregation and a 15-fold
increase to ADP, determined by both aggregometry and ^{14}C-serotonin
release. This procedure produces platelets similar to those in
type II patients. Cholesterol-normal lipid dispersions had no
effect on platelet lipids or function.

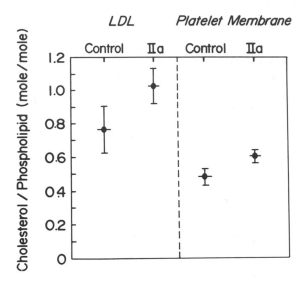

Fig. 2. Cholesterol-phospholipid ratio in low density lipoprotein
(LDL) and platelet membranes in normal and hyperbetalipoproteinemia
(IIa) patients. The mean and two standard errors (bars) are dis-
played in 23 controls (-●-) and 19 IIA (-●-). Adapted from J.
Lab. Clin. Med. (1977) 89, 341-353.

        Platelet cell membranes probably consist of bimolecular layers
of phospholipid and free cholesterol in which are embedded globular
proteins. The major role of lipids is to maintain a fluid matrix
for the function of specialized membrane structures and for the
plasticity of the cell.

        One determinant of membrane fluidity is the C/PL. Incorpora-
tion of cholesterol into the platelet membrane results in an increase in platelet microviscosity as measured by fluorescence polar-
ization (7). There is an excellent correlation between C/PL ratio
and microviscosity. Exactly how the more rigid membrane leads to
greater sensitivity to epinephrine and ADP is not yet known.

        Incorporation of cholesterol in platelet membrane may also
alter membrane-associated enzymes. Of special importance is the
interaction of the cholesterol-enriched platelet membrane with the
cyclic AMP (cAMP) system known to inhibit platelet function (8).
Prostaglandin E_1 is known to stimulate membrane bound enzyme adeny-

late cyclase raising platelet cAMP. Cyclic AMP is in turn degraded by phosphodiesterases. The cAMP content of platelets incubated with cholesterol-rich dispersions gradually increased, and at 5 hours had increased by 56%. The increased level of cAMP in cholesterol-rich platelets suggested further that the activity of enzymes responsible for the synthesis and/or degradation of cAMP might be altered by cholesterol incorporation.

The kinetic constants of cAMP phosphodiesterases in cholesterol-rich platelets were similar to those of normal platelets (Table 1). Therefore, the elevated cAMP content of cholesterol-rich platelets could not be accounted for by defective catabolism. In contrast, consistent abnormalities of adenylate cyclase were observed in cholesterol-rich platelets. Basal adenylate cyclase activity demonstrated a progressive increase during the 5 hour incubation of platelets with cholesterol-rich dispersions, and this increase was proportional to the extent of cholesterol incorporation (Fig. 3). At 5 hours, cholesterol-rich platelets had a basal adenylate cyclase activity 2.5-fold higher than that of platelets incubated for the same period of time with either Tyrode's buffer or cholesterol-normal dispersions. To demonstrate further the effect of cholesterol on basal adenylate cyclase activity, normal platelets were partially depleted of cholesterol by incubating them for 5 hours with cholesterol-poor lecithin dispersions. Platelets lost 21% cholesterol and their basal adenylate cyclase activity decreased 40%. Thus, basal adenylate cyclase is a direct function of the cholesterol/phospholipid ratio in platelet membranes. The increased activity may be due to a direct effect on the enzyme or to the increase in microviscosity altering the environment of the enzyme.

Table 1

Kinetic Constants for Platelet cAMP Phosphodiesterases

	K_m	V_{max}
	μM	nmol/mg protein/min
Low K_m		
Normal platelets	50	0.020
Cholesterol-rich platelets	60	0.030
High K_m		
Normal platelets	232	2.8
Cholesterol-rich platelets	243	3.3

Reprinted from J. Biol. Chem.
(1977) 252, 3310-3314.

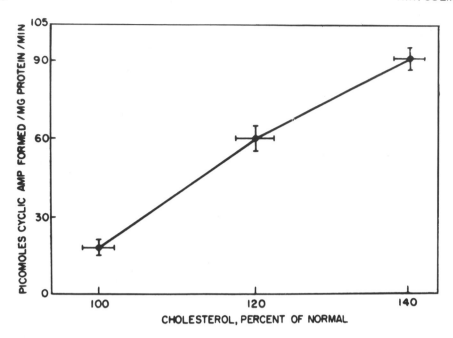

Fig. 3. Relationship between amount of cholesterol incorporated and basal adenylate cyclase activity of platelets. Bars represent + S.E. Reprinted from J. Biol. Chem. (1977) 252, 3310-3314.

The hormonal responsiveness of adenylate cyclase to PGE_1 was studied next (Fig. 4). PGE_1, 0.1 μM, stimulated the adenylate cyclase activity of platelets incubated 5 hours with Tyrode's buffer by 2-fold and PGE_1, 1.0 μM, stimulated the enzyme 3.5-fold. A 4.5-fold stimulation of the enzyme was observed with sodium fluoride (2.0 mM). In contrast, the adenylate cyclase activity of cholesterol-rich platelets was not stimulated by PGE_1, sodium fluoride, or a combination of both. Concomitant with this, platelets became refractory to the inhibitory effect of PGE_1 on epinephrine-induced aggregation and the mean minimal concentration of PGE_1 required to inhibit aggregation was 5-10 fold higher than normal (Fig. 5). Adenylate cyclase solubilized from other sources requires phospholipid for optimal stimulation by hormones and this regulatory role for phospholipids also operates in intact membranes. In platelets, cholesterol might inhibit the interaction of membrane phospholipid and adenylate cyclase by competing directly with cyclase for interaction with critical phospholipids. Alternatively, cholesterol might restrict the fluidity of phospholipid fatty acids and thus

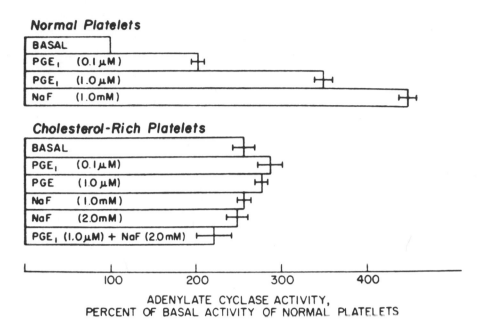

Fig. 4. Adenylate cyclase activity of platelets incubated for 5 h with Tyrode's buffer (normal platelets) or with cholesterol-rich dispersions (cholesterol-rich platelets). All data are compared to basal activity of normal platelets, which was normalized to 100% activity for each experiment. The data represent the mean + 2 S.E. for three experiments performed in triplicate. Reprinted from J. Biol. Chem. (1977), 252, 3310-3314.

impair the transmembrane event necessary for hormonal stimulation of the enzyme. The increased sensitivity of cholesterol-rich platelets to aggregating agents and their increased levels of inhibitory cAMP appears to be independent effects of cholesterol on membrane components which affect the process of platelet aggregation in opposite directions.

To explore whether the increase in platelet sensitivity could be modified by drugs, clofibrate, a drug which in some studies has decreased morbidity or mortality in type IIa individuals, was studied (9). Clofibrate did not alter the plasma or low density lipoprotein cholesterol levels. However, clofibrate, given orally to IIa subjects, returned platelet sensitivity to normal with ADP, toward normal with epinephrine, but failed to alter the hypersensitivity to collagen (Fig. 6). Clofibrate (200 µg/ml) in vitro inhibited the release of ^{14}C-serotonin from normal platelets when ADP,

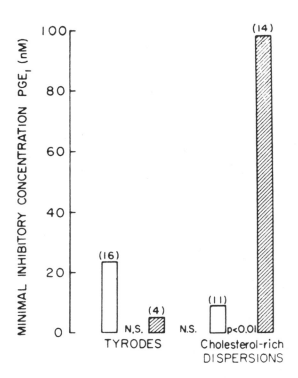

Fig. 5. Effect of cholesterol incorporation on the inhibitory
potency of PGE$_1$ on epinephrine-induced platelet aggregation. The
height of the bars represents the geometric mean. Open bars represent unincubated platelets, whereas hatched bars represent platelets incubated for 5 h at 37°. The number in parentheses above
each bar indicates the number of experiments performed. The significance of the difference between the means was calculated by Stu-
dent's t test. Since the data are distributed lognormally, standard errors of the mean cannot be calculated. Reprinted from J.
Biol. Chem. (1977), 252, 3310-3314.

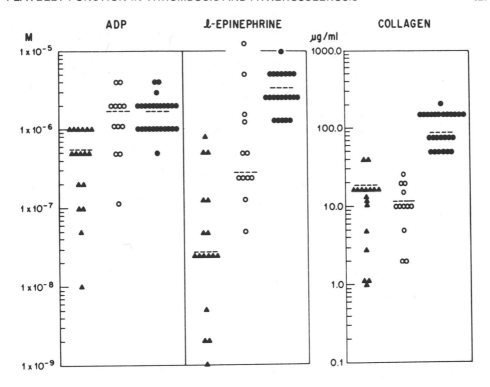

Fig. 6. Platelet Aggregation Studies. The minimum concentration of each aggregating agent (ADP, 1-epinephrine, collagen) to give a full response is plotted for each patient. Note the logarithmic scale. The triangles represent type II hyperlipoproteinemia patients; open circles, clofibrate-treated type II patients; filled circles, normal subjects. Reprinted from Circulation (1974), 50, 570-574.

epinephrine, and collagen were used as aggregating agents. However, this was not due to an aspirin-like effect since the inhibition could be reversed by a higher concentration of epinephrine.

In searching for a more potent agent, we have studied a congener of clofibrate, halofenate, with similar lipid lowering ability (10). The effect of the two drugs was compared in vitro in 11 different subjects. In these studies, platelets were incubated with clofibrate and halofenate at their therapeutic concentrations in vivo. Because of its higher molecular weight molar concentrations require halofenate concentrations at 300 μg/ml (0.96 mM) and clofibrate, 200 μg/ml (0.82 mM). Both drugs caused an increase in the

Table 2

Platelet Sensitivity to Aggregating Agents as
Modified by Clofibrate and Halofenate

	Drug added		
Aggregating agent	None	Clofibrate (200 µg/ml.)	Halofenate (400 µg/ml.)
Epinephrine (µM):			
Geometric mean*	4.2	10.0	245†
95% range	(1-15)	(1-50)	(200-250)
ADP (µM):			
Geometric mean	1.8	1.6	3.2‡
95% range	(1-5)	(1-5)	(2-10)
Collagen (µg/ml):			
Geometric mean	36	38	50§
95% range	(30-90)	(30-90)	(30-120)

*Eleven separate subjects tested.
†p < 0.001 compared to no drug or clofibrate.
‡p < 0.05 compared to no drug; <0.01 compared to clofibrate.
§p < 0.02 compared to no drug; >0.1 compared to clofibrate.

Reprinted from J. Lab. Clin. Med. (1977) 88, 282-291.

Table 3

Effect of Halofenate Concentration on
Sensitivity of Platelets

	Halofenate (µg/ml.)				
Aggregating agent	0	100	200	300	400
Epinephrine (µM):					
Geometric mean*	1.7	4.0	5.0	68	250
95% range †	(1-5)	(2.5-10)	(2.5-10)	(25-250)	(250)
ADP (µM):					
Geometric mean	1.3	1.0	1.3	1.7	5.8
95% range	(0.5-2.5)	(0.5-2.0)	(0.5-5)	(1-5)	(5-8)
Collagen (µg/ml.):					
Geometric mean	30	47	60	47	60
95% range	(30)	(30-60)	(60)	(30-60)	(60)

*Eleven individuals were tested. The logarithms of the concentration of the aggregating agent needed to
produce a full response were recorded, the mean of logarithms calculated, and the geometric mean which is
antilog of that mean is recorded.
†The 95 per cent range of the actual concentration of aggregating agent is used since standard deviations are
not a valid measure of a log normal distribution.

Reprinted from J. Lab. Clin. Med. (1977) 88, 282-291.

threshold concentration of epinephrine. The threshold concentrations for ADP and collagen were also increased by halofenate but not with clofibrate (Table 2).

The mechanism of action of halofenate has been studied in detail. Halofenate inhibits platelet secretion as measured by ^{14}C serotonin release (Table 3). In addition, it inhibits epinephrine induced prostaglandin synthesis. Malondealdehyde (MDA) is a by-product when arachidonic acid is metabolized to prostaglandin endoperoxides (PGG_2 and PGH_2) as well as thromboxane A_2. Epinephrine stimulated MDA is inhibited by halofenate (11). However, this is not due to an aspirin-like action. When arachidonate (1 mM) is used to stimulate platelet aggregation and MDA formation, halofenate fails to inhibit the process. Thus, halofenate appears to act prior to the conversion of arachidonate to prostaglandin endoperoxide. The effect of halofenate could be due to inhibition of phospholipase A which hydrolyzes arachidonic acid from phosphatidylcholine in the platelet membrane, to stimulation of adenylate cyclase or to a direct effect on membrane fluidity.

Using a model membrane, dipalmitoyl phosphatidylcholine bilayers, we have shown that halofenate induces phase separation as measured by differential scanning calorimetry. In a series of substituted amantadines, we found a close correlation of ability to induce phase separation with platelet inhibitory activity (12). Amantadine at therapeutic concentrations inhibits platelet aggregation with 50% inhibition (ID_{50}) at 1.5 mM. Amantadine also induces phase separation as seen by differential scanning calorimetry. The phase transition profile for pure dipalmitoyl phosphatidylcholine liposomes shows a sharp symmetrical transition commencing at 41.0° (T_C) which is essentially complete at 1.6°C (Fig. 7, top). It was found that all of the amantadine derivatives in this study produced another sharp transition at a lower temperature (Fig. 7, bottom). As the concentration of the amantadine was increased, the area of a parent peak decreased and the area of the new peak increased.

Thus, as the concentration of the amantadine derivative is increased, T_C decreases and the combined half-height-width (HHW') of the two transition increases. To compare the relative potencies of the amantadine derivatives, we have defined an arbitrary constant, HHW'$_{100}$, which is the concentration of drug at which the HHW' of the phase transition profile of pure dipalmitoyl phosphatidylcholine liposomes increased by 100%. The HHW'$_{100}$ values obtained from the differential scanning calorimetry curves for 11 amantadine derivatives examined are plotted against the ID_{50} values for these compounds from the platelet aggregation studies (Fig. 8). The correlation coefficient (r) is 0.70 (p<0.02). Thus, there is a significant relationship between the relative potencies of various amantadines in inhibiting platelet aggregation in vitro and the abilities of these compounds including phase separation in dipalmitoyl

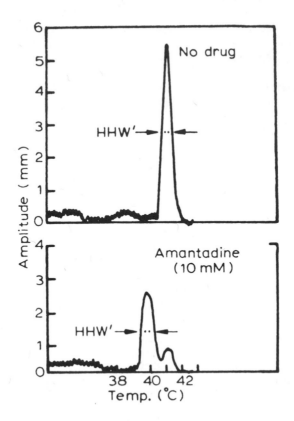

Fig. 7. Differential scanning calorimetry profiles of pure dipalmitoyl phosphatidylcholine liposomes (70 mM) and of such liposomes doped with amantadine (10.67 mM). The half-height widths (HHW') are noted. Reprinted from <u>Biochem. Biophys. Acta</u> (1977) 467, 273-279.

phosphatidylcholine bilayers. The action of halofenate in inducing phase separation in model membranes may indicate a similar action on the platelet membrane lipids.

Cholesterol-rich platelets are appropriate for a variety of studies of possible mechanisms on control of platelet hypersensitivity. We studied the effect of halofenate and clofibrate on seven

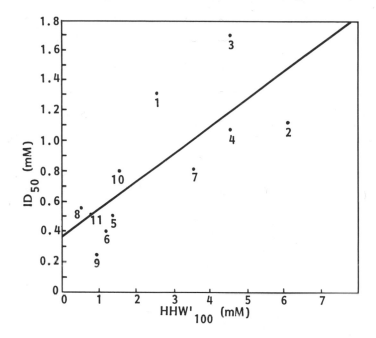

Fig. 8. Plot of ID_{50} vs. HHW_{100} for eleven amantadine derivatives. The equation of the line obtained by linear regression analysis of the data is $y = 0.38 + 0.18x$ with $r = 0.70$ and $p < 0.02$. Reprinted from Biochem. Biophys. Acta (1977) 467, 273-279.

separate normal subjects whose platelets had been rendered hyper-sensitive by cholesterol incorporation (Table 4). Cholesterol-rich platelets were 114-fold more sensitive to epinephrine and two-fold more sensitive to ADP than normal platelets but after incubation with halofenate became even less sensitive than normal. Clofibrate inhibited the extent of aggregation of hypersensitive platelets but did not alter the threshold concentration of epinephrine necessary for aggregation. Thus, halofenate is more potent than clofibrate in reducing the sensitivity of normal platelets to aggregating agents in vitro and can completely reverse experimentally produced platelet hypersensitivity.

Cholesterol incorporation into blood platelets increases the microviscosity of the platelet membrane, increases the sensitivity

Table 4. Cholesterol-induced platelet hypersensitivity as modified by clofibrate and halofenate

Aggregating agent	Incubation of platelets with			
	Tyrode's	Cholesterol-rich liposomes	Cholesterol-rich liposomes + clofibrate	Cholesterol-rich liposomes - halofenate
Epinephrine (μM): Geometric mean* 95% range	143 (50-250)	1.3** (0.25-5.0)	1.5 (0.25-5.0)	250§ (250)
ADP (μM): Geometric mean 95% range	1.4 (1-5)	0.6† (0.5-1.0)	0.5 (0.5)	1.7¶ (1-5)
Collagen (μg/ml): Geometric mean 95% range	25 (12-30)	11 (1.2-30)	3.3# (1.2-12)	36¶¶ (30-60)

*Seven separate subjects tested.
**$p < 0.001$ compared with Tyrode's.
†$p < 0.05$ compared with Tyrode's.
§$p < 0.001$ compared with cholesterol-rich liposomes alone: $p < 0.001$ compared with clofibrate.
¶$p < 0.02$ compared with cholesterol-rich liposomes alone: $p < 0.01$ compared with clofibrate.
¶¶$p < 0.02$ compared with cholesterol-rich liposomes alone: $p < 0.01$ compared with clofibrate.
#$p < 0.02$ compared with cholesterol-rich liposomes alone.
Reprinted from J. Lab. Clin. Med. (1977) 88, 282-291.

of the platelets to ADP and epinephrine and alters platelet cyclic AMP metabolism. It may follow that a drug-induced increase in the fluidity of the membrane and/or the formation of border domains between gel and liquid crystalline regions in the membrane lead to decreased platelet aggregation.

In this paper, I have explored the interaction of plasma lipoproteins, platelet membranes and lipid soluble anti-platelet agents. It appears clear that the physical state of membrane lipids can alter the membrane proteins including both the externally oriented receptors and the intracellular regulatory proteins such as adenylate cyclase. While cholesterol increases membrane microviscosity, the action of lipid soluble drugs may reverse the process by inducing phase separation. This class of drugs may therefore possess unique application in disorders such as type II hyperlipoproteinemia.

REFERENCES

1. French, J.E. (1971) Semin. Hematol. 8, 84-94.

2. Kannel, W.B., Castelli, W.P., and McNamara, P.M. (1967) J. Occup. Med. 9, 611-621.

3. Carvalho, A.C.A., Colman, R.W., and Lees, R.S. (1974) N. Engl. J. Med. 290, 434-348.

4. Cooper, R.A., Arner, E.C., Wiley, J.S., and Shattil, S.J. (1975) J. Clin. Invest. 55, 115-126.

5. Shattil, S.J., Bennett, J.S., Colman, R.W., and Cooper, R.A. (1977) J. Lab. Clin. Med. 89, 341-353.

6. Shattil, S.J., Anaya-Galindo, R., Bennett, J., Colman, R.W., and Cooper, R.A. (1975) J. Clin. Invest. 55, 636-643.

7. Shattil, S.J., and Cooper, R.A. (1976) Biochemistry 15, 4832-4837.

8. Sinha, A.K., Shattil, S.J., and Colman, R.W. (1977) J. Biol. Chem. 252, 3310-3314.

9. Carvalho, A.C.A., Colman, R.W., and Lees, R.S. (1974) Circulation 50, 570-574.

10. Colman, R.W., Bennett, J.S., Sheridan, J.F., Cooper, R.A., and Shattil, S.J. (1976) J. Lab. Clin. Med. 88, 282-291.

11. Favis, G.R., and Colman, R.W. (1977) <u>Thromb. and Hemostasis</u>
     38, 64.

12. Colman, R.W., Kuchibhotla, J., Jain, M.K., and Murray, R.K.,
     Jr. (1977) <u>Biochem. Biophys. Acta</u> 467, 273-279.

     Acknowledgments: I wish to thank the following journals
for allowing me to use the tables and figures that appear in my
paper:
     Journal of Biological Chemistry - table 1, figures 3, 4, and
     5;
     Biochem. Biophys. Acta - figures 7 and 8;
     Journal of Laboratory and Clinical Medicine - tables 2, 3,
     and 4 and figure 2;
     Circulation - figure 6.

PLATELET SURVIVAL DETERMINATION IN ATHEROSCLEROSIS

Edward Genton

Faculty of Health Sciences
McMaster University
Hamilton, Ontario, Canada

It has been convincingly established that the blood platelet
plays a key and often primary role in thrombosis, especially in
the arterial circulation. Mounting evidence indicates that the
thrombotic process plays a major role in atherosclerosis. Whether
the process is involved with the initiation of atherosclerotic
lesions, as increasing evidence suggests, is not firmly established;
but there seems no doubt that thromboembolism contributes greatly
to the progression of atherosclerosis and to the clinical complications of the process, such as stroke or myocardial infarction.
The blood platelet may contribute to degenerative vascular disease
in a number of ways, including that the substances they release
upon stimulation actually cause vessel injury or produce a response
of the vessel to injury; that they constitute a major component of
the thrombi which form on an area of arterial damage or atherosclerotic plaque which may lead to vessel occlusion or serve as a
source of emboli that contributes to organ ischemia (1).

Data which incriminate the platelet as a major factor in arterial thrombosis and in atherosclerosis have led to the development of great interest in identifying methods to detect alteration
in platelet function in patients with thrombosis, atherosclerosis,
or other conditions associated with a high incidence of arterial
thromboembolism. Of the numerous in vitro tests designed to detect
alteration in platelet function none have proven reliable to detect
thrombosis or predict thrombosis proneness, and it appears likely
that such tests fail to reflect accurately the activity of platelets
in vivo. If platelets are involved in the sequence of events following vessel injury, and this entails the alteration in their
shape, structure, or contents, or if they are incorporated into
thrombotic masses which form in association with vessel injury,

437

their destruction or accelerated rate of removal from the circulation should occur and this might be detectable by an increased rate
of turnover of platelets or a shortened platelet survival time.

MEASUREMENT OF PLATELET SURVIVAL TIME

Several approaches have been developed for the measurement of
platelet survival time, of which those involving the isotopic labeling of circulating platelets are the most practical. Of the several
isotopes which can be used for platelet labeling and methods of
doing so, the technique most widely employed involves the in vitro
labeling of platelets with chromium, using the technique described
by Aster and Jandl with minor modifications (2,3). The effect of
numerous variables on labeling and platelet viability have been
evaluated (4). The procedure currently being employed involves the
isotopic labeling of platelets separated from freshly drawn citrated,
usually autologous, whole blood which are concentrated in a platelet
button by differential centrifugation at room temperature after pH
adjustment of the platelet rich plasma to approximately 6.5 to prevent aggregation during the processing. Ordinarily 300-400 milliliters of blood is processed, but reliable results may be obtained
with the use of platelets from as little as 100-150 milliliters of
blood in adult patients. Labeling is accomplished with 200-400
microcuries of high specific activity chromate sodium during incubation for 30-60 minutes. The efficiency of labeling is approximately 10-20%, and upon intravenous injection of the resuspended
platelets, there is recovery into the circulation of approximately
55-75% of the labeled platelets. Disappearance of the platelets
is followed for 5-10 days by withdrawal of daily blood samples.
In most instances whole blood may be used for counting unless there
has been contamination with labeled red blood cells in sufficient
amount to produce interference or too little platelet activity, in
which case washed platelet buttons must be prepared for counting.
Determination of the platelet survival time is calculated by least
squares analysis of the series of daily counts, preferably utilizing a computer-assisted program to avoid bias. It is probably
preferable to express results as a gamma function although calculation as a linear or exponential decay function may be satisfactory.
Platelet consumption or "turnover" per microliter of blood per
day may be calculated by dividing peripheral blood platelet count
by platelet survival time, after correcting for the recovery rate
of labeled platelets.

Extensive experience with the modified Aster and Jandl method
indicates that the results yield a reliable and reproducible estimate (+ 5-10%) of platelet survival. Comparison of platelet survival calculated by this method with other techniques indicate good
correlation. Normal $T_{1/2}$ is 3.3 to 4.2 days, and platelet survival
time 8 to 10 days.

MECHANISM OF ALTERED PLATELET SURVIVAL TIME

It seems logical to assume that reduction in platelet survival time and increase in turnover of platelets in patients with vascular disease would reflect the consequence of the platelet interaction with an abnormal surface. Simplistically this sequence would involve adherence of platelets to the damaged vessel wall surface and release of constituents. Platelets which were incorporated into a thrombus or platelet aggregate and remained there would disappear from the circulation, as would those which broke away from the platelet aggregate and reentered the circulation, which would be removed by the reticuloendothelia system because of the damage that had occurred to them in their involvement with the thrombotic event. That the process is not this straightforward is demonstrated by a number of studies. For example, it has been shown that platelets that have been aggregated in response to ADP exposure or have been degranulated by thrombin have normal survival time in experimental animals (5, 6). Similarly, the stripping of endothelial cells from the aorta of rabbits by the balloon catheter technique was not associated with detectable alteration in platelet survival time (7). Thus there are unanswered questions concerning precise factors which are associated with reduction in platelet survival time.

Recently reported studies describing the development of atherosclerotic lesions in sub-human primates have contributed important information on this subject. In these experiments, atherosclerotic lesions were produced in baboons by homocystine infusion, or in pigtail monkeys by feeding of a lipid rich diet alone or in combination with balloon injury of arteries (3, 8). In both studies platelet survival time was shortened significantly, and the degree of shortening from normal correlated directly with the degree of endothelial damage that was produced (Tables 1 and 2). Evidence that the reduction in platelet survival resulted from the interaction of platelets with the damaged surface was obtained by injection of isotopically labeled platelets from a normal donor into the hyperlipemic animals and observing a shortening of their survival time, while platelets taken from hyperlipemic animals were demonstrated to have normal survival in a normal lipemic recipient. In these elegant studies additional information concerning the contribution made by platelets to the development of the atherosclerotic lesion was obtained by treating a group of animals with dipyridamole simultaneously with homocystine infusion. These animals had platelet survival and turnover which was significantly different than in homocystinemic animals not given dipyridamole (Table 1). At sacrifice they demonstrated the same endothelial damage as did homocystinemic animals not receiving dipyridamole. However, there was striking, although not total, prevention of the atherosclerotic lesion in the damaged vessel, suggesting that the platelet surface interaction had been modified to a major extent, presumably by

prevention of release of mitogenic factor from platelets at the
site of vessel damage (Table 3). These data provide strong evidence
to suggest that the platelet survival time, if shortened in patients
with vascular disease, would indicate the presence of a damaged
vascular surface and suggest that the degree of the shortening may
have a direct correlation with the extensiveness of vascular damage.
Similarly, it suggests that the return to normal of platelet survival time might parallel a change in vessel wall damage.

Table 1. Platelet survival - Correlation with endothelial damage
          in homocystinemic baboons (Harker et al. - JCI, 1976)

Baboons	No.	Homocystine (mM)	Endothelial Cell Loss %	Platelet Survival Days
Control	8	0.00	0	5.4 (+ 0.1)
Homocystinemic	15	0.17 (+ 0.02)	9.6 (+ 2.2)	2.8 (+ 0.3)
Dipyridamole + Homocystinemia	11	0.13 (+ 0.01)	7.0 (+ 0.9)	4.8 (+ 0.2)

Table 2. Platelet survival - Correlation with endothelial damage
          in hyperlipemic monkeys (Ross, Harker - Science, 1976)

Diet	No.	Cholesterol (mgm %)	Endothelial Loss (%)	Platelet Survival Days
Normal	8	88 + 5	0	8 + 0.3
Lipid Rich	6	223 + 22	5 + 1.2	5.8 + 0.5

Table 3. Platelet suppressant therapy - Dipyridamole effect in
          homocystinemic baboons (Harker et al. - JCI, 1976)

Baboons	No.	Endothelial Loss (%)	Intimal Lesion (Score)
Control	8	0	4 (+ 1)
Homocystinemic	15	9.6 (+ 2.2)	63 (+ 5)
Dipyridamole Rx	11	7.0 (+ 0.9)	16 (+ 2)

PLATELET SURVIVAL

Platelet survival measurement has been made in a variety of disease states. Most of the conditions in which shortened platelet survival time has been reported are listed (Table 4). In the acute column are listed conditions in which platelet survival time is limited in most cases to the acute phase of the process and clinical recovery is usually associated with return of platelet survival to normal. Although the number of cases studied in these groups is not great, the reports would suggest that virtually all patients in these groups will have shortened survival time (9). It seems likely that in these conditions a variety of factors may contribute to the shortened platelet survival time, and it seems doubtful that the test offers much specificity in terms of pathophysiologic processes or therapeutic implications in this setting.

In the chronic column are shown conditions associated with prolonged shortening of platelet survival. In several of these conditions available data indicate that virtually all afflicted patients have shortened platelet survival time throughout their course, such as those with active vasculitis, thrombotic thrombocytopenic purpura, marked hypoxemia, or homocystinemia. In other of these conditions some but not all patients show shortened platelet survival. This group would include patients with placement of intravascular prosthetic materials (heart valves, arterial grafts, etc.), neoplasia, recurrent arterial thromboembolism, or widespread atheroclerosis. In most groups the available information is not sufficient to exclude the possibility that there are intermittent abnormalities in the platelet survival time.

Table 4. Platelet survival time - Conditions associated with shortened values

Acute	Chronic
Myocardial Infarction	Vasculitis
Stroke	Thrombotic Thrombocytopenic Purpura
Venous Thromboembolism	Hypoxemia
Postoperative	Homocystinuria
Febrile Illness	Intravascular Prosthesis
Consumption Coagulopathy	Neoplasia
	Arterial Thromboembolism
	Atherosclerosis
	Hypertension
	Venous Thromboembolism

In patients with peripheral atherosclerosis usually in association with the symptom of intermittent claudication, platelet
survival time measurement performed during a stable period in their
course has usually shown some reduction in platelet survival, of
mild degree (Table 5) (10, 11, 12, 13). There is some suggestion
that the value correlates with the severity of the disease, with
greatest shortening in those patients who have rapidly progressing
disease. In the study by Harker, simultaneous fibrinogen survival
was measured and found slightly reduced from normal, suggesting
that there may be low grade intravascular coagulation involving
both fibrin formation as well as platelet deposition. The small
group of patients reported by Harker with artery to artery embolism
are particularly interesting. These were patients who had recurrent
episodes of embolization into various arterial beds where diagnostic studies suggested that the emboli had arisen from the wall of
major arteries, usually the aorta. In these patients, the platelet
survival time showed much greater shortening than in patients with
a stable claudication picture.

Platelet survival measurements have been made in patients with
coronary artery disease by a number of investigators (Table 6) (10,
11, 14, 15). In one of the earliest reports (16) Mustard et al.
measured platelet survival using the DFP 32 method in patients with
a variety of atherosclerotic lesions, including coronary artery
disease. The patients had a significantly shortened platelet survival compared to a normal group. These authors made the important
observation that some patients in the control group had a strong
family history of atherosclerotic disease and shorter platelet survival than the other controls. When the difference in platelet
survival was made between the clinically symptomatic atherosclerotic
group and the control group with negative family history for coronary disease, the statistical significance was increased.

Table 5. Platelet survival - Results in peripheral atherosclerosis

	Patients (#)	Shortened Survival (%)
O'Neill 1964	5	0 - PS by early technique
Abrahamsen 1968	18	50 - Claudication
1974	9	100 - Claudication
Harker 1974	6	100 - Claudication; fibrinogen survival slightly reduced
	8	100 - Artery-artery embolism - Marked PS shortening - Fibrinogen survival reduced

Table 6. Platelet survival - Results in coronary artery disease

	Patients (#)	Shortened Survival (%)
O'Neill 1964	5	0 - PS by early technique
Abrahamsen 1968	36	50 - Clinical Dx (post M.I.)
Steele 1974	68	60 - Angio Dx; Incidence highest with type IV HLP
Ritchie 1977	58	53 - Angio Dx

More recent studies have been carried out in patients who have coronary artery disease documented by angiography. The results in these cases are remarkably similar and indicate that approximately half of patients with clinically symptomatic coronary disease will have shortened platelet survival. In most instances this shortening is not marked in degree, but significantly below the normal range for that laboratory. Where mentioned, no correlation was recognized between platelet survival and such clinical factors as the age or sex of patient, presence or absence of angina pectoris, history of myocardial infarction, or with the location of angiographically-demonstrated narrowing of coronary vessels or their severity. It has been noted, however, that hyperlipidemia may be related to platelet survival time. Thus, in the study by Steele et al., a higher percentage of patients with type IV hyperlipidemia had demonstrable shortening of platelet survival compared to patients with normal lipid patterns. Similarly, Jonker et al. reported shortened platelet survival in type IV hyperlipoproteinemia and in patients with type IIb patterns (17).

It appears, therefore, that coronary artery disease is associated with shortened platelet survival in a significant percentage of patients, although the significance of this finding as regards the degree or activity of vascular damage is unclear. It has been suggested that the platelet survival time result is stable in patients who have undergone serial determinations (14, 17). It has also been observed that the degree of platelet survival shortening may vary with the clinical status of the patient in that a shortened platelet survival time has become even further reduced with worsening of angina, and the platelet survival was observed to have returned toward normal upon improvement of angina or following aortocoronary bypass surgery (15, 18). In several studies where it has been commented upon, the platelet survival time has not correlated with the result of other platelet function tests such as platelet adhesion and platelet aggregation to various agents (13, 14, 19).

Observations of this kind are interesting and expand our knowledge about the dynamic process of thrombosis and atherosclerosis, but do not establish a value for platelet survival determinations in the clinical management of patients. In some patient groups such a role for platelet survival has been suggested. Thus, in patients with prosthetic heart valves constructed from currently available low thrombogenic materials, the majority of patients have normal platelet survival, time and the incidence of thromboembolic events in such cases is extremely low. In contrast, a varying percentage of patients with a particular valve will demonstrate shortened platelet survival, and it is from this sub-group that those with thromboembolism will derive, and practically all patients who develop thromboembolism have chronic shortening of platelet survival (20). In patients with non-operated rheumatic mitral value disease a similar association between shortened platelet survival and propensity to systemic thromboembolism has been reported (21).

In coronary disease patients an interesting correlation between platelet survival time and the incidence of occlusion of aortocoronary bypass grafts has been reported (22). In that study 35 patients underwent follow-up coronary arteriography a minimum of three months following coronary surgery, in most cases for the evaluation of symptoms suggesting graft occlusion. In 16 of these patients platelet survival had been performed pre-operatively and there was no significant change in values at the post-operative study. Thus, two-thirds of the patients had shortened platelet survival both pre- and post-operatively and the remainder had normal values at both determinations. Twenty of the patients had one or more of the vein grafts occluded, and the average platelet survival for this group was shortened and significantly different from those with patency of the saphenous vein grafts (Figure 1). Ninety-five percent of patients with occluded grafts had shortened platelet survival. In contrast, 15 patients had patency of all their grafts and the average survival time was normal in that group, and 60 percent of the patients had normal survival time.

These data suggest that the measurement of platelet survival in patients scheduled to undergo aortocoronary bypass surgery may be useful to identify those at particular risk of developing late graft closure. This would presume that the shortened platelet survival identifies patients with platelet reactivity that increases the likelihood of graft occlusion, probably through the pathway of progressive intimal proliferation to which platelets may contribute significantly.

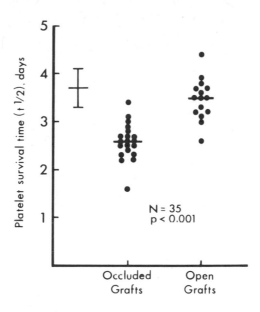

Figure 1

ROLE OF PLATELET SURVIVAL FOR IDENTIFICATION
OF CLINICALLY USEFUL PLATELET SUPPRESSANT DRUGS

In addition to the interest in defining the role of platelets in the genesis of degenerative vascular disease there has been much interest in identifying drugs that would be effective clinically as antithrombotic agents through their effect on platelet function. Progress in this field has been significantly hampered by the lack of a method other than difficult, time consuming, and expensive clinical trials, to identify a clinically useful platelet suppressant drug. Although there are many compounds which alter one or more of the in vitro "platelet function tests," it is not presently known which platelet function(s) is of significance in thrombosis or what drug action would correlate with clinical effectiveness. The observation that platelet survival may predict thrombosis proneness in man, and in experimental models correlates with endothelial damage or its reversal, suggests that the platelet survival test

may be useful to identify promising platelet suppressant drugs.
This is not to say that a drug which failed to improve shortened
platelet survival might not be effective in clinical circumstances
where the provocation to thrombosis was slight, but a drug which
consistently improved or completely corrected a shortened platelet
survival time would certainly have potential clinical value.

A number of drugs have been administered to patients with
atherosclerotic disease and shortened platelet survival time. These
include aspirin, dipyridamole alone or in combination with aspirin,
clofibrate, and sulfinpyrazone. Aspirin, when used alone in doses
in excess of one gram per day, has not lengthened or shortened platelet survival time in a small number of patients with coronary artery
disease, peripheral atherosclerosis, or arterial thromboembolism
(9, 13). Results with dipyridamole (400 mg daily) alone or in combination with aspirin (dipyridamole 100 and aspirin 1 g daily) have
been conflicting. In one study of five patients with arterial
thromboembolism and shortened platelet survival a return to normal
of survival time was seen in each patient. In contrast, patients
with stable peripheral vascular disease and slightly reduced platelet survival time had no significant change with dipyridamole-aspirin treatment (13). In another study of nine patients with peripheral vascular disease and somewhat more marked shortening of
platelet survival, similar results were obtained, e.g., no reversal
of the shortened platelet survival after treatment with a combination of dipyridamole-aspirin (23). In patients with coronary artery
disease and reduced platelet survival time, treatment with dipyridamole-aspirin combination, sulfinpyrazone (800 mg daily), or clofibrate (2,000 mg daily) prolonged a shortened platelet survival time
in the majority, and returned it to normal in more than half the
patients. Again, aspirin in a small number of patients has not been
shown to be effective (9, 13, 17). From the available studies it
is not possible to determine with certainty the rapidity with which
the platelet survival time is affected. With dipyridamole-aspirin
an effect may be measured after a few days of treatment, but
followup studies with other agents have usually been delayed for
several weeks or months making it difficult to determine when
change in platelet survival occurred. The mechanism by which the
drugs alter shortened platelet survival time is also uncertain.
Whether the effect is entirely related to direct action of the drugs
on platelets, indirectly by effect on vessel wall, a combination
of these, or through other pathways is at present uncertain.

SUMMARY

Platelet survival presently represents a useful method for the
study of atherosclerosis and its consequences in patients and in
animal models. The currently used technique, while time consuming,

appears to be reliable and reproducible for the measurement of platelet survival and turnover rate. The test offers promise to detect and perhaps quantify the degree of active vessel wall damage. In addition, it might prove useful to identify drugs with potential as platelet suppressants. Finally, the test might be used to compare with new techniques developed or used to identify vessel damage or thrombosis proneness.

REFERENCES

1. Mustard, J.F. (1976) Transactions of American Clinical and Climatological Association 87, 104-127.

2. Aster, R.H., and Jandl, J.H. (1964) J. Clin. Invest. 43, 843-855.

3. Harker, L.A., Ross, R., Slichter, S.J., and Scott, C.R. (1976) J. Clin. Invest. 58, 731-741.

4. Abrahamsen, A.F. (1968) Scand. J. Hemat. 5, 53-63.

5. Cazenave, J.P., Packham, M.A., Guccione, M.A., and Mustard, J.F. (1974) J. Lab. Clin. Med. 86, 551-563.

6. Reimers, H.J., Kinlough-Rathbone, R.L., Cazenave, J.P., Senyi, A.F., Hirsh, J., Packham, M.A., and Mustard, J.F. (1976) Thrombosis and Haemost. 35, 151-166.

7. Groves, H.M., Kinlough-Rathbone, R.L., Richardson, M., and Mustard, J.F. Blood. In press.

8. Ross, R., and Harker, L. (1976) Science 193, 1094-1100.

9. Genton, E. (1976) Proceedings of Int'l Symposium on Platelets and Thrombosis, Milan, Italy.

10. O'Neill, B., and Firkin, B. (1964) J. Lab. Clin. Med. 64, 188-201.

11. Abrahamsen, A.F. (1968) Scand. J. Hemat. 5, Suppl. 3, 1-53.

12. Abrahamsen, A.F., Eika, C., Godal, H.C., and Lorentsen, E. (1974) Scand. J. Hemat. 13, 241-245.

13. Harker, L.A., and Slichter, S.J. (1974) Thromb. Diath. Haemorrh. 31, 188-203.

14. Steele, P.P., Battock, D., and Genton, E. (1975) <u>Circulation</u>
    52, 473-476.

15. Ritchie, J.L., and Harker, L.A. (1974) <u>Circulation</u> 50, Suppl. 3,
    285.

16. Murphy, E.A., and Mustard, J.F. (1962) <u>Circulation</u> 25, 114-125.

17. Jonker, J.J., Veen, M.R., Schopman, W., and den Ottolander,
    G.J.G. (1974) <u>Thromb. Res.</u> 4, 65-67.

18. Ritchie, J.L., and Harker, L.A. (1977) <u>Am. J. Cardiol.</u> 39,
    595-598.

19. Salky, N., and Dugdale, M. (1973) <u>Am. J. Cardiol.</u> 32, 612-
    617.

20. Weily, H.S., Steele, P.P., Davies, H., Pappas, G., and Genton,
    E. (1974) <u>N. Engl. J. Med.</u> 290, 534-537.

21. Steele, P.P., Weily, H.S., Davies, H., and Genton, E. (1974)
    <u>N. Engl. J. Med.</u> 290, 537-539.

22. Steele, P.P., Battock, D., Pappas, G., and Genton, E. (1976)
    <u>Circulation</u> 53, 685-687.

23. Abrahamsen, A.F., Eika, C., Godal, H.C., and Lorentsen, E.
    (1974) <u>Scand. J. Hemat.</u> 13, 241-245.

ASSAYS FOR HYPERCOAGULABILITY

Robert D. Rosenberg, Herbert Lau,
David Beeler, and Judith S. Rosenberg

Harvard Medical School, Sidney Farber Cancer Clinic,
Department of Medicine of Beth Israel Hospital,
Boston, Massachusetts

Many investigators have attempted to determine whether a relationship exists between excessive activity of the hemostatic mechanism and the atherosclerotic process. A major difficulty encountered in unraveling this puzzle has been the lack of reliable
techniques for quantifying pertinent changes in blood coagulability.
We have focused our attention on detecting alterations in the
zymogens and protease inhibitors of the coagulation system which
might occur prior to the development of overt thrombotic phenomena.
Measurement of these early changes may be critical, if we wish to
dissect the molecular events which are ultimately responsible for
the atherosclerotic lesion and intervene with appropriate therapy
prior to the onset of gross pathologic changes. In the sections
below, we outline the difficulties associated with developing this
methodology. Furthermore, we describe two new radioimmunoassays
that may serve as prototype techniques for monitoring the activity
of the hemostatic mechanism.

BIOCHEMICAL ASPECTS

Protein components of the hemostatic mechanism are termed zymogens if they can be converted to proteolytic enzymes (serine proteases). The relevant species included in this category are pro-

This work was supported by the National Institutes of Health
(HL91931, HL20079, and HL21602) and the American Heart Association
(75-952). One of the authors (R.D.R.) is a recipient of an
American Heart Association Established Investigatorship Award.

thrombin, Factor VII, Factor IX, Factor X, Factor XI and Factor XII. In almost all instances, activation is accomplished by cleavage of peptide bonds and subsequent release of a portion of the molecule. We shall consider the conversion of prothrombin to thrombin as an example of this type of process.

Using purified human preparations of prothrombin, Factor Xa, and Factor V, we have studied the pathways of thrombin generation in the presence and absence of naturally occurring inhibitors (1). In the absence of these antagonists, prothrombin (P_1) ($\sim$70,000) is cleaved to form the thrombin precursor P_2 ($\sim$51,700) and the fragment F_A ($\sim$19,500). Subsequently, P_2 is converted to the thrombin precursor P_3 ($\sim$38,000) as well as a second fragment F_B ($\sim$11,500). In the presence of these antagonists, an additional pathway emerges. Prothrombin is cleaved directly to P_3 and a single fragment (F_{A+B}) ($\sim$31,000). In both pathways, the single chain polypeptide P_3 is proteolyzed to form the heavy (T_H) ($\sim$30,000) and light (T_L) ($\sim$6,500) chains of thrombin. This activation sequence is similar to that published by Hanahan and his coworkers (2).

Thus, we have demonstrated the existence of two human prothrombin activation sequences similar to those identified by Stenn et al. (3), Jackson et al. (4) and Mann et al. (5) for the bovine zymogen. More recently, Mann et al. (6) have shown that a small polypeptide of 13 amino acid residues is removed from the N-terminal region of P_3 prior to or immediately after its conversion to the active enzyme. It is unclear whether this step would take place in vivo. Therefore, P_3 and thrombin may exist within the blood with an extended T_L chain (T_L^{ext}). The sequence of transformations responsible for thrombin generation are summarized in Figure 1.

It should be obvious that the above transitions must occur to only a limited extent in vivo since a vast excess of prothrombin is present within blood. Indeed, the conversion of 0.3% of the plasma's content of this zymogen would result in the immediate generation of a fibrin cast throughout the vasculature. These conclusions are similar for other zymogen activation processes. The levels of these components within blood appear to be controlled in large measure by general catabolic pathways.

Thus, attempts to monitor prethrombotic states by measuring the ambient levels of zymogens or by determining their catabolic rates within the circulatory system are doomed to failure. New techniques must be devised for directly assaying these conversion processes. Unfortunately, the final enzyme products of these pathways are evanescent species rapidly neutralized by naturally occurring protease inhibitors and therefore unavailable for quantitation. Faced with this obstacle, we have focused our attention on the measurement of activation fragments such as F_B (see above) that are

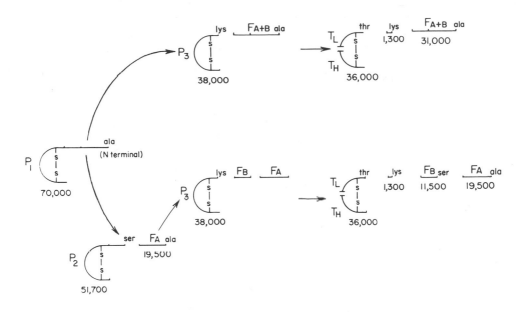

Figure 1. The sequence of transformations responsible for thrombin generation.

produced _pari passu_ with enzyme generation. These by-products of zymogen transformation are stable entities which may circulate for prolonged periods of time.

Protease inhibitors normally circulate within the blood and serve to dampen as well as restrict the activity of the hemostatic mechanism. These species include antithrombin, α_2-plasmin inhibitor, α_2-macroglobulin, C^1 esterase inhibitor, and α_1-antitripsin (7-11). Antithrombin appears to be of prime importance in the modulation of coagulation system activity. This component is able to neutral-ize the action of virtually all of the serine proteases of the coagulation system, i.e., thrombin, Factor IXa, Factor Xa, Factor XIa and Factor XIIa (12-16). Inactivation is accomplished by form-ation of a 1:1 complex between enzyme and inhibitor (12-16). Fur-thermore, congenital reductions in antithrombin result in inherited

thrombotic diatheses (17). This latter phenomenon does not occur
when the plasma concentrations of other protease inhibitors are
reduced by a similar mechanism.

The levels of antithrombin within the blood are greater than
the levels of zymogens whose enzymes this component serves to neu-
tralize. Furthermore, the survival of antithrombin within the circulation is largely determined by a general catabolic pathway.
Therefore, one would expect that measurement of this substance would
not reveal the extent of zymogen activation. This is due to the
fact that only small amounts of the coagulation system enzymes will
be generated and complexed by this inhibitor. Thus, even rapid
removal of enzyme-inhibitor products should not significantly reduce
the plasma levels of antithrombin. If the prethrombotic state is
to be detected, direct quantifying of enzyme-antithrombin complexes
must be attempted.

In the sections below, we describe two new radioimmunoassays
that are capable of measuring prothrombin activation fragments and
thrombin-antithrombin complexes. The central difficulty encountered
in the development of these techniques stems from the fact that
nanogram quantities of these species must be measured in the presence
of hundreds of micrograms of parent zymogen and protease inhibitor
which normally circulate in the blood. This dilemma can be resolved
in one of two ways. On the one hand, the cross-reacting species
can be eliminated by extensive sample processing prior to the initiation of assay procedures. In this case, the antibody preparation
utilized in the radioimmunoassay need not be highly specific for
the fragments of complexes. Of course, sample processing is difficult to standardize, could introduce a variety of potential artifacts, and would significantly increase the time as well as labor
involved in conducting the assay procedures. On the other hand, one
can attempt to obtain an antibody population that recognizes antigenic sites on the activation fragment or complex then are hidden
in the parent zymogen or inhibitor. Provided that the necessary
degree of antibody specificity is attained, this technique would
obviate the requirement for sample processing. We have used the
latter approach in designing assays which are potentially capable
of directly measuring thrombin generation and inhibition within
blood.

RADIOIMMUNOASSAY OF ACTIVATION FRAGMENTS

We have injected human F_B fragment into 10 rabbits and goats
and obtained antisera directed against this component. The IgG
portion of each antiserum was isolated and individually filtered
through columns of prothrombin-sepharose as well as P_2-sepharose.
The effluent from each set of fractionations was concentrated and

subsequently applied to a column of F_B - sepharose. The specific
antibody population bound to the insolubilized antigen was eluted
with 1M acetic acid and immediately brought to neutral pH. This
specific fraction, in conjunction with ^{125}I-labeled F_B, was used
to develop a double antibody radioimmunoassay. The technique
detects as little as 0.5 ng/ml of F_B and has permitted us to explore the specificity of our antibody preparation. In the discussion below, we cite data obtained from a single bleeding of one
rabbit that exhibited the highest affinity for F_B and the most
restricted specificity for this antigen. In all instances, antisera generated in other rabbits and goats was decidedly inferior
to the fraction utilized with respect to one or the other of these
parameters.

The extent of interaction of our specific F_B antibody preparation with components of the prothrombin activation sequence was carefully examined. First, molecular species that do not contain the
F_B segment as a part of their covalent structure, such as F_A or
thrombin, exhibit no immunoreactivity in our assay system. Second,
components whose primary structure may include an F_B region, such
as prothrombin or P_2, only interact to a minimal degree with our
specific antibody fraction. Based upon the 50% displacement point
for F_B and prothrombin, we have determined that a ∼5000-fold molar
excess of zymogen as compared to activation fragment is required
to register an equivalent signal in our radioimmunoassay. This
estimate represents the average obtained for 10 different preparations of prothrombin. The minor degree of residual immunoreactivity
does not appear to be due to generation of the F_B fragment from the
zymogen during the radioimmunoassay procedure. However, quantitative conversion of prothrombin to thrombin and activation fragments
via the addition of Factor Xa permits the theoretically predicted
amounts of F_B immunoreactivity to be released. A similar analysis
of the data at the 50% displacement point, indicates that a 7000-
fold molar excess of P_2 as compared to F_B is needed to produce an
identical reading in our assay procedure. Our estimate is based
upon data obtained for 10 different preparations of P_2. This minor
extent of immunoreactivity is surprising since the F_B segment is at
the N-terminal of the P_2 intermediate. However, quantitative conversion of this component to thrombin and activation fragment by
the addition of Factor Xa results in the release of the theoretically
predicted amount of F_B immunoreactivity. Third, preliminary data
suggests that the F_{A+B} fragment has a similar reactivity to F_B.
This result appears to be due to an intrinsic property of this component and is not secondary to the conversion of F_{A+B} to F_B during
the radioimmunoassay procedure.

We have further defined the specificity of our antibody fraction by determining whether increased exposure of the F_B region
within the P_2 intermediate would alter the immunoreactivity of this
component. This was accomplished by converting P_2 to P_2^* with puri-

fied Echis carinatus venom (18). In this species, the F_B fragment
is covalently attached to the T_L^{ext} chain which, in turn, is linked
to the T_H chain by an S-S bridge. The immunoreactivity of this
component is surprisingly minimal. Based upon a 50% displacement
point, we have determined that a 2000-fold molar excess of P_2^* as
compared to F_B is required to produce an equivalent signal in our
radioimmunoassay. This estimate represents data obtained from an
average of 10 different preparations of P_2^*. Furthermore, quantity
conversion of P_2^* to thrombin and activation fragments via the addition of Factor Xa results in the generation of the theoretically
predicted amounts of F_B immunoreactivity.

The cloistered nature of this F_B determinant within P_2 or P_2^*
may either be due to interactions of the T_H chain with the F_B region or to the attachment of the T_L^{ext} chain to the C-terminal end
of the F_B fragment. To explore this issue, we isolated the carboxy-
methylated T_L^{ext} - F_B polypeptide chain of P_2^* and determined
its immunoreactivity. Based upon a 50% displacement point, we estimate that a 200-fold molar excess of T_L^{ext} - F_B as compared to
F_B is required to produce an equivalent signal in our radioimmunoassay. Furthermore, the conversion of the T_L^{ext} - F_B polypeptide
to F_B fragment and T_L chain via the addition of Factor Xa results
in the generation of the theoretically predicted level of F_B
immunoreactivity.

In summary, we have developed a radioimmunoassay that will
measure nanogram quantities of F_B or F_{A+B}, but is insensitive to
prothrombin, P_2 or P_2^*. This technique will permit us to quantify
the extent of thrombin formation within whole blood at levels likely
to occur during prethrombotic states. These measurements should
be independent of the activation pathway employed to generate thrombin. Furthermore, processing of samples to remove cross-reacting
species such as prothrombin or P_2 will not be required due to the
remarkable specificity of our antibody fraction.

RADIOIMMUNOASSAY OF THROMBIN-ANTITHROMBIN COMPLEXES

The purified thrombin-antithrombin complex was injected into
10 rabbits and goats, and antisera directed against this component
was obtained. The IgG fractions of each preparation were isolated
by standard techniques and the products were individually adsorbed
to columns of thrombin-antithrombin complex-sepharose. In each
instance, specific antibody preparations were harvested with 1M
acetic acid and rapidly titrated to neutral pH. Depending upon
the specificity of individual preparations, the specific antibody
fractions were subsequently filtered through columns of antithrom-
bin-sepharose or thrombin-sepharose. Optimal quantities of these
immunoadsorbents were used for each antibody preparation. If too
little immunoadsorbent was employed, antibodies which are directed

against prothrombin or antithrombin were preserved within the
final product. If too much immunoadsorbent was used, high titer
antibody directed against the thrombin-antithrombin complex was
also removed from the final preparation.

The specific antibody pool directed against the enzyme-inhibitor complex was employed in conjunction with ^{125}I-labeled thrombin-antithrombin to develop a double antibody radioimmunoassay.
Our procedure can measure as little as 10 ng/ml of thrombin-antithrombin complex. The experiments presented below use selected
antibody preparations from two rabbits and one goat that exhibit
the highest affinity as well as the most restricted selectivity
for thrombin-antithrombin complexes. Antisera obtained from other
rabbits or goats had reduced affinity and/or selectivity with
respect to this antigen.

We have compared the immunoreactivity of prothrombin, antithrombin and P_2 to the thrombin-antithrombin complex. All of
these components react only minimally in our radioimmunoassay.
The degree of immunoreactivity of these species is difficult to
quantify since component concentrations required to achieve 50%
displacement of ^{125}I-labeled thrombin-antithrombin complex could
not be attained. However, we would estimate from an 80% displacement point that 8000-20,000-fold molar excess of these proteins
as compared with thrombin-antithrombin complex would be required
to produce an equivalent signal in our assay procedure. Thrombin
or P_3 intermediate cross react more strongly with our specific
antibody fraction. Based upon a 50% displacement point, we estimate that a 500-fold molar excess of these two species as compared
with thrombin-antithrombin complex would be needed to generate an
identical signal in our radioimmunoassay. As previously pointed
out, essentially no free thrombin can exist within the blood;
therefore this species should not be present in our plasma samples.
The occurence of P_3 intermediate at high concentrations is also
unlikely. However, trace amounts of either component could be
quickly and easily removed from plasma samples by filtration through
columns of hirudin-sepharose. This leech protein reacts specifically with thrombin or P_3 but does not bind to thrombin-antithrombin complex (18).

We have also determined the immunoreactivity of other enzyme-
antithrombin complexes such as plasmin-antithrombin, Factor Xa -
antithrombin or Factor IXa - antithrombin. Based upon a 50% displacement point, we estimate that the various complexes must be
present in amounts that range from 250-fold to 2000-fold molar
excess as compared to thrombin-antithrombin to produce an equivalent
signal in our radioimmunoassay. Thus, generation of these complexes will not appreciably distort data obtained with this assay
technique.

In summary, we have developed a radioimmunoassay that is capable of measuring thrombin-antithrombin complexes at the nanogram level, but is only minimally perturbed by plasma concentrations of prothrombin and antithrombin. The procedure should allow us to quantitate thrombin inhibitor under in vivo conditions and therefore may permit us to monitor excessive generation of this enzyme prior to the development of thrombotic phenomena.

REFERENCES

1. Rosenberg, J.S., Beeler, D.F., and Rosenberg, R.D. (1975) J. Biol. Chem. 250, 1607-1617.

2. Kisiel, W., and Hanahan, D.J. (1973) Biophys. Acta 329, 221-232.

3. Stenn, K., Blout, E.R. (1972) Biochemistry 11, 4502-4515.

4. Esmon, C.T., Owen, W.G., Jackson, C.M. (1974) J. Biol. Chem. 249, 594.

5. Bajaj, S.P., Butkowski, R.J., and Mann, K.G. (1975) J. Biol. Chem. 250, 2150-2156.

6. Downing, M.R., Butkowski, R.J., Clark, M.M., Mann, K.G. (1975) J. Biol. Chem. 250, 8897.

7. Waugh, D.F., Fitzgerald, M.A. (1956) Am. J. Physiol. 184, 627-639.

8. Janoff, A. (1972) Am. Rev. Respir. Dis. 105, 121-122.

9. Schultze, H.E., Glollner, I., Heide, K., et al. (1955) Z Naturforsch (B) 10, 463-473.

10. Donaldson, V.H., and Evans, R.R. (1963) Am. J. Med. 35, 37-44.

11. Eriksson, S. (1965) Acta Med. Scand. 177 (Suppl. 432), 1-85.

12. Rosenberg, R.D., and Damus, P.S. (1973) J. Biol. Chem. 238, 7149-7163.

13. Rosenberg, J.S., McKenna, P.W., Rosenberg, R.D. (1975) J. Biol. Chem. 250, 8883-8888.

14. Kurachi, K., Fujikawa, K., Schmier, G., and Davie, E.W. (1976) Biochem. 15, 373-377.

15. Damus, P.S., Hicks, M., and Rosenberg, R.D. (1973) Nature
     246, 355-357.

16. Stead, N.W., Kaplan, A., and Rosenberg, R.D. (1976) J. Biol.
     Chem. 251, 6481-6488.

17. Egeberg, O. (1965) Thromb. Diath. and Haemorrh. 13, 516-530.

18. Aronson, D.L. (1975) J. Biol. Chem. 250, 7057.

ASSAY OF FIBRINOPEPTIDES A AND B AND OF RELEASED PLATELET PROTEINS AS A MEASURE OF ACTIVATION OF HEMOSTASIS

Hymie L. Nossel

Columbia University
College of Physicians and Surgeons
New York, New York

Our understanding of relationships between atherosclerosis and the hemostatic system would be greatly enhanced, if tests were available which would reproducibly and clearly demonstrate perturbations of the system in association with atherosclerosis. Tests of the hemostatic mechanism may be divided into two general types, those which measure the functional status of different components and those which measure the products of specific reactions. Functional status tests have been particularly useful in distinguishing, diagnosing and monitoring therapy in the bleeding disorders but have been of very limited usefulness in studying thromboembolism. The results of studies with functional tests in which patients with atherosclerosis were compared with patients with other disease are not available. The newly developed tests which measure the products of hemostatic reactions appear to be useful in studying thromboembolism and await application to the study of atherosclerosis. The present manuscript will review the theoretical basis for these tests and summarize the limited available clinical data. The results of studies on patients with hyperlipidemia will also be discussed.

ASSAYS BASED ON FIBRINOGEN PROTEOLYSIS

Fibrinogen-Fibrin Conversion and Dissolution

The central event in the coagulation of blood is the transformation of the soluble plasma protein fibrinogen into an insoluble plasma protein fibrinogen and then into an insoluble polymeric gel termed fibrin. A great deal of information has been acquired about the structure of fibrinogen but there is uncertainty concerning a

number of critical questions such as the shape of the molecule
and the location of the fibrinopeptides. There is general agreement that the molecular weight is 340,000 + 20,000 and that the
native molecule is a dimer each half of which consists of 3 polypeptide chains termed A-alpha, B-beta and gamma (1).

The conversion of fibrinogen to fibrin results from the action
of the serine protease thrombin. Thrombin cleaves bonds between
arginine (16) and glycine (17) on the A-alpha chain and between
arginine (14) and glycine (15) on the B-beta chain to produce two
molecules of fibrinopeptide A (FPA), two molecules of fibrinopeptide B (FPB) and one of fibrin monomer (2-5) (Figure 1). Fibrin
monomer forms complexes with both fibrin and fibrinogen. When the
concentration of fibrin is low relative to that of fibrinogen (ratio
less than 1:5) fibrin-fibrinogen complexes are formed and the fib-

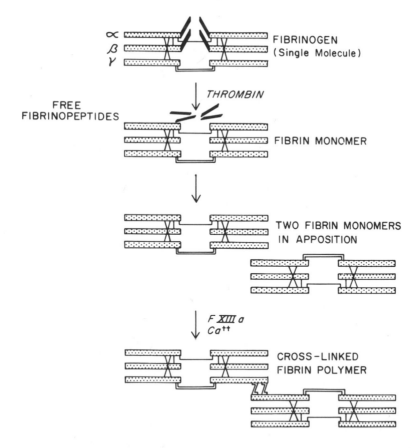

Fig. 1. Conversion of Fibrinogen to Fibrin.

rin remains in solution. When the ratio of fibrin to fibrinogen
exceeds 1:5 fibrin dimers and polymers form and precipitate from
solution to form fibrin clots (6-7). These clots are hemostati-
cally ineffective until the fibrin molecules are cross-linked by
the action of Factor XIIIa in the presence of calcium. Six covalent intermolecular cross-links involving glutamic and lysine
residues are formed by each fibrin molecule. Two cross-links occur
between the gamma chains of adjacent molecules and the other four
cross-links involve the alpha chains (8-10). Plasmin, the clot-
dissolving enzyme, may act on fibrinogen or fibrin. Plasmin has
proteolytic specificity intermediate between that of thrombin and
trypsin and it produces sequential degradation of fibrinogen and
fibrin. Two early products of plasmin action on fibrinogen are
peptides from the carboxy-terminal half of the A-alpha (11-12) and
B-beta 1-42 from the amino-terminal end of the B-beta chain (13-14).
Antisera have developed to some of these peptides (12).

        Late degradation products include a fragment from the amino-
terminal end (fragment E) and one from the carboxyterminal end
(Fragment D) and detailed immunological studies of these two fragments have been made (15-16).

        Most clinical tests which reflect fibrinogen proteolysis are
based on measurement of fibrinogen antigen and degradation products
in serum derived from blood clotted by thrombin in vitro (17) although more specific antisera have been used and are available (18).
Tests based on these techniques may reflect the action of plasmin
or of other proteases (19). A number of attempts have been made
to develop tests specific for thrombin action in vivo based on the
detection of fibrin monomer (20-25). These tests have the advantage in that the clearance rate from the blood of fibrin monomer
is appreciably slower than the clearance rate for FPA (26). The
discussion in this presentation will, however, focus on the FPA
assay.

ASSAYS OF FIBRINOPEPTIDES A AND B

        Fibrinopeptide A, which is composed of 16 amino acids (Fig. 2),
is measured with use of two reagents: A radiolabeled tracer, prepared by coupling tyrosine to the fibrinopeptide and labeling the
produce with iodine-125 by the chloramine T technique; and fibrinopeptide A-specific antibodies, prepared by immunizing rabbits with
peptide covalently linked to albumin. Fibrinopeptide A is measured by competitive inhibition of binding of tracer to antibody
(27). The assay can detect 0.013 pmoles of fibrinopeptide A. Free
fibrinopeptide A, fibrinogen and portions of the fibrinogen molecule that contain fibrinopeptide A all inhibit tracer binding by
antiserum.

For use as a tracer in the assay for fibrinopeptide B (Fig. 2), a fibrinopeptide B analogue is prepared by substitution of glutamic acid for N-terminal pyroglutamine. Solid-phase synthesis of fibrinopeptide B analogue and coupling of tyrosine to N-terminal glutamic acid produce a tyrosine-fibrinopeptide B analogue. The methods for radiolabeling of this analogue, raising of specific antisera and development of the assay are similar to those used in the assay for fibrinopeptide A (28). Since it is of primary importance to establish the specificity of the product measured by these assays, detailed studies of the immunochemistry of fibrinopeptide A were undertaken.

Immunochemistry of Fibrinopeptide A

The degree of inhibition by fibrinogen of binding of ^{125}I fibrinopeptide A to antiserum varies with the antiserum used. With most antisera, the molar cross-reactivity of fibrinogen is similar to its fibrinopeptide A content, but some antisera exhibit significant selectivity towards FPA. The selective antisera (R2 type) exhibit the same degree of low cross-reactivity with other fibrinopeptide-A-containing antigens, such as the amino terminal disulfide knot of fibrinogen, fibrinogen fragment E, A-alpha chain 1-51 and even A-alpha chain 1-23 (29, 30).

```
                           1   2   3   4   5   6   7   8
FIBRINOPEPTIDE A   H2N-ALA-ASP-SER-GLY-GLU-GLY-ASP-PHE-

                           9  10  11  12  13  14  15  16
                   LEU-ALA-GLU-GLY-GLY-GLY-VAL-ARG-

                           1   2   2   4   5   6   7
FIBRINOPEPTIDE B   PYR-GLY-VAL-ASN-ASP-ASN-GLU-

                           8   9  10  11  12  13  14
                   GLU-GLY-PHE-PHE-SER-ALA-ARG-
```

Figure 2. Amino Acid Sequences of Fibrinopeptides A and B.

In experiments with synthetic partial fibrinopeptide-A-sequences, the antigenic determinant for the selective antiserum was found to reside in the 10 amino acid sequence A-alpha 7-16; arginine (16), aspartic acid (7) and phenylalanine (8) were specifically necessary. The antigenic determinants for the nonselective antisera were different (31).

A practical application of these immunochemical findings is the use of the R2 antiserum to detect the presence, in samples tested before and after treatment with thrombin, of any fibrinopeptide-A-containing fragments the size of A-alpha 1-23 or larger. It is important to distinguish fragments of this size from A 1-16 (fibrinopeptide A) because plasmin produces A-alpha 1-23 by cleavage of arginine (23)-histidine (24), but does not produce fibrinopeptide A (29). Thrombin treatment does not increase immunoreactivity if fibrinopeptide A is present alone but it causes a 100-fold increase if fibrinogen or fibrinopeptide-A-containing fragments the size of A-alpha 1-23 or larger are present. In clinical studies, fibrinopeptide A immunoreactivity was not increased after thrombin treatment of plasma extracts. This result provides strong evidence that the immunoreactivity was caused by fibrinopeptide A itself, and not by larger fragments that might have been produced by other proteases (32).

In Vitro Application of Fibrinopeptide Assays

When the assays were used to measure the rates at which various enzymes cleaved fibrinopeptides from fibrinogen, thrombin cleaved fibrinopeptide A much faster than fibrinopeptide B (Fig. 3a) (28, 30). Plasmin cleaved portions of the B-beta chain that contained fibrinopeptide B more rapidly than peptides that contained fibrinopeptide A (Fig. 3b). The initial rate of FPA cleavage by thrombin at varying fibrinogen concentrations showed little change between 2 and 4 mg/ml with a Km of 2.99 M. At a fibrinogen concentration of 2.5 mg/ml the FPA cleavage rate was 49.2 nmol/ml/min. per unit of thrombin (33).

CLINICAL APPLICATION OF FIBRINOPEPTIDE ASSAYS

The principal potential of fibrinopeptide assays is to provide information about fibrinopeptide production in clinical blood samples (34). For this purpose methods were devised to measure fibrinopeptide concentrations in whole blood and to prevent in vitro generation and degradation. In vitro cleavage or loss of fibrinopeptide immunoreactivity can be prevented with use of an anticoagulant mixture that contains heparin and aprotinin (Trasylol - a proteinase inhibitor). In the presence of these inhibitors, the fibrinopeptide

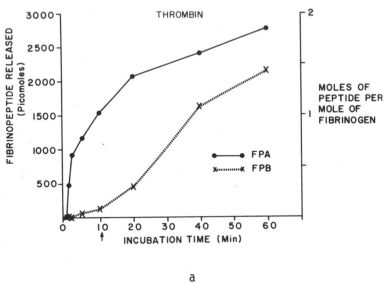

a

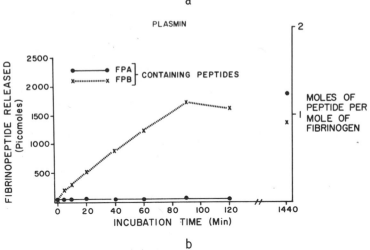

b

Figure 3. Cleavage of Fibrinopeptide A (FPA) and Fibrinopeptide B (FPB) by thrombin (in a) and by plasmin (in b). Reproduced from Bilezikian et al. (28).

A level remains stable for many months in plasma samples stored at
-40°C (35). Although fibrinogen cross-reactivity is relatively low
with the R2 antiserum, its concentration is so much higher than that
of the fibrinopeptides that fibrinogen must be completely removed
before the blood fibrinopeptide content is measured. Removal of
fibrinogen with reproducible recovery of fibrinopeptide is accomplished by precipitation with ethanol or trichloroacetic acid (32,
36). These methods are very time-consuming and delay the results
for several days. Recently, promising results have been obtained
by bentonite absorption of fibrinogen permitting the results to be
obtained the same day.

Fibrinopeptide A Levels in Patients

In 100 normal individuals, the mean fibrinopeptide A level
was 0.6 pmoles per milliliter, with a range of 0.1 to 1.3 pmoles
per milliliter (32, 35-40). Artificially high levels were present
when blood flow was obstructed. In an acute-care hospital ward,
approximately one patient in four had an elevation of fibrinopeptide
A. In patients with levels in the normal range (< .13 pmoles per
milliliter), the mean level was 1.1 pmoles -- higher than the mean
level in normal subjects.

Grossly elevated levels (> 7 pmoles per milliliter) have been
found in patients with acute pulmonary embolism, acute thrombophlebitis or acute disseminated intravascular coagulation. Moderately elevated levels (1.4 to 7 pmoles per milliliter) have been
found in patients with these disorders in subactue forms and in
patients with acute infections such as septicemia, lobar pneumonia,
cellulitis, carcinomatosis without clinically evident thrombosis,
systemic lupus erythematosus, renal-transplant rejection and aortic
aneurysm (39).

In studies on patients with acute symptomatic thrombo-embolism
as evidenced by positive venography or lung scan, elevated FPA
levels were present in 42 out of 47 patients. Patients with recent
onset of symptoms had higher levels (40). Fibrinopeptide A levels
have been elevated in all patients with disseminated intravascular
coagulation diagnosed on the basis of hypofibrinogenemia, elevated
serum fibrin-degradation products and thrombocytopenia. The degree
of elevation did not correlate with the levels of fibrin-degradation products or with the severity of hypofibrinogenemia.

In Vivo Clearance of Fibrinopeptide A

Intravenous injection of up to 5 nmoles of fibrinopeptide A
per kilogram of body weight, a quantity without known physiologic

effect, produced markedly elevated levels in normal subjects, and comparison of the plasma volume with the amount of injected peptide indicated that 70 to 100 per cent was recovered in the blood. The fibrinopeptide A level declined rapidly. Since the rate of decline was equivalent to a half time of three minutes, it was estimated that in 24 hours 7 pmoles per milliliter could be produced by thrombin proteolysis of 800 mg of fibrinogen. This amount represents 36 per cent of the total fibrinogen catabolism in a normal person who weighs 70 kg. The mean fibrinopeptide A level in normal subjects (0.6 pmoles per milliliter) could be produced by thrombin proteolysis of a maximum of 3 per cent of total fibrinogen catabolism per 24 hours. Since the half time of fibrinopeptide A within the normal range could be more than three minutes, normal thrombin proteolysis may be responsible for substantially less than 3 per cent of total fibrinogen catabolism (32).

Effects of Heparin Infusion

In patients with elevated FPA levels and acute thromboembolism heparin infusion (mean dose 100 units/kg) given intravenously in 1 minute resulted in a rapid fall in FPA concentration reaching the normal range within 15 minutes in 24 of 25 patients studied. The initial rate of fall was consistent with a t-1/2 of 3 minutes (41). In normal individuals heparin infusion reduced the FPA level very slightly from 0.69 to 0.54 pmol/ml (32).

Studies in Hyperlipidemia

There have been no FPA measurements specifically related to atherosclerosis. In planning such studies the most critical issue appears to be that of finding appropriate groups of atherosclerotic and control patients for comparison. However, there have been a number of studies in patients with hyperlipidemia. Carvalho and colleagues (41) have reported major increases in high molecular weight fibrinogen derivatives in patients with type II hyperlipidemia (mean 31.6%) and lesser increases in patients with type IV hyperlipidemia (mean 19.8%) as compared with normal individuals (mean level 3.2%). Following 6 weeks treatment with clofibrate the percentage of high molecular weight fibrinogen derivatives in the type II hyperlipidemic patients decreased to 11% and in the type IV hyperlipidemic patients increased to 26%. Serum fibrinogen degradation products in patients with type II hyperlipidemia were 1.93 g/ml before treatment with clofibrate and 31.4 µg/ml after treatment. The data were interpreted to signify intravascular coagulation in type II hyperlipidemia which was reduced by treatment with clofibrate (42). Our data with the fibrinopeptide A assay appear to be inconsistent with increased intravascular coagulation in hyperlipidemia. In 32 controls (mean + SEM cholesterol (c) 238 + 7 mg/dl, triglyceride (T) 112 + 10) matched for age mean + S.D. FPA levels (pmol/ml) were 0.65 + 0.38. Twenty-seven patients with elevated cholesterol (c 344 + 18, T 113 + 9) had FPA levels of 0.74 + 0.49. Twenty-nine patients with elevated cholesterol and triglyceride (c 304 + 12, T 271 + 33) had FPA levels of 0.89 + 0.81. Forty-two patients with elevated triglyceride levels (c 222 + 7, T 322 + 16) had FPA levels of 0.69 + 0.5. In 56 of these patients (12 control, 10 hypercholesterolemic, 15 combined hyper-lipidemic and 19 hypertriglyceridemic) coagulation factors II, VII and X were measured. Small statistically significant increases in Factor II were found in hypercholesterolemia and in Factor X in hypertriglyceridemia.

These results indicate that there is no sustained state of increased intravascular thrombin action as detected by plasma FPA measurements in the group of hyperlipidemic patients studied.

PROTEINS SECRETED BY PLATELETS

Just as new tests are being developed which reflect activation rather than the functional status of the coagulation system, tests are being developed which indicate platelet activation in vivo. A major focus for such tests is the platelet release reaction in which specific platelet constituents are released into the ambient fluid following an appropriate stimulus. Among the proteins released or secreted are 3 platelet-specific proteins which have promise as indices of the platelet release reaction occurring in vivo. The potential usefulness of these tests in studying athero-sclerosis is that if platelets are reacting with atherosclerotic regions of the arterial wall it might be anticipated that they would secrete these proteins into the surrounding fluid producing increased plasma concentrations of these proteins.

The three platelet-specific proteins are platelet factor 4, beta-thromboglobulin and the platelet-derived smooth muscle growth factor. The smooth muscle growth factor, platelet-derived growth factor (Pt-DGF), has been discussed in detail earlier in this conference and several detailed reviews concerning platelet factor 4 and beta-thromboglobulin are available (43-45). Both platelet factor 4 and beta-thromboglobulin are well characterized proteins. The complete primary structure of platelet factor 4 has been deter-mined in several different laboratories (46-48) and studies are under way to determine that of beta-thromboglobulin. Specific antisera and immunoassays have been developed for these proteins. The radioimmunoassay technique appears to be the only one which has the requisite sensitivity for clinical application.

In vitro studies have demonstrated parallel release of platelet factor 4 and beta-thromboglobulin and in response to stimulation by ADP, collagen or epinephrine and no cleavage of FPA under
such circumstances. Thrombin releases the 3 platelet proteins in
parallel and also of course cleaves FPA. Aspirin or indomethacin
inhibit release of the 3 platelet proteins induced by ADP or epinephrine in vitro.

Clinical application thus far has been limited. Plasma levels
of platelet factor 4 and beta-thromboglobulin have been measured
in several different laboratories. Normal levels of beta-thromboglobulin appear to be in the range of 15-30 ng/ml and platelet
factor 4 levels appear to be below 10 ng/ml. Elevated levels of
platelet factor 4 have been reported in patients with acute myocardial infarction (49) or with prosthetic heart valves (50).
Elevated levels of beta-thromboglobulin have been reported in
patients with acute thromboembolism (51-52) and in patients with
prosthetic heart valves (51). Studies in hyperlipidemia or atherosclerosis have not been reported.

REFERENCES

1. Doolittle, R.F. (1973) Advances in Protein Chemistry 27, 1-109.

2. Herzig, R.H., Ratnoff, O.D., and Shainoff, J.R. (1970) J. Lab.
    Clin. Med. 76, 451-465.

3. Blombäck, B. (1967) in Blood Clotting Enzymology (Seegers,
    W.H., Ed.), Academic Press, New York, pp. 143-215.

4. Bailey, K., Bettelheim, F.R., Lorand, L., and Middlebrook,
    W.R. (1951) Nature 167, 233-234.

5. Blombäck, B., Blombäck, M., Edman, P., and Hessel, B. (1966)
    Biochim. Biophys. Acta 115, 371-396.

6. Shainoff, J.R., Page, I.H. (1962) J. Exp. Med. 116, 687-707.

7. Yudelman, I., Spanondis, K., and Nossel, H.L. (1974) Thromb.
    Res. 5, 495-509.

8. Pisano, J.J., Bronzert, T.J., Peyton, M.P., and Finlayson,
    J.S. (1972) Ann. N.Y. Acad. Sci. 202, 98-113.

9. Chen, R., and Doolittle, R.F. (1970) Proc. Nat. Acad. Sci.
    USA 63, 420-427.

10. Chen, R., and Doolittle, R.F. (1971) Biochemistry 10, 4486-4491

11. Harfenist, E., and Canfield, R.E. (1975) Biochemistry 14, 4110-4117.

12. Blombäck, M., Blombäck, B., and Holmquist, H. (1976) Thromb. Res. 8, 567-578.

13. Lahiri, B., and Shainoff, J.R. (1973) Biochim. Biophys. Acta 303, 161-170.

14. Takagi, T., and Doolittle, R.F. (1975) Biochem. 14, 940-946.

15. Plow, E., and Edgington, T.S. (1973) J. Clin. Invest. 52, 273-282.

16. Plow, E.F., and Edgington, T.S. (1975) J. Biol. Chem. 150, 3386-3392.

17. Merskey, C., Kleiner, G.J., and Johnson, A.J. (1966) Blood 28, 1-18.

18. Gordon, Y.B., Martin, M.J., McNeile, A.T., Chard, T. (1973) Lancet 2, 1168-1170.

19. Merskey, C. (1973) Blood 41, 599.

20. Fletcher, A.P., Alkjaersig, N., O'Brien, J., and Tulevski, V. G. (1970) Trans. Assoc. Am. Physicians Phila. 83, 159-167.

21. Niewiarowski, S., and Gurewich, V. (1971) J. Lab. Clin. Med. 77, 665-676.

22. Kisker, C.T., and Rush, R. (1971) J. Clin. Invest. 50, 2235-2251.

23. Fletcher, A.P., Alkjaersig, N.K., O'Brien, J.R., and Tulevski, F. (1977) J. Lab. Clin. Med. 89, 1349-1366.

24. Matthias, R., Reinicke, R., Heene, D. (1977) Thromb. Res. 10, 365-384.

25. Reinicke, R., Matthias, F.R., and Lasch, H.G. (1977) Thromb. Res. 11, 365-375.

26. Müller-Berghaus, G., and Mahn, I. (1977) Thromb. and Haemos. 38, 220.

27. Nossel, H.L., Younger, L.R., Wilner, G.D., Procupez, T., Canfield, R.E., and Butler, Jr., V.P. (1971) Proc. Natl. Acad. Sci. USA 68, 2350-2353.

28. Bilezikian, S.B., Nossel, H.L., Butler, V.P., Jr., and Canfield, R.E. (1975) J. Clin. Invest. 56, 438-445.

29. Nossel, H.L., Butler, V.P., Jr., Wilner, G.D., Canfield, R.E., and Harfenist, E.J. (1976) Thromb. Diath. Haemorrh. 35, 101-109.

30. Canfield, R.E., Dean, J., Nossel, H.L., Butler, V.P., Jr., and Wilner, G.D. (1976) Biochemistry 15, 1203-1209.

31. Wilner, G.D., Nossel, H.L., Canfield, R.E., and Butler, V.P., Jr. (1976) Biochemistry 15, 1209-1213.

32. Nossel, H.L., Yudelman, I., Canfield, R.E., Butler, V.P., Jr., Spanondis, K., Wilner, G.D., and Qureshi, G.D. (1974) J. Clin. Invest. 54, 43-53.

33. Nossel, H.L., Ti, M., Kaplan, K.L., Spanondis, K., Soland, T., and Butler, V.P., Jr. (1976) J. Clin. Invest. 58, 1136-1144.

34. Teger-Nilsson, A.-C. (1968) Acta Physiol. Scand. (Suppl.) 319, 1-40.

35. Kockum, C. (1976) Thromb. Res. 8, 225-236.

36. Cronlund, M., Hardin, J., Burton, J., Lee, L., Haber, E., and Bloch, K.J. (1976) J. Clin. Invest. 58, 142-151.

37. Gerrits, W.B.J., Flier, O.T.N., and Van Der Meer, J. (1974) Thromb. Res. 5, 197-212.

38. Budzynski, A.Z., and Marder, V.J. (1975) Thromb. Diath. Haemorrh. 34, 709-717.

39. Hofmann, V., and Straub, P.W. (1977) Thromb. Res. 11, 171-181.

40. Yudelman, I., Nossel, H.L., Kaplan, K.L., and Hirsh, J. (1977) Thromb. and Haemos. 38, 74.

41. Carvalho, A.C., Lees, R.S., Vaillancourt, R.A., Cabral, R.B., Weinberg, R.M., and Colman, R.W. (1976) Thromb. Res. 8, 843-857.

42. Carvalho, A.C., Lees, R.S., Vaillancourt, R.A., Colman, R.W. (1977) Circulation 56, 114-118.

43. Moore, S., and Pepper, D.S. (1976) in Platelets in Biology and Pathology (Gordon, J.L., Eds.), North Holland Publishing Co., p. 293.

44. Niewiarowski, S., Rucinski, B., Millman, M., and Hawiger, J. (1976) in Proceedings from the Workshop on Platelets in Philadelphia (Day, Holmsen and Zucker, Eds.) U.S. Government Press. In press.

45. Kaplan, K.L., Nossel, H.L., Drillings, M., and Lesznik, G. (1978) Br. J. Haemat. In press.

46. Deuel, T.F., Keim, P.S., Farmer, M., and Heinrikson, R.L. (1977) Proc. Natl. Acad. Sci. USA 74, 2256-2258.

47. Morgan, F.J., Chesterman, C.N., McGready, J.R., and Begg, G.S. (1977) Haemostasis 6, 53-58.

48. Hermodsen, M., Schmer, G., and Kurachi, K. J. Biol. Chem. In press.

49. Handin, R.I., McDonough, M., and Lesch, M. (1976) Circulation 54 (Suppl. II), 198.

50. Bolton, A.E., Ludlam, C.A., Pepper, D.S., Moore, S., and Cash, J.D. (1976) Thromb. Res. 8, 51-58.

51. Ludlam, C.A., Bolton, A.E., Moore, S., and Cash, J.D. (1975) Lancet 2, 259-260.

52. Smith, R.C., Ruckley, C.V., Duncanson, J., Allan, N.C., Dawes, J., Pepper, D.S., and Cash, J.D. (1977) Thromb. Haemost. 38, 166.

DISCUSSION FOLLOWING THIRD PLENARY SESSION:
CLINICAL ASSESSMENT OF THE THROMBOTIC PROCESS
IN RELATION TO ATHEROSCLEROSIS

R.S. Lees: Dr. Nossel, one of the reasons for the differences
in the results in various laboratories may be not only the different
tests and the different things that they measure, not only the
heterogeneity of the patients, whose genetic makeup varies widely
from patient group to patient group, but also the "normal subjects."
Your normal subjects had a mean plasma cholesterol concentration
of 220 mg %, I believe. I and most of the epidemiologists present,
I expect, feel that 220 mg % is the upper limit of normal for plasma cholesterol, so that half of your "normal" population is hyperlipidemic. It may not be surprising, therefore, not to find differences between these subjects and those with a greater degree of
hyperlipidemia. By exchanging subjects and by performing all of
the pertinent coagulation studies on the same well-defined groups
of truly normal and hyperlipidemic subjects, I think we will eventually resolve the apparent difference between the results in different laboratories and learn which tests will guide us best as to
the relationships between hyperlipidemia and coagulation and what
those relationships are.

H. Stormorken: I am somewhat confused about platelet survival,
particularly as to the effect of normalizing a shortened survival.
As it appeared from the multicenter Canadian study, comparing the
effect of ASA, sulfinpyrazone, and placebo on TIA/stroke, the drug,
ASA, that had a significant effect on thromboembolytic events did
not normalize platelet survival; whereas sulfinpyrazone, which did
normalize shortened survival, had no such effect. How can this be
explained?

E. Genton: The question is very relevant and identifies the
type of issues that remain unresolved. It is correct that aspirin
reduced stroke and death in both the Canadian and American cerebral
vascular disease trials, and in the former, sulfinpyrazone had no
apparent effect. As noted, shortened platelet survival is lengthened by sulfinpyrazone but not by aspirin. Conceivably, the effect of aspirin in cerebral vascular disease is through a mechanism

other than one which involves platelet vessel wall interaction. Alternately, of course, the data may indicate the lack of correlation between effect of a drug on platelet survival time and therapeutic benefit. A similar issue is raised in relationship to clofibrate in coronary artery disease. This drug has been shown to improve shortened platelet survival time, and in clinical trial has not affected the endpoints of myocardial infarction or death.

A. Nordøy: I think it is very important that we, in these discussions, underline the heterogenity of patients belonging to the one or the other of the various types of hyperlipoproteinemias. In 1969, we observed PF-3 hypersensitivity of platelets in patients with type II hyperlipoproteinemia. In 1975, we investigated another group of type II subjects with plasma cholesterol levels about 500 mg/dl, whereas the controls had a cholesterol level of about 270 mg/dl. In this study, we could not confirm any difference between patients and controls with regard to platelet sensitivity to various aggregating agents.

I thus would like to ask Dr. Colman what he knows about the heterogeneity of his patients with type II hyperlipoproteinemia. Was there any correlation between plasma cholesterol level and platelet reactivity?

In addition, I would like to ask a question about his study where he incubated platelets in a cholesterol/phosphatidylcholine (PC) dispersion, where the PC had two palmitic fatty acids. Could it be that the palmitic acid or the phospholipid by itself could affect the platelet reactivity?

R.W. Colman: In answer to Dr. Nordøy's first question, our patients were all type IIa by the WHO classification and did not include IIb. Our normals had mean cholesterols of 160 mg/dl and the IIa patients 330 mg/dl. Clearly, these are different groups than those studied by Dr. Nordøy. The hypersensitivity of IIa platelets has been demonstrated by Carvalho et al. and Shattil et al. and confirmed in unpublished results by Mielke et al. and Jaffe et al. We found no correlation between total or LDL cholesterol and platelet sensitivity. From our recent studies the important variable to correlate is the cholesterol/phospholipid ratio of LDL and/or platelet membranes and these studies are in progress in our laboratory.

In regard to the second question, our controls include dispersions of dipalmitoyl lecithin with cholesterol at the same concentration as in the platelet membranes. These control dispersions do not induce hypersensitivity, although they contain exactly the same phospholipid with the same fatty acid as the cholesterol-rich dispersions which transfer cholesterol to platelet membranes and induce hypersensitivity to epinephrine and ADP.

B.A. Kottke: I would like to make a plea for the more precise definition of type II patterns surveyed for thrombosis and coagulation defects. It is only a historic accident that types II_A and II_B hyperlipoproteinemia both have the Roman numeral II in their definition. They are totally different clinical entities in terms of apolipoproteins and in terms of cholesterol and lipoprotein metabolism. In addition, they have been officially designated as separate entities by the World Health Organization.

D.J. Hanahan: Dr. Colman, have you measured the actual amount of dipalmitoyl lecithin taken by the platelets?

R.W. Colman: Yes, we measured dipalmitoyl lecithin per 10^8 platelets in platelets incubated with buffer for 5 hours and in the platelets incubated with cholesterol-rich liposomes. In the former, there were 35 micrograms of phospholipid per 10^8 platelets and in the latter a mean of 36. Since the standard error of the mean on these determinations was $\pm$ 2, this does not represent a significant difference (Shattil, et al. (1975) J. Clin. Invest. 55, 636-643.

D.J. Hanahan: Would you care to comment on the possibility that the dipalmitoyl lecithin is the component influencing the cyclic AMP formation?

R.W. Colman: Since there was no net incorporation of dipalm-itoyl lecithin as compared with the cholesterol which increased 40% (Shattil, et al. (1975) J. Clin. Invest. 55), it does not appear that the increase in cyclic AMP could be attributed to the phospho-lipid (Sinha, et al. (1977) J. Biol. Chem. 252, 3310-3314.)

D.J. Hanahan: Can you remove the cholesterol from the choles-terol-rich platelets by mixing with phospholipid dispersions? Does it affect the platelet behavior?

R.W. Colman: Yes, when we incubated normal platelets with cholesterol-poor liposomes, they underwent a selective loss of 21.4% cholesterol. This change was associated with an 18-fold reduction in their sensitivity to epinephrine (Shattil, et al. (1975) J. Clin. Invest. 55) and a decrease in adenylate cyclase activity of 40% (Sinha, et al. (1977) J. Biol. Chem. 252).

EPILOGUE

The Workshop on the Thrombotic Process in Atherogenesis reflected an enthusiasm for interdisciplinary research and facilitated
an extensive exchange of information. The format of the Workshop
provided an opportunity to examine the problems of atherogenesis
from many points of view. Several months were devoted to developing
the appropriate sequencing of presentations. Special attention was
given to the inclusion of topics that could effectively catalyze
discussions concerning the thrombotic process in atherogenesis.
During the Workshop, it became clear that what happens in atherogenesis at the vessel wall is not caused by any single process, but
is related to a subtle interplay of several complex processes.

Successful investigation of atherogenesis requires meaningful
cooperation between scientists working in different fields, both in
basic science and in clinical areas. Opportunities for cooperative
work were developed by the workshop participants. At the conclusion
of the meeting, many of the investigators reviewed the proceedings
and identified areas for collaborative research that included both
the sharing of ideas, and the sharing of resources such as assays,
animal models, and specialized facilities. Future investigative
efforts may be furthered by encouraging multidisciplinary programs
that relate the thrombotic process to atherogenesis. This Workshop
represents a positive effort in this direction.

Curtis B. Nelson

APPENDIX A

BIBLIOGRAPHY
ENDOTHELIUM 1977

Guido Majno and Isabelle Joris

ENDOTHELIUM 1977: A REVIEW

1. Majno, G. (1965): Ultrastructure of the vascular membrane.
    In Handbook of Physiology, Sect. 2/III (Hamilton, W.F. and Dow,
    P., Eds.), American Physiological Society, Washington, D.C.,
    pp. 2293-2375.

2. Dikstein, S. (1973): Efficiency and survival of the corneal
    endothelial pump. Exp. Eye Res. 15, 639-644.

3. Kephalides, N.A., Cameron, J.D., Tomichek, E.A., and Yanoff, M.
    (1976): Biosynthesis of basement membrane collagen by rabbit
    corneal endothelium in vitro. J. Biol. Chem. 251, 730-733.

4. Jennings, M.A., and Florey, H.W. (1967): An investigation of
    some properties of endothelium related to capillary permeabil-
    ity. Proc. Roy. Soc. Lond. Biol. 167, 39-63.

5. Florey, H.W., and Sheppard, B.L. (1970): The permeability of
    arterial endothelium to horseradish peroxidase. Proc. Roy.
    Soc. Lond. Biol. 174, 435-443.

6. Zweifach, B.W., Grant, L., and McCluskey, R.T. (Eds.), (1973):
    The Inflammatory Process, Vol. 2, 2nd Ed., Academic Press, New
    York.

7. Gabbiani, G., and Majno, G. (1976): Fine structure of endo-
    thelium. In Microcirculation, Vol. 1 (Kaley, G. and Altura,
    B.M., Eds.), University Park Press, Baltimore, pp. 133-144.

8. Gimbrone, M.A., Jr. (1976): Culture of vascular endothelium.
    In Progress in Hemostasis and Thrombosis, Vol. III (Spaet,
    T.H., Ed.), Grune & Stratton, Inc., New York, pp. 1-28.

9. Folkman, J., and Cotran, R.S. (1976): Relation of vascular
    proliferation to tumor growth. Int. Rev. Exp. Pathol. 16,
    207-248.

10. Simionescu, N., Simionescu, M., and Palade, G.E. (1976): Structural-functional correlates in the transendothelial exchange of water-soluble macromolecules. Thromb. Res. 8 (Suppl. II), pp. 257-269.

11. Simionescu, N., Simionescu, M., and Palade, G.E. (1976): Recent studies on vascular endothelium. Ann. N.Y. Acad. Sci. 275, 64-75.

12. Simionescu, N., and Simionescu, M. (1977): The cardiovascular system. In Histology (Weiss, L. and Greep, R.O., Eds.), 4th Ed., McGraw-Hill Book Co., New York, pp. 373-431.

13. Mason, R.G., Sharp, D., Chuang, H.Y.K., and Mohammad, S.F. (1977) The endothelium. Arch. Pathol. Lab. Med. 101, 61-64.

14. Kaley, G., and Altura, B.M. (Eds.), (1977): Microcirculation, Vol. I, University Park Press, Baltimore.

15. Ryan, J.W., and Ryan, U.S. (1977): Pulmonary endothelial cells. Fed. Proc. 36, 2683-2691.

16. Crone, C., and Lassen, N.A. (Eds.), (1970): Capillary Permeability. Alfred Benzon Symposium II, Munksgaard, Copenhagen and Academic Press, New York.

17. Bell, F.P., Adamson, I.L., and Schwartz, C.J. (1974): Aortic permeability to albumin: focal and regional patterns of uptake and transmural distribution of ^{131}I-albumin in the young pig. Exp. Mol. Pathol. 20, 57-68.

18. Huttner, I., Boutet, M., and More, R.H. (1973): Studies on protein passage through arterial endothelium. II. Regional differences in permeability to fine structural protein tracers in arterial endothelium of normotensive rats. Lab. Invest. 28, 678-685.

19. Giacomelli, F., and Wiener, J. (1974): Regional variation in the permeability of the rat thoracic aorta. Am. J. Pathol. 75, 513-528.

20. Giacomelli, F., Anversa, P., and Wiener, J. (1975): Interendothelial gap size of subendocardial vs. subepicardial capillaries. Microvasc. Res. 10, 38-42.

21. Korneliussen, H. (1975): Fenestrated blood capillaries and lymphatic capillaries in rat skeletal muscle. Cell Tissue Res. 163, 169-174.

22. Forssmann, W.G. (1976): Die normale Gefasswand und Transportphanomene. Med. Welt 27, 1606-1610.

23. Simionescu, N., and Palade, G.E. (1971): Dextrans and glycogens as particulate tracers for studying capillary permeability. J. Cell Biol. 50, 616-624.

24. Karnovsky, M.J. (1967): The ultrastructural basis of capillary permeability studied with peroxidase as a tracer. J. Cell Biol. 35, 213-236.

25. Simionescu, N., Simionescu, M., and Palade, G.E. (1973): Permeability of muscle capillaries to exogenous myoglobin. J. Cell Biol. 57, 424-452.

26. Karnovsky, M.J., and Rice, D.F. (1969): Exogenous cytochrome C as an ultrastructural tracer. J. Histochem. Cytochem. 17, 751-753.

27. Feder, N. (1970): A heme-peptide as an ultrastructural tracer. J. Histochem. Cytochem. 18, 911-913.

28. Simionescu, N., Simionescu, M., and Palade, G.E. (1975): Permeability of muscle capillaries to small heme-peptides. Evidence for the existence of patent transendothelial channels. J. Cell Biol. 64, 586-607.

29. Plattner, H., Wachter, E., and Grobner, P. (1977): A heme-nonapeptide tracer for electron microscopy. Preparation, characterization and comparison with other heme-tracers. Histochemistry 53, 223-242.

30. Schurer, J.W., Hoedemaeker, P.J., and Molenaar, I. (1977): Polyethyleneimine as tracer for (immuno) electron microscopy. J. Histochem. Cytochem. 25, 384-387.

31. Vegge, T., and Haye, R. (1977): Vascular reactions to horseradish peroxidase in the guinea pig. Histochem. 53, 217-222.

32. Clark, J.M., and Glagov, S. (1976): Evaluation and publication of scanning electron micrographs. Science 192, 1360-1361.

33. Davies, P.F., and Bowyer, D.E. (1975): Scanning electron microscopy: arterial endothelial integrity after fixation at physiological pressure. Atherosclerosis 21, 463-469.

34. Clark, J.M., and Glagov, S. (1976): Luminal surface of distended arteries by scanning electron microscopy: eliminating configurational and technical artefacts. Br. J. Exp. Pathol. 57, 129-135.

35. Sade, R.M., and Folkman, J. (1972): En face stripping of vascular endothleium. Microvasc. Res. 4, 77-80.

36. Morrison, A.D., Berwick, L., Orci, L., and Winegrad, A.I. (1976): Morphology and metabolism of an aortic intima-media preparation in which an intact endothelium is preserved. J. Clin. Invest. 57, 650-660.

37. Wagner, R.C., and Matthews, M.A. (1975): The isolation and culture of capillary endothelium from epididymal fat. Microvasc. Res. 10, 286-297.

38. Simionescu, M., and Simionescu, N. (1977): Isolation of endothelial cells of the heart microvasculature. J. Cell Biol. 75 (Part 2), 248a.

39. Prasad, N. (1970): Sex chromatin in cells of the endothelial lining of aorta and heart. Acta Cytol. 14, 607-608.

40. Luft, J.H. (1966): Fine structure of capillary and endocapillary layer as revealed by ruthenium red. Fed. Proc. 25, 1773-1783.

41. Weber, G., Fabbrini, P., and Resi, L. (1973): On the presence of a Concanavalin-A reactive coat over the endothelial aortic surface and its modifications during early experimental cholesterol atherogenesis in rabbits. Virchows Arch. Abt. A Path. Anat. 359, 299-307.

42. Weber, G., Fabbrini, P., and Resi, L. (1974): Scanning and transmission electron microscopy observations on the surface lining of aortic intimal plaques in rabbits on a hypercholesterolic diet. Virchows Arch. A Path. Anat. Histol. 364, 325-331.

43. Stein, O., Chajek, T., and Stein, Y. (1976): Ultrastructural localization of Concanavalin-A in the perfused rat heart. Lab. Invest. 35, 103-110.

44. Shirahama, T., and Cohen, A.S. (1972): The role of mucopolysaccharides in vesicle architecture and endothelial transport. An electron microscope study of myocardial blood vessels. J. Cell Biol. 52, 198-206.

45. Klynstra, F.B. (1974): On the passage-restricting role of acid mucopolysaccharides in the endothelium of pig aortas. Atherosclerosis 19, 215-220.

46.   Loudon, M.F., Michel, C.C., and White, I.F. (1975): Proceed-
      ings: some observations upon the rate of labeling of endothe-
      lial vesicles by ferritin in frog mesenteric capillaries.
      J. Physiol. (Lond.) 252, 79P-80P.

47.   Palade, G.E., and Bruns, R.R. (1968): Structural modulations
      of plasmalemmal vesicles. J. Cell Biol. 37, 633-649.

48.   Hiebert, L.M., and Jaques, L.B. (1976): Heparin uptake on
      endothelium. Artery 2, 26-37.

49.   Hiebert, L.M., and Jaques, L.B. (1976): The observation of
      heparin on endothelium after injection. Thromb. Res. 8, 195-
      204.

50.   Latta, H., and Johnston, W.H. (1976): The glycoprotein inner
      layer of glomerular capillary basement membrane as a filtration
      barrier. J. Ultrastruct. Res. 51, 65-67.

51.   Latta, H., Johnston, W.H., and Stanley, T.M. (1975): Sialogly-
      coproteins and filtration barriers in the glomerular capillary
      walls. J. Ultrastruct. Res. 51, 354-376.

52.   Bignon, J., Chahinian, P., Feldmann, G., and Spain, C. (1975)
      Ultrastructural immunoperoxidase demonstration of autologous
      albumin in the alveolar capillary membrane and in the alveolar
      lining material in normal rats. J. Cell Biol. 64, 503-509.

53.   Bignon, J., Jaubert, F., and Jaurand, M.C. (1976): Plasma pro-
      tein immunocytochemistry and polysaccharide cytochemistry at
      the surface of alveolar and endothelial cells in the rat lung.
      J. Histochem. Cytochem. 24, 1076-1084.

54.   Stone, F.J., Cohen, H.A., and Frisch, D. (1974): The ultra-
      structural localization of fibrinogen at the erythrocyte sur-
      face and in the capillary endothelium. Cell Tissue Res. 153,
      253-260.

55.   Copley, A.L. (1974): Hemorheological aspects of the endothe-
      lium-plasma interface. Microvasc. Res. 8, 192-212.

56.   dé Bono, D. (1976); Endothelial-lymphocyte interactions in
      vitro. I. Adherence of nonallergised lymphocytes. Cell. Im-
      munol. 26, 78-88.

57.   Lackie, J.M., and de Bono, D. (1977): Interactions of neutro-
      phil granulocytes (PMNs) and endothelium in vitro. Microvasc.
      Res. 13, 107-112.

58. Lentnek, A.L., Schreiber, A.D., and MacGregor, R.R. (1976):
     The induction of augmented granulocyte adherence by inflam-
     mation. J. Clin. Invest. 57, 1098-1103.

59. MacGregor, R.R., Macarak, E.J., and Kefalides, N.A. (1978):
     Comparative adherence of granulocytes to endothelial monolayers
     and nylon fiber. J. Clin. Invest. In press.

60. MacGregor, R.R. (1976): The effect of anti-inflammatory agents
     on granulocyte adherence. Am. J. Med. 61, 597-6U7.

61. Rennke, H.G., Cotran, R.S., and Venkatachalam, M.A. (1975):
     Role of molecular charge in glomerular permeability. Tracer
     studies with cationized ferritins. J. Cell Biol. 67, 638-646.

62. Skutelsky, E., Rudich, Z., and Danon, D. (1975): Surface
     charge properties of the luminal front of blood vessel walls.
     An electron microscopical analysis. Thromb. Res. 7, 623-634.

63. Skutelsky, E., and Danon, D. (1976): Redistribution of surface
     anionic sites on the luminal front of blood vessel endothelium
     after interaction with polycationic ligand. J. Cell Biol. 71,
     232-241.

64. Danon, D., and Skutelsky, E. (1976): Endothelial surface
     charge and its possible relationship to thrombogenesis. Ann.
     N.Y. Acad. Sci. 275, 47-63.

65. Sawyer, P.N., Stanczewski, B., Ramasamy, N., Ramsey, W.S., Jr.,
     and Srinivasan, S. (1973): Electrochemical interactions at
     the endothelial surface. J. Supramolecular Struct. 1, 417-436.

66. Gurtner, G.H., Song, S.H., and Farhi, L.E. (1969): Alveolar
     to mixed venous $^PCO_2$ difference under conditions of no gas
     exchange. Resp. Physiol. 7, 173-187.

67. Gabbiani, G., and Majno, G. (1969): Endothelial microvilli in
     the vessels of the rat gasserian ganglion and testis. Z. Zell-
     forsch. 97, 111-117.

68. Fujimoto, S., Yamamoto, K., and Takeshige, Y. (1975): Elec-
     tron microscopy of endothelial microvilli of large arteries.
     Anat. Rec. 183, 259-266.

69. Smith, U., Ryan, J.W., Michie, D.D., and Smith, D.S. (1971):
     Endothelial projections as revealed by scanning electron
     microscopy. Science 173, 925-927.

70. Lemeunier, A., Burri, P.H., and Weibel, E.R. (1969): Absence of acid phosphatase activity in specific endothelial organelles. Histochemie 20, 143-149.

71. Sengel, A., and Stoebner, P. (1970): Golgi origin of tubular inclusions in endothelial cells. J. Cell Biol. 44, 223-226.

72. Steinsiepe, K.F., and Weibel, E.R. (1970): Electronenmikroskopische Untersuchungen an spezifischen Organellen von Endothelzellen des Frosches (Rana temporaria). Z. Zellforsch. 108, 105-126.

73. Fuchs, A., and Weibel, E.R. (1966): Morphometrische Untersuchung der Verteilung einer spezifischen Cytoplasmatischen Organelle in Endothelzellen der Ratte. Z. Zellforsch. 73, 1-9.

74. Santolaya, R.C., and Bertini, F. (1970): Fine structure of endothelial cells of vertebrates. Distribution of dense granules. Z. Anat. Entwickl.-Gesch. 131, 148-155.

75. Bertini, F., and Santolaya, R. (1970): A novel type of granules observed in toad endothelial cells and their relationship with blood pressure active factors. Experientia 26, 522-523.

76. Burri, P.H., and Weibel, E.R. (1968): Beeinflussung einer spezifischen cytoplasmatischen Organelle von Endothelzellen durch Adrenalin. Z. Zellforsch. 88, 426-440.

77. Zelickson, A.S. (1966): A tubular structure in the endothelial cells and pericytes of human capillaries. J. Invest. Dermatol. 46, 167-171.

78. Bruns, R.R., and Palade, G.E. (1968): Studies on blood capillaries. I. General organization of blood capillaries in muscle. J. Cell Biol. 37, 244-276.

79. Simionescu, M., Simionescu, N., and Palade, G.E. (1974): Morphometric data on the endothelium of blood capillaries. J. Cell Biol. 60, 128-152.

80. Casley-Smith, J.R. (1969): The dimensions and numbers of small vesicles in cells, endothelial and mesothelial and the significance of these for endothelial permeability. J. Microscopy 90, 251-269.

81. Casley-Smith, J.R., Green, H.S., Harris, J.L., and Wadey, P.J. (1975): The quantitative morphology of skeletal muscle capillaries in relation to permeability. Microvasc. Res. 10, 42-64.

82. Smith, U., and Ryan, J.W. (1972): Substructural features of pulmonary endothelial caveolae. Tissue Cell 4, 49-54.

83. Smith, U., Ryan, J.W., and Smith, D.S. (1973): Freeze-etch studies of the plasma membrane of pulmonary endothelial cells. J. Cell Biol. 56, 492-499.

84. Sun, C.N., and Ghidoni, J.J. (1973): The ultrastructure of aortic endothelial cells of normal dogs. Cytologia (Tokyo) 38, 667-675.

85. Friend, D.S., and Farquhar, M.G. (1967): Functions of coated vesicles during protein absorption in the rat vas deferens. J. Cell Biol. 35, 357-376.

86. De Bruyn, P.P.H., Michelson, S., and Becker, R.P. (1975): Endocytosis, transfer tubules, and lysosomal activity in myeloid sinusoidal endothelium. J. Ultrastruct. Res. 53, 133-151.

87. Simionescu, N., Simionescu, M., and Palade, G.E. (1978): Structural basis of permeability in sequential segments of the microvasculature. I. Bipolar microvascular fields in the diaphragm. Microvasc. Res. In press.

88. Simionescu, N., Simionescu, M., and Palade, G.E. (1978): Structural basis of permeability in sequential segments of the microvasculature. II. Pathways followed by microperoxidase across the endothelium. Microvasc. Res. In press.

89. Williams, M.C., and Wissig, S.L. (1975): The permeability of muscle capillaries to horseradish peroxidase. J. Cell Biol. 66, 531-555.

90. Simionescu, N., Simionescu, M. and Palade, G.E. (1977): Open junctions of venular endothelium: size limit of permeant molecules. J. Cell Biol. 75, 373a.

91. Simionescu, M., Simionescu, N., and Palade, G.E. (1975): Segmental differentiations of cell junctions in the vascular endothelium. The microvasculature. J. Cell Biol. 67, 863-885.

92. McNutt, N.S., and Weinstein, R.S. (1973): Membrane ultrastructure at mammalian intercellular junctions. Progr. Biophys. Molec. Biol. 26, 45-101.

93. Simionescu, M., Simionescu, N., and Palade, G.E. (1976): Segmental differentiations of cell junctions in the vascular endothelium. Arteries and veins. J. Cell Biol. 68, 705-723.

94. Hüttner, I., Boutet, M., and More, R.H. (1973): Gap junctions in arterial endothelium. J. Cell Biol. 57, 247-252.

95. Stehbens, W.E. (1966): The basal attachment of endothelial cells. J. Ultrastruct. Res. 15, 389-399.

96. Ts'ao, C., and Glagov, S. (1970): Basal endothelial attachment. Tenacity at cytoplasmic dense zones in the rabbit aorta. Lab. Invest. 23, 510-516.

97. Tyson, G.E., and Bulger, R.E. (1972): Endothelial detachment sites in glomerular capillaries of vinblastine-treated rats. Anat. Rec. 172, 669-674.

98. Baumgartner, H.R., Stemerman, M.B., and Spaet, T.H. (1971): Adhesion of blood platelets to subendothelial surface: distinct from adhesion to collagen. Experientia 27, 283-285.

99. Huang, T.W., Lagunoff, D., and Benditt, E.P. (1974): Nonaggregative adherence of platelets to basal lamina in vitro. Lab. Invest. 31, 156-160.

100. Vracko, R. (1974): Basal lamina scaffold: anatomy and significance for maintenance of orderly tissue structure. Am. J. Pathol. 77, 314-346.

101. Yen, A., and Braverman, I.M. (1976): Ultrastructure of the human dermal microcirculation: the horizontal plexus of the papillary dermis. J. Invest. Dermatol. 66, 131-142.

102. Wisse, E. (1970): An electron microscopic study of the fenestrated endothelial lining of rat liver sinusoids. J. Ultrastruct. Res. 31, 125-150.

103. Weiss, L. (1974): A scanning electron microscopic study of the spleen. Blood 43, 665-691.

104. Chen, L-T., and Weiss, L. (1973): The role of the sinus wall in the passage of erythrocytes through the spleen. Blood 41, 529-537.

105. Heusermann, U., and Stutte, H.J. (1975): Comparative histochemical and electron microscopic studies of the sinus and venous walls of the human spleen with special reference to the sinus-venous connections. Cell Tissue Res. 163, 519-533.

106. Heusermann, U., and Stutte, H.J. (1974): Intercellular junctions of sinus lining cells in the human spleen. Cell Tissue Res. 151, 337-342.

107. Cho, Y., and De Bruyn, P.P.H. (1975): Passage of red blood
     cells through the sinusoidal wall of the spleen. Am. J. Anat.
     142, 91-106.

108. Muto, M. (1976): A scanning and transmission electron micro-
     scopic study on rat bone marrow sinuses and transmural migra-
     tion of blood cells. Arch. Histol. Jpn. 39, 51-66.

109. Bankston, P.W., and De Bruyn, P.P.H. (1974): The permeability
     to carbon of the sinusoidal lining cells of the embryonic rat
     liver and rat bone marrow. Am. J. Anat.. 141, 281-290.

110. De Bruyn, P.P.H., Michelson, S., and Becker, R.P. (1975):
     Endocytosis, transfer tubules, and lysosomal activity in mye-
     loid sinusoidal endothelium. J. Ultrastruct. Res. 53, 133-151.

111. De Bruyn, P.P.H., Michelson, S., and Becker, R.P. (1977):
     Phosphotungstic acid as a marker for the endocytic-lysosomal
     system (vacuolar apparatus) including transfer tubules of the
     lining cells of the sinusoids in the bone marrow and liver.
     J. Ultrastruct. Res. 58, 87-95.

112. Fahimi, H.D. (1970): The fine structural localization of endo-
     genous and exogenous peroxidase activity in Kupffer cells of
     rat liver. J. Cell Biol. 47, 247-262.

113. Widmann, J-J., Cotran, R.S., and Fahimi, H.D. (1972): Mononu-
     clear phagocytes (Kupffer cells) and endothelial cells. Iden-
     tification of two functional cell types in rat liver sinusoids
     by endogenous peroxidase activity. J. Cell Biol. 52, 159-170.

114. Fahimi, H.D., Gray, B.A., and Herzog, V.K. (1976): Cytochem-
     ical localization of catalase and peroxidase in sinusoidal
     cells of rat liver. Lab. Invest. 34, 192-201.

115. Knook, D.L., Blansjaar, N., and Sleyster, E.C. (1977): Isola-
     tion and characterization of Kupffer and endothelial cells
     from rat liver. Exp. Cells Res. 109, 317-330.

116. Motta, P. (1975): A scanning electron microscopic study of
     the rat liver sinusoid. Cell Tissue Res. 164, 371-385.

117. Nopanitaya, W., Lamb, J.C., Grisham, J.W., and Carson, J.L.
     (1976): Effect of hepatic venous outflow obstruction on pores
     and fenestration in sinusoidal endothelium. Br. J. Exp. Pathol
     57, 604-609.

118. De Bruyn, P.P.H., Michelson, S., and Thomas, T.B. (1971): The
     migration of blood cells of the bone marrow through the
     sinusoidal wall. J. Morphol. 133, 417-438.

119. Becker, R.P., and De Bruyn, P.P.H. (1976): The transmural passage of blood cells into myeloid sinusoids and the entry of platelets into the sinusoidal circulation; a scanning electron microscopic investigation. Am. J. Anat. 145, 183-206.

120. Muto, M. (1976): A scanning and transmission electron microscopic study on rat bone marrow sinuses and transmural migration of blood cells. Arch. Histol. Jpn. 39, 51-66.

121. Weiss, L. (1977): Bone marrow. In Histology (Weiss, L. and Greep, R.O., Eds.), 4th Ed., McGraw-Hill Book Co., New York, pp. 487-502.

122. De Bruyn, P.P.H., Becker, R.P., Michelson, S. (1977): The transmural migration and release of blood cells in acute myelogenous leukemia. Am. J. Anat. 149, 247-268.

123. Schoefl, G.I. (1972): The migration of lymophocytes across the vascular endothemlium in lymphoid tissue. J. Exp. Med. 136, 568-588.

124. Anderson, A.O., and Anderson, N.D. (1975): Studies on the structure and permeability of the microvasculature in normal rat lymph nodes. Am. J. Pathol. 80, 387-418.

125. Anderson, N.D., Anderson, A.O., and Wyllie, R.G. (1976): Specialized structure and metabolic activities of high endothelial venules in rat lymphatic tissues. Immunology 31, 455-473.

126. Anderson, A.O., and Anderson, N.D. (1976): Lymphocyte emigration from high endothelial venules in rat lymph nodes. Immunology 31, 731-748.

127. Wenk, E.J., Orlic, D., Reith, E.J., and Rhodin, J.A.G. (1974): The ultrastructure of mouse lymph node venules and the passage of lymphocytes across their walls. J. Ultrastruct. Res., 47, 214-241.

128. Umetani, Y. (1977): Postcapillary venule in rabbit tonsil and entry of lymphocytes into its endothelium: a scanning and transmission electron microscope study. Arch. Histol. Jpn. 40, 77-94.

129. Farr, A.G., and De Bruyn, P.P.H. (1975): The mode of lymphocyte migration through postcapillary venule endothelium in lymph node. ·Am. J. Anat. 143, 59-92.

130. van Deurs, B., Röpke, C., and Westergaard, E. (1975): Perme-
     ability properties of the postcapillary high-endothelial ven-
     ules in lymph nodes of the mouse. Lab. Invest. 32, 201-208.

131. Bradfield, J.W.B. (1973): Altered venules in the stimulated
     human thymus as evidence of lymphocyte recirculation. Clin.
     Exp. Immunol. 13, 243-252.

132. Smith, J.B., McIntosh, G.H., and Morris, B. (1970): The migra-
     tion of cells through chronically inflamed tissues. J. Pathol.
     100, 21-28.

133. Röpke, C., Jørgensen, O., and Claesson, M.H. (1972): Histo-
     chemical studies of high-endothelial venules of lymph nodes and
     Peyer's patches in the mouse. Z. Zellforsch. 131, 287-297.

134. Anderson, N.D., Anderson, A.O., and Wyllie, R.G. (1975):
     Microvascular changes in lymph nodes draining skin allografts.
     Am. J. Pathol. 81, 131-160.

135. Aumüller, G., Rauterberg, E., and Brühl, U. (1975): Feinstruk-
     tur und Funktion der postcapillaren Venolen im Lymphknoten.
     Verh. Anat. Ges. 69, 125-130.

136. Sedgley, M., and Ford, W.L. (1976): The migration of lympho-
     cytes across specialized vascular endothelium. I. The entry
     of lymphocytes into the isolated mesenteric lymph-node of the
     rat. Cell Tissue Kinet. 9, 231-243.

137. Stamper, H.B., Jr., and Woodruff, J.J. (1976): Lymphocyte
     homing into lymph nodes: in vitro demonstration of the selec-
     tive affinity of recirculating lymphocytes for high-endothelial
     venules. J. Exp. Med. 144, 828-833.

138. Stamper, H.B., Jr., and Woodruff, J.J. (1977): An in vitro
     model of lymphocyte homing. I. Characterization of the inter-
     action between thoracic duct lymphocytes and specialized high-
     endothelial venules of lymph nodes. J. Immunol. 119, 772-780.

139. Woodruff, J.J., Katz, I.M., Lucas, L.E., and Stamper, H.B.
     (1978): Binding of lymphocytes to HEV in vitro. J. Immunol.
     In press.

140. Clementi, F., and Palade, G.E. (1969): Intestinal capillaries.
     I. Permeability to peroxidase and ferritin. J. Cell Biol.
     41, 33-58.

141. Simionescu, N., Simionescu, M., and Palade, G.E. (1972): Per-
     meability of intestinal capillaries. Pathway followed by dex-
     trans and glycogens. J. Cell Biol. 53, 365-392.

142. Caulfield, J.P., and Farquhar, M.G. (1974): The permeability of glomerular capillaries to graded dextrans. Identification of the basement membrane as the primary filtration barrier. J. Cell Biol. 63, 883-903.

143. Casley-Smith, J.R. (1971): Endothelial fenestrae in intestinal villi: differences between the arterial and venous ends of the capillaries. Microvasc. Res. 3, 49-68.

144. Field, J., Hurley, J.V., and McCallum, N.E.W. (1976): The mechanism of escape of plasma protein from small blood vessels in the mucosa of the small intestine of the rat. J. Pathol. 121, 51-58.

145. Majno, G. (1970): Two endothelial "novelties": endothelial contraction; collagenase digestion of the basement membrane. In Vascular Factors and Thrombosis (Koller, F. et al., Eds.), F.K. Schattauer Verlag, Stuttgart, New York, pp. 23-30.

146. Jaffe, E.A., Minick, C.R., Adelman, B., Becker, C.G., and Nachman, R. (1976): Synthesis of basement membrane collagen by cultured human endothelial cells. J. Exp. Med. 144, 209-225.

147. Macarak, E.J., Howard, B.V., and Kefalides, N.A. (1976): Biosynthesis of collagen and metabolism of lipids by endothelial cells in culture. Ann. N.Y. Acad. Sci. 275, 104-113.

148. Howard, B.V., Macarak, E.J., Gunson, D., and Kefalides, N.A. (1976): Characterization of the collagen synthesized by endothelial cells in culture. Proc. Natl. Acad. Sci. USA 73, 2361-2364.

149. Buonassisi, V. (1973): Sulfated mucopolysaccharide synthesis and secretion in endothelial cell cultures. Exp. Cell Res. 76, 363-368.

150. Slater, D.N. (1976): The synthesis of lipids from $[1-^{14}C]$ acetate by human venous endothelium in tissue culture. Atherosclerosis 25, 237-244.

151. Evensen, S.A., and Henriksen, T. (1975): Sterol synthesis in human endothelial cells. Thromb. Diath. Haemorrh. 34, 330.

152. Gimbrone, M.A., Jr., and Alexander, R.W. (1975): Angiotensin II stimulation of prostaglandin production in cultured human vascular endothelium. Science 189, 219-220.

153. Weksler, B.B., Marcus, A.J., and Jaffe, E.A. (1977): Synthesis of prostaglandin I_2 (prostacyclin) by cultured human and bovine endothelial cells. Proc. Natl. Acad. Sci. USA 74, 3922-3926.

154. Jaffe, E.A. (1977): Endothelial cells and the biology of Factor VIII. N. Engl. J. Med. 296, 377-383.

155. Jaffe, E.A., Hoyer, L.W., and Nachman, R.L. (1973): Synthesis of antihemophilic factor antigen by cultured human endothelial cells. J. Clin. Invest. 52, 2757-2764.

156. Jaffe, E.A., and Nachman, R.L. (1975): Subunit structure of factor VIII antigen synthesized by cultured human endothelial cells. J. Clin. Invest. 56, 698-702.

157. Macarak, E.J., Howard, B.V., and Kefalides, N.A. (1977): Properties of calf endothelial cells in culture. Lab. Invest. 36, 62-67.

158. van Tilburg, N.H., and Pauwels, E.K. (1974): Extrahepatic factor VIII synthesis. Lung transplants in hemophilic dogs. Transplantation 18, 56-62.

159. Jaffe, E.A., Hoyer, L.W., and Nachman, R.L. (1974): Synthesis of von Willebrand factor by cultured human endothelial cells. Proc. Natl. Acad. Sci. USA 71, 1906-1919.

160. Caen, J.P., and Sultan, Y. (1975): von Willebrand disease as an endothelial-cell abnormality. Lancet 2, 1129.

161. Giddings, J.C., Shearn, S.A.M., and Bloom, A.L. (1975): The immunological localization of Factor V in human tissue. Br. J. Haematol. 29, 57-65.

162. Stemerman, M.B., Pitlick, F.A., and Dembitzer, H.M. (1976): Electron microscopic immunohistochemical identification of endothelial cells in the rabbit. Circ. Res. 38, 146-156.

163. Maynard, J.R., Dreyer, B.E., Stemerman, M.B., and Pitlick, F.A. (1977): Tissue-factor coagulant activity of cultured human endothelial and smooth muscle cells and fibroblasts. Blood 50, 387-396.

164. Saba, S.R., and Mason, R.G. (1974): Studies of an activity from endothelial cells that inhibits platelet aggregation, serotonin release, and clot retraction. Thromb. Res. 5, 747-757.

165. Fishman, A.P., and Pietra, G.G. (1974): Handling of bioactive materials by the lung. N. Engl. J. Med. 291, 884-890, 953-959.

166. Junod, A.F. (1977): Metabolism of vasoactive agents in lung. Am. Rev. Resp. Dis. 115 (Part 2), 51-57.

167. Johnson, A.R., and Erdos, E.G. (1977): Inactivation of sub-
     stance P by cultured human endothelial cells. In Substance P
     (von Euler, U.S. and Pernow, B., Eds.), Raven Press, New York,
     pp. 253-260.

168. Cross, S.A.M., Alabaster, V.A., Bakhle, Y.S., and Vane, J.R.
     (1974): Sites of uptake of ^{3}H-5-hydroxytryptamine in rat iso-
     lated lung. Histochemistry 39, 83-91.

169. White, M.K., Hechtman, H.B., and Shepro, D. (1975): Canine
     lung uptake of plasma and platelet serotonin. Microvasc. Res.
     9, 230-241.

170. Strum, J.M., and Junod, A.F. (1972): Radioautographic demon-
     stration of 5-hydroxytryptamine-^{3}H uptake by pulmonary endo-
     thelial cells. J. Cell Biol. 54, 456-467.

171. Block, E.R., and Fisher, A.B. (1977): Depression of serotonin
     clearance by rat lungs during oxygen exposure. J. Appl. Phy-
     siol. 42, 33-38.

172. Shepro, D., Batbouta, J.C., Robblee, L.S., Carson, M.P., and
     Belamarich, F.A. (1975): Serotonin transport by cultured
     bovine aortic endothelium. Circ. Res. 36, 799-806.

173. Bevan, J.A., and Duckles, S.P. (1975): Evidence for alpha-
     adrenergic receptors on intimal endothelium. Blood Vessels
     12, 307-310.

174. Matre, R. (1977): Similarities of Fcγ receptors on tropho-
     blasts and placental endothelial cells. Scand. J. Immunol.
     6, 953-958.

175. Buonassisi, V., and Venter, J.C. (1976): Hormone and neuro-
     transmitter receptors in an established vascular endothelial
     cell line. Proc. Natl. Acad. Sci. USA 73, 1612-1616.

176. Northover, B.J. (1975): Interaction of mono- and divalent
     metallic cations and of indomethacin on the membrane potential
     of vascular endothelial cells in vitro. Br. J. Pharmacol. 55,
     105-110.

177. Ryan, J.W., Ryan, U.S., Schultz, D.R., Whitaker, C., and Chung,
     A. (1975): Subcellular localization of pulmonary angiotensin-
     converting enzyme (kininase II). Biochem. J. 146, 497-499.

178. Ryan, U.S., Ryan, J.W., Whitaker, C., and Chiu, A. (1976):
     Localization of angiotensin-converting enzyme (kininase II).
     II. Immunocytochemistry and immunofluorescence. Tissue & Cell
     8, 125-145.

179. Ryan, U.S., Ryan, J.W., and Chiu, A. (1976): Kininase II (angiotensin-converting enzyme) and endothelial cells in culture. In Kinins: Pharmacodynamics and Biological Roles (Sicuteri, F., Back, N. and Haberland, G.L., Eds.), Plenum Publishing Corporation, New York, pp. 217-227.

180. Ryan, J.W., and Ryan, U.S. (1976): Biochemical and morphological aspects of the actions and metabolism of kinins. In Chemistry and Biology of the Kallikrein-Kinin System in Health and Disease (Pisano, J.J. and Austen, K.F., Eds.), Fogarty Int. Center Proc., U.S. Govt. Printing Office, Washington, D.C., pp. 315-333.

181. Ryan, U.S., and Ryan, J.W. (1977): Correlations between the fine structure of the alveolar-capillary unit and its metabolic activities. In Metabolic Functions of the Lung (Bakhle, Y.S. and Vane, J.R., Eds.), Vol. 4 of Lung Biology in Health and Disease (Lenfant, C., Ed.), Marcel Dekker, New York, pp. 197-232.

182. Ody, C., and Junod, A.F. (1977): Converting enzyme activity in endothelial cells isolated from pig pulmonary artery and aorta. Am. J. Physiol. 232, C95-C98.

183. Ryan, J.W., and Smith, U. (1971): Metabolism of adenosine 5'-monophosphate during circulation through the lungs. Trans. Assoc. Am. Physicians 134, 297-306.

184. Stein, O., Chajek, T., and Stein, Y. (1976): Transport of lipoprotein lipase in the endothelium of rat heart. Paroi Arterielle 3, 136.

185. Olivecrona, T., Bengtsson, G., Marklund, S., Lindahl, U., and Höök, M. (1977): Heparin-lipoprotein lipase interactions. Fed. Proc. 36, 60-65.

186. Dicorleto, P.E., and Zilversmit, D.B. (1975): Lipoprotein lipase activity in bovine aorta. Proc. Soc. Exp. Biol. Med. 148, 1101-1105.

187. Olivecrona, T., Bengtsson, G., Höök, M., and Lindahl, U. (1976): Physiologic implications of the interaction between lipoprotein lipase and some sulfated glycosaminoglycans. In Lipoprotein Metabolism (Greten, H., Ed.), Springer, Berlin, pp. 13-19.

188. Bengtsson, G., Olivecrona, T., Höök, M., and Lindahl, U. (1977): Interaction of heparin with proteins. Demonstration of different binding sites for antithrombin and lipoprotein lipase. FEBS Letters 79, 59-63.

189. Bengtsson, G., and Olivecrona, T. (1977): Interaction of lipo-
     protein lipase with heparin-sepharose. Biochem. J. 167, 109-
     119.

190. Tőkés, Z.A., and Sorgente, N. (1976): Cell surface-associated
     and released proteolytic activities of bovine aorta endothelial
     cells. Biochem. Biophys. Res. Commun. 73, 965-971.

191. Becker, C.G., and Harpel, P.C. (1976): Alpha 2-macro-globulin
     on human vascular endothelium. J. Exp. Med. 144, 1-9.

192. Pugatch, E.M.J., and Poole, J.C. (1969): Studies on the fi-
     brinolytic activity of an extract from vascular endothelium.
     Quart. J. Exp. Physiol. 54, 80-84.

193. Pugatch, E.M.J., Foster, E.A., MacFarlane, D.E., and Poole,
     J.C. (1970): The extraction and separation of activators and
     inhibitors of fibrinolysis from bovine endothelium and meso-
     thelium. Br. J. Haematol. 18, 669-681.

194. Todd, A.S. (1973): Endothelium and fibrinolysis. Bibl. Anat.
     12, 98-105.

195. Nicolaides, A.N., Clark, C.T., Thomas, R.D., and Lewis, J.D.
     (1976): Fibrinolytic activator in the endothelium of the veins
     of the lower limb. Br. J. Surg. 63, 881-884.

196. Warren, B.A., and Khan, S. (1974): The ultrastructure of the
     lysis of fibrin by endothelium in vitro. Br. J. Exp. Pathol.
     55, 138-149.

197. Hegt, V.N. (1976): Distribution and variation of fibrinolytic
     activity in the walls of human arteries and veins. Haemostasis
     5, 355-372.

198. Yao, J.S., Bergan, J.J., and Kwaan, H.C. (1974): Quantitation
     of fibrinolytic activity in venous and prosthetic arterial
     grafts. Arch. Surg. 109, 163-167.

199. Joris, I., and Majno, G. (1974): Cellular breakdown within
     the arterial wall. An ultrastructural study of the coronary
     artery in young and aging rats. Virchows Arch. A Path. Anat.
     Histol. 364, 111-127.

200. Hecht, A., Hackensellner, H.A., and Sajkiewicz, K. (1965):
     Comparative enzyme-histochemical studies on the wall and on
     the endothelium of the aorta and the pulmonary artery. Z.
     Zellforsch. 68, 611-617.

201. Hollis, T.M., and Rosen, L.A. (1972): Histidine decarboxylase activity of bovine aortic endothelium and intima-media. Proc. Soc. Exp. Biol. Med. 141, 978-981.

202. Gottlob, R., and Hoff, H.F. (1968): Histochemical investigations on the nature of large blood vessel endothelial and medial argyrophilic lines and on the mechanism of silver staining. Histochemie 13, 70-83.

203. Majno, G., Shea, S.M., and Leventhal, M. (1969): Endothelial contraction induced by histamine-type mediators. J. Cell Biol. 42, 647-672.

204. Matsusaka, T. (1975): Tridimensional views of the relationship of pericytes to endothelial cells of capillaries in the human choroid and retina. J. Electron Microsc. (Tokyo) 24, 13-18.

205. Beacham, W.S., Konishi, A., and Hunt, C.C. (1976): Observations on the microcirculatory bed in rat mesocecum using differential interference contrast microscopy in vivo and electron microscopy. Am. J. Anat. 146, 385-426.

206. Rhodin, J.A.G. (1974): Histology: a text and atlas. Oxford University Press, New York, pp. 348-352.

207. Rennels, M.L., and Nelson, E. (1975): Capillary innervation in the mammalian central nervous system: an electron microscopic demonstration. Am. J. Anat. 144, 233-241.

208. Saba, S.R., and Mason, R.G. (1975): Effects of platelets and certain platelet components on growth of cultured human endothelial cells. Thromb. Res. 7, 807-812.

209. D'Amore, P., and Shepro, D. (1977): Stimulation of growth and calcium influx in cultured, bovine, aortic endothelial cells by platelets and vasoactive substances. J. Cell. Physiol. 92, 177-184.

210. Cotran, R.S. (1965): Endothelial phagocytosis: an electron-microscopic study. Exp. Mol. Pathol. 4, 217-231.

211. Hausmann, K., Wulfhekel, U., Düllmann, J., and Kuse, R. (1976): Iron storage in macrophages and endothelial cells. Histochemistry, ultrastructure and clinical significance. Blut 32, 289-295.

212. Renkin, E.M. (1978): Transport pathways through capillary endothelium. (Eugene M. Landis Award Lecture), Microvasc. Res. In press.

213. Renkin, E.M. (1977): Multiple pathways of capillary permeability. Circ. Res. 41, 735-743.

214. Bruns, R.R., and Palade, G.E. (1968): Studies on blood capillaries. II. Transport of ferritin molecules across the wall of muscle capillaries. J. Cell Biol. 37, 277-299.

215. Wissig, S.L. (1964): The transport by vesicles of protein across the endothelium of muscle capillaries. Anat. Rec. 148, 411.

216. Shea, S.M., and Karnovsky, M.J. (1966): Brownian motion: a theoretical explanation for the movement of vesicles across the endothelium. Nature 212, 353-355.

217. Tomlin, S.G. (1969): Vesicular transport across endothelial cells. Biochim. Biophys. Acta 183, 559-564.

218. Shea, S.M., Karnovsky, M.J., and Bossert, W.H. (1969): Vesicular transport across endothelium: simulation of a diffusion model. J. Theor. Biol. 24, 30-42.

219. Casley-Smith, J.R., and Clark, H.I. (1972): The dimensions and numbers of small vesicles in blood capillary endothelium in the hind legs of dogs, and their relation to vascular permeability. J. Microscopy 96:263-267.

220. Green, H.S., and Casley-Smith, J.R. (1972): Calculations on the passage of small vesicles across endothelial cells by Brownian motion. J. Theor. Biol. 35, 103-111.

221. Casley-Smith, J.R., Green, H.S., and Wadey, H.J.L. (1975): The quantitative morphology of skeletal muscle capillaries in relation to permeability. Microvasc. Res. 10:43-64.

222. Heinrich, D., Metz, J., Raviola, E., and Forssmann, W.G. (1976) Ultrastructure of perfusion-fixed fetal capillaries in the huma placenta. Cell Tissue Res. 172, 157-169.

223. Dieterich, C.E., Dieterich, H.J., and Hildebrand, R. (1976): Comparative electron-microscopic studies on the conus papillaris and its relationship to the retina in night and day active geckos. Albrecht v. Graefes Arch. Klin. Exp. Opthalmol. 200, 279-292.

224. Marquart, K.H., and Caesar, R. (1970): Quantitative Untersuchungen über die sogenannten Pinocytosebläschen im Capillarendothel. Virchows Arch. Abt. B Zellpath. 6, 220-233.

225. Reyners, H., Gianfelici de Reyners, E., Jadin, J.M., and
     Maisin, J.R. (1975): An ultrastructural quantitative method
     for the evaluation of the permeability to horseradish perox-
     idase of cerebral cortex endothelial cells of the rat. Cell
     Tissue Res. 157, 93-99.

226. De Fouw, D.O., and Berendsen, P.B. (1977): The air-blood
     barrier of isolated-perfused dog lungs in stable and edematous
     conditions. Fed. Proc. 36, 428.

227. Weihe, E., Aoki, A., Aumüller, G., Greenberg, J., Metz, J.,
     Hartschuh, W., and Forssmann, W.G.: Experimentelle Untersuch-
     ungen zur terminalen Strombahn des Hodens. In preparation.

228. Ishimura, K., Okamoto, H., and Fujita, H. (1976): Freeze-
     etching studies on ultrastructural changes of endothelial
     cells in the thyroid of normal, TSH-treated and thyradin-
     treated mice. Cell Tissue Res. 175, 313-317.

229. Westergaard, E. (1975): Enhanced vesicular transport of exoge-
     nous peroxidase across cerebral vessels, induced by serotonin.
     Acta Neuropathol. 32, 27-42.

230. Eto, T., Oniki, H., Onoyama, K., Omae, T., and Yamamoto, T.
     (1977): Increased capillary permeability in muscularis layer
     of rat intestine caused by kidney extract. Virchows Arch. B
     Cell Pathol. 25, 83-93.

231. Wagner, R.C., Andrews, S.B., and Matthews, M.A. (1977): A
     fluorescence assay for micropinocytosis in isolated capillary
     endothelium. Microvasc. Res. 14, 67-80.

232. Pappenheimer, J.R., Renkin, E.M., and Borrero, L.M. (1951):
     Filtration, diffusion and molecular sieving through peripheral
     capillary membranes. A contribution to the pore theory of
     capillary permeability. Am. J. Physiol. 167, 13-46.

233. Renkin, E.M. (1952): Capillary permeability to lipid-soluble
     molecules. Am. J. Physiol. 168, 538-544.

234. Renkin, E.M. (1953): Capillary and cellular permeability to
     some compounds related to antipyrine. Am. J. Physiol. 173,
     125-129.

235. Chinard, F.P., Perl, W., and Ritter, A.R. (1976): Interaction
     of aqueous and lipid pathways in the pulmonary endothelium.
     Microcircul. 2, 71-74.

236. Stein, Y., and Stein, O. (1972): Lipid synthesis and degrada-
     tion and lipoprotein transport in mammalian aorta. In Athero-
     genesis: Initiating Factors, Ciba Foundation Symposium, Else-
     vier-Excerpta Medica, North-Holland, Amsterdam, pp. 165-179.

237. Stein, O., Stein, Y., and Eisenberg, S. (1973): A radio-auto-
     graphic study of the transport of ^{125}I-labeled serum lipopro-
     teins in rat aorta. Z. Zellforsch. 138, 223-237.

238. Christensen, S., and Nielsen, H. (1977): Permeability of arte-
     rial endothelium to plasma macromolecules. The concomitant
     transfer to plasma phosphatidylethanolamine, phosphatidylchol-
     ine, sphingomyelin and phosphoprotein across the aortic endo-
     thelial surface in normal cockerels following the injection
     of labelled, hyperlipidemic, plasma. With a note on carbon
     monoxide. Atherosclerosis 27, 447-463.

239. Pietra, G.G., Spagnoli, L.G., Capuzzi, D.M., Sparks, C.E.,
     Fishman, A.P., and Marsh, J.B. (1976): Metabolism of ^{125}I-
     labeled lipoproteins by the isolated rat lung. J. Cell Biol.
     70, 33-46.

240. Stein, O., and Stein, Y. (1976): High density lipoproteins
     reduce the uptake of low density lipoproteins by human endo-
     thelial cells in culture. Biochim. Biophys. Acta 431, 363-368.

241. Howard, B.V. (1977): Uptake of very low density lipoprotein
     triglyceride by bovine aortic endothelial cells in culture.
     J. Lipid Res. 18, 561-571.

242. Scow, R.O., Blanchette-Mackie, E.J., and Smith, L.C. (1976):
     Role of capillary endothelium in the clearance of chylomicrons.
     A model for lipid transport from blood by lateral diffusion in
     cell membranes. Circ. Res. 39, 149-162.

243. Blanchette-Mackie, E.J., and Scow, R.O. (1971): Sites of
     lipoprotein lipase activity in adipose tissue perfused with
     chylomicrons. Electron microscope cytochemical study. J.
     Cell Biol. 51, 1-25.

244. Wolff, J.R. (1977): Ultrastructure of the terminal vascular
     bed as related to function. In Microcirculation (Kaley, G.
     and Altura, B.M., Eds.), Univ. Park Press, Baltimore, pp. 95-
     130 (see Tab. 1).

245. Rhodin, J.A.G. (1968): Ultrastructure of mammalian veins,
     capillaries, venules, and small collecting veins. J. Ultra-
     struct. Res. 25, 452-500.

246. Majno, G., Palade, G.E., and Schoefl, G.I. (1961): Studies on
     inflammation. II. The site of action of histamine and sero-
     tonin along the vascular tree: a topographic study. J. Bio-
     phys. Biochem. Cytol. 11, 607-626.

247. Cotran, R.S., Suter, E.R., and Majno, G. (1967): The use of
     colloidal carbon as a tracer for vascular injury. A review.
     Vasc. Dis. 4:107-127.

248. Siflinger, A., Parker, K., and Caro, C.G. (1975): Uptake of
     ^{125}I albumin by the endothelial surface of the isolated dog
     common carotid artery: effect of certain physical factors and
     metabolic inhibitors. Cardiovasc. Res. 9, 478-489.

249. Ryan, G.B., and Majno, G. (1977): Acute inflammation. A
     review. Am. J. Pathol. 86, 183-276.

250. Caro, C.G., Lewis, C.T., and Weinbaum, S. (1975): A mechanism
     by which mechanical disturbances can increase the uptake of
     macromolecules by the artery wall. J. Physiol. (Lond.) 246,
     71P-73P.

251. Perl, W., Silverman, F., Delea, A.C., and Chinard, F.P. (1976):
     Permeability of dog lung endothelium to sodium, diols, amides,
     and water. Am. J. Physiol. 230, 1708-1721.

252. Michel, R.P., Inoue, S., and Hogg, J.C. (1977): Pulmonary
     capillary permeability to HRP in dogs: a physiological and
     morphological study. J. Appl. Physiol. 42, 13-21.

253. Inoue, S., Michel, R.P., and Hogg, J.C. (1976): Zonulae occlu-
     dentes in alveolar epithelium and capillary endothelium in dog
     lungs studied with the freeze-fracture technique. J. Ultrastr.
     Res. 56, 215-225.

254. Fishman, A.P., and Pietra, G.G. (1976): Permeability of pulmo-
     nary vascular endothelium. In Lung Liquids, Ciba Foundation
     Symposium #38, Elsevier-Excerpta Medica, North-Holland, Amster-
     dam, pp. 3-28.

255. Schneeberger, E.E. (1976): Ultrastructural basis for alveolar-
     capillary permeability to protein. In Lung Liquids, Ciba Foun-
     dation Symposium #38, Elsevier-Excerpta Medica, North-Holland,
     Amsterdam, pp. 3-28.

256. Reese, T.C., and Karnovsky, M.J. (1976): Fine structural
     localization of a blood-brain barrier to exogenous peroxidase.
     J. Cell Biol. 34, 207-217.

257. Brightman, M.W., and Reese, T.S. (1969): Junctions between intimately apposed cell membranes in the vetebrate brain. J. Cell Biol. 40, 648-677.

258. Sørensen, S.C. (1974): The permeability to small ions of tight junctions between cerebral endothelial cells. Brain Res. 70, 174-178.

259. Dermietzel, R. (1975): Junctions in the central nervous system of the cat. IV. Interendothelial junctions of cerebral blood vessels from selected areas of the brain. Cell Tissue Res. 164, 45-62.

260. Rapoport, S.I. (1976): Blood-brain Barrier in Physiology and Medicine. Raven Press, New York.

261. Yudilevich, D.L., and Barry, D.I. (1977): Indicator diffusion and other non-destructive methods for the study of experimental modifications of the blood-brain barrier. Exp. Eye Res. 25 (Suppl.), 511-521.

262. Pardridge, W.M., and Oldendorf, W.H. (1977): Transport of metabolic substrates through the blood-brain barrier. J. Neurochem. 28, 5-12.

263. Westergaard, E., and Brightman, M.W. (1973): Transport of proteins across normal cerebral arterioles. J. Comp. Neurol. 152, 17-44.

264. Majno, G., and LaGattuta, M. (1966): Über die durch chemische Mediatoren induzierte Gefäss-durchlässigkeit: eine in-vivo-Untersuchung mit "Russmarkierung." In Die Entzündung (Heister, R. and Hofmann, H.F., Eds.), Urban & Schwarzenberg, München., pp. 3-6.

265. Majno, G., and Leventhal, M. (1967): Pathogenesis of "histamine-type" vascular leakage. Lancet 2, 99.

266. Majno, G., and Joris, I.: Endothelial contractility. In The Circulation (Schwartz, C.J., Ed.), Plenum Press. In preparation.

267. Joris, I., Majno, G., and Ryan, G.B. (1972): Endothelial contraction in vivo: a study of the rat mesentery. Virchows Arch. Abt. B Zellpath. 12, 73-83.

268. Cecio, A. (1967): Ultrastructural features of cytofilaments within mammalian endothelial cells. Zeitschr. Zellforsch. 83, 40-48.

269. Röhlich, P., and Oláh, I. (1967): Cross-striated fibrils in the endothelium of the rat myometral arterioles. J. Ultrastruct. Res. 18, 667-676.

270. Becker, C.G., and Murphy, G.E. (1969): Demonstration of contractile protein in endothelium and cells of the heart valves, endocardium, intima, arteriosclerotic plaques, and Aschoff bodies of rheumatic heart disease. Am. J. Pathol. 55, 1-37.

271. Becker, C.G. (1976): Contractile and relaxing proteins of smooth muscle and platelets: their presence in the endothelium. Ann. N.Y. Acad. Sci. 275, 78-86.

272. Moore, A., Jaffe, E.A., Becker, C.G., and Nachman, R.L. (1977): Myosin in cultured human endothelial cells. Br. J. Haematol. 35, 71-79.

273. Lauweryns, J.M., Baert, J., and De Loecker, W. (1976): Fine filaments in lymphatic endothelial cells. J. Cell Biol. 68, 163-167.

274. Yohro, T., and Burnstock, G. (1973): Filament bundles and contractility of endothelial cells in coronary arteries. Z. Zellforsch. 138, 85-95.

275. De Bruyn, P.P.H., and Cho, Y. (1974): Contractile structures in endothelial cells of splenic sinusoids. J. Ultrastruct. Res. 49, 24-33.

276. Giacomelli, F., Wiener, J., and Spiro, D. (1970): Cross-striated arrays of filaments in endothelium. J. Cell Biol. 45, 188-192.

277. Gabbiani, G., Badonnel, M-C., and Rona, G. (1975): Cytoplasmic contractile apparatus in aortic endothelial cells of hypertensive rats. Lab Invest. 32, 227-234.

278. Lauweryns, J.M., and Boussauw, L. (1973): Striated filamentous bundles associated with centrioles in pulmonary lymphatic endothelial cells. J. Ultrastruct. Res. 42:25-28.

279. Blose, S.H., and Chacko, S. (1976): Rings of intermediate (100 Å) filament bundles in their perinuclear region of vascular endothelial cells. Their mobilization by colcemid and mitosis. J. Cell Biol. 70, 459-466.

280. Blose, S.H. (1976): Contractile proteins and cytoplasmic filaments in cloned venous endothelial cells. Fed. Proc. 35, 154a.

281. Blose, S.H., Shelanski, M.L., and Chacko, S. (1977): Localization of bovine brain filament antibody on intermediate (100 Å) filaments in guinea pig vascular endothelial cells and chick cardiac muscle cells. Proc. Natl. Acad. Sci. USA 74, 662-665.

282. Pollard, T.D. (1976): Cytoskeletal functions of cytoplasmic contractile proteins. J. Supramolec. Struct. 5, 317(269)-334 (286).

283. Robertson, A.L., Jr., and Khairallah, P.A. (1973): Arterial endothelial permeability and vascular disease. The "trap door" effect. Exp. Molec. Pathol. 18, 2412-2460.

284. Hammersen, F. (1976): Endothelial contractility - an undecided problem in vascular research. Beitr. Path. Bd. 157, 327-348.

285. Shimamoto, T. (1975): Drugs and foods on contraction of endothelial cells as a key mechanism in atherogenesis and treatment of atherosclerosis with endothelial-cell relaxants (cyclic AMP phosphodiesterase inhibitors). Adv. Exp. Med. Biol. 60, 77-105.

286. Johansson, B.B. (1976): Cerebrovascular permeability to protein in spontaneously hypertensive rats (SHR) after acute blood pressure elevation. Clin. Exp. Pharm. Physiol. Suppl. 3, 97-100.

287. Wojcik, J.D., Van Horn, D.L., Webber, A.J., and Johnson, S.A. (1969): Mechanism whereby platelets support the endothelium. Transfusion 9, 324-335.

288. Elgjo, R.F. (1976): Platelets, endothelial cells and macrophages in the spleen. An ultrastructural study on perfusion-fixed organs. Am. J. Anat. 145, 101-120.

289. Nachman, R.L., and Jaffe, E.A. (1976): The platelet-endothelial cell--VIII axis. Thromb. Haemostas. 35, 120-123.

290. Van Horn, D.L., and Johnson, S.A. (1966): The mechanism of thrombocytopenic bleeding. Am. J. Clin. Pathol. 46, 204-213.

291. Van Horn, D.L., and Johnson, S.A. (1968): The escape of carbon from intact capillaries in experimental thrombocytopenia. J. Lab. Clin. Med. 71, 301-311.

292. Dale, C., and Hurley, J.V. (1977): An electron-microscope study of the mechanism of bleeding in experimental thrombocytopenia. J. Pathol. 121, 193-212.

293. Kitchens, C.S., and Weiss, L. (1975): Ultrastructural changes of endothelium associated with thrombocytopenia. Blood 46, 567-578.

294. Kitchens, C.S. (1977): Amelioration of endothelial abnormalities by prednisone in experimental thrombocytopenia in the rabbit. J. Clin. Invest. 60, 1129-1134.

295. Gimbrone, M.A., Jr., Aster, R.H., Cotran, R.S., Corkery, J., Jandl, J.H., and Folkman, J. (1969): Preservation of vascular integrity in organs perfused in vitro with a platelet-rich medium. Nature 222, 33-36.

296. Folkman, J., and Gimbrone, M.A., Jr. (1971): Perfusion of the thyroid. In Karolinska Symposia on Research Methods in Reproductive Endocrinology, IV Symposium, Perfusion Techniques (Diczfalusy, E., Ed.), Karolinska Institutet, Stockholm, pp. 237-248.

297. Wasteson, Å, Höök, M., and Westermark, B. (1976): Demonstration of a platelet enzyme degrading heparan sulphate. FEBS Letters 64, 218-221.

298. Mustard, J.F., and Packham, M.A. (1975): The role of blood and platelets in atherosclerosis and the complications of atherosclerosis. Thromb. Diath. Hemorrh. 33, 444-456.

299. Rafelson, M.E., Jr., Hoveke, T.P., and Booyse, F.M. (1973): The molecular biology of platelet-platelet and platelet-endothelial interactions. Ser. Haematol. 6, 367-381.

300. Payling-Wright, H. (1968): Endothelial mitosis around aortic branches in normal guinea pigs. Nature 220, 78-79.

301. Payling-Wright, H. (1970): Endothelial turnover. In Vascular Factors and Thrombosis (Koller, F. et al., Eds.), F.K. Schattauer Verlag, Stuttgart, New York, pp. 79-84.

302. Payling-Wright, H. (1971): Areas of mitosis in aortic endothelium of guinea pigs. J. Pathol. 105, 65-67.

303. Payling-Wright, H. (1972): Mitosis patterns in aortic endothelium. Atherosclerosis 15, 93-100.

304. Payling-Wright, H. (1973): Endothelial injury and repair. Bibl. Anat. 12, 87-91.

305. Schwartz, S.M., and Benditt, E.P. (1973): Cell replication in the aortic endothelium: a new method for study of the problem. Lab. Invest. 28, 699-707.

306. Schwartz, S.M., and Benditt, E.P. (1976): Clustering of repli-
     cating cells in aortic endothelium. Proc. Natl. Acad. Sci. USA
     73, 651-653.

307. Schwartz, S.M., and Benditt, E.P. (1977): Aortic endothelial
     cell replication. I. Effects of age and hypertension in the
     rat. Circ. Res. 41, 248-255.

308. Caplan, B.A., and Schwartz, C.J. (1973): Increased endothelial
     cell turnover in areas of in vivo Evans blue uptake in the pig
     aorta. Atherosclerosis 17, 401-417.

309. Engerman, R.L., Pfaffenbach, D., and Davis, M.D. (1967): Cell
     turnover of capillaries. Lab Invest. 17, 738-743.

310. Jaffe, E.A., Nachman, R.L., Becker, C.G., and Minick, C.R.
     (1973): Culture of human endothelial cells derived from um-
     bilical veins. Identification by morphologic and immunologic
     criteria. J. Clin. Invest. 52, 2745-2756.

311. Gimbrone, M.A., Jr., Cotran, R.S., and Folkman, J. (1974):
     Human vascular endothelial cells in culture. Growth and DNA
     synthesis. J. Cell Biol. 60, 673-684.

312. Haudenschild, C.C., Cotran, R.S. Gimbrone, M.A., Jr., and
     Folkman, J. (1975): Fine structure of vascular endothelium
     in culture. J. Ultrastruct. Res. 50, 22-32.

313. Gimbrone, M.A., Jr., (1976): Culture of vascular endothelium.
     In Progress in Hemostasis and Thrombosis, Vol. III (Spaet, T.H.,
     Ed.), Grune & Stratton, Inc., New York, pp. 1-28.

314. Macarak, E.J., Howard, B.V., and Kefalides, N.A. (1977): Pro-
     perties of calf endothelial cells in culture. Lab. Invest.
     36, 62-67.

315. Sholley, M.M., Gimbrone, M.A., Jr., and Cotran, R.S. (1977):
     Cellular migration and replication in endothelial regeneration.
     A study using irradiated endothelial cultures. Lab. Invest.
     36, 18-25.

316. Blose, S.H., and Chacko, S. (1975): In vitro behavior of
     guinea pig arterial and venous endothelial cells. Develop.
     Growth Different. 17, 153-165.

317. Sedlak, B.J., Booyse, F.M., Bell, S., and Rafelson, M.E., Jr.,
     (1976): Comparison of two types of endothelial cells in long
     term culture. Thromb. Haemostas. 35, 167-177.

318. de Bono, D. (1975): En face organ culture of vascular endothe-
     lium. Br. J. Exp. Pathol. 56, 8-13.

319. Chemnitz, J., Christensen, B.C., and Tkocz, I. (1977): En face
     organ cultures of rabbit aortic segments after a single dila-
     tion trauma in vivo. A new model in the study of endothelial
     regeneration. Virchows Arch. A Path. Anat. and Histol. 375,
     257-262.

320. Deem, C.W., Futterman, S., and Kalina, R.E. (1974): Induction
     of endothelial cell proliferation in rat retinal venules by
     chemical and indirect physical trauma. Invest. Ophthalmol. 13,
     580-585.

321. Schaper, J., König, R., Franz, D., and Schaper, W. (1976):
     The endothelial surface of growing coronary collateral arteries.
     Intimal margination and diapedesis of monocytes. A combined
     SEM and TEM study. Virchows Arch. A Pathol. Anat. Histol.
     370, 193-205.

322. Florentin, R.A., Nam, S.C., Lee, K.T., and Thomas, W.A. (1969):
     Increased ^{3}H-thymidine incorporation into endothelial cells of
     swine fed cholesterol for 3 days. Exp. Mol. Pathol. 10, 250-
     255.

323. Widmann, J-J., and Fahimi, H.D. (1976): Proliferation of endo-
     thelial cells in estrogen-stimulated rat liver. A light and
     electron microscopic cytochemical study. Lab. Invest. 34, 141-
     149.

324. Sholley, M.M., and Cotran, R.S. (1976): Endothelial DNA syn-
     thesis in the microvasculature of rat skin during the hair
     growth cycle. Am. J. Anat. 147, 243-254.

325. Polverini, P.J., Cotan, R.S., and Sholley, M.M. (1977): Endo-
     thelial proliferation in the delayed hypersensitivity reaction:
     an autoradiographic study. J. Immunol. 118, 529-532.

326. Folkman, J. (1976): The vascularization of tumors. Scientific
     American 234, 58-73.

327. Cavallo, T., Sade, R., Folkman, J., and Cotran, R.S. (1973):
     Ultrastructural autoradiographic studies of the early vaso-
     proliferative response in tumor angiogensis. Am. J. Pathol.
     70, 345-362.

328. Ausprunk, D.H., and Folkman, J. (1977): Migration and prolif-
     eration of endothelial cells in preformed and newly formed
     blood vessels during tumor angiogenesis. Microvasc. Res. 14,
     53-65.

329. Haudenschild, C.C., Zahniser, D., Folkman, J., and Klagsbrun, M. (1976): Human vascular endothelial cells in culture. Lack of response to serum growth factors. Exp. Cell Res. 98, 175-183.

330. Fenselau, A., and Mello, R.J. (1976): Growth stimulation of cultured endothelial cells by tumor cell homogenates. Cancer Res. 36, 3269-3273.

331. Kelly, P.J., Suddith, R.L., Hutchison, H.T., Werrbach, K., and Haber, B. (1976): Endothelial growth factor present in tissue culture of CNS tumors. J. Neurosurg. 44, 342-346.

332. Atherton, A. (1977): Growth stimulation of endothelial cells by simultaneous culture with sarcoma 180 cells in diffusion chambers. Cancer Res. 37, 3619-3622.

333. Hoffman, H., McAuslan, B., Robertson, D., and Burnett, E. (1976): An endothelial growth-stimulating factor from salivary glands. Exp. Cell Res. 102, 269-275.

334. Gospodarowicz, D., Moran, J., Braun, D., and Birdwell, C. (1976): Clonal growth of bovine vascular endothelial cells: fibroblast growth factor as a survival agent. Proc. Natl. Acad. Sci. USA 73, 4120-4124.

335. Knudtzon, S., and Mortensen, B.T. (1975): Growth stimulation of human bone marrow cells in agar culture by vascular cells. Blood 46, 937-943.

336. Eisenstein, R., Kuettner, K.E., Neapolitan, C., Soble, L.W., and Sorgente, N. (1975): The resistance of certain tissues to invasion. III. Cartilage extracts inhibit the growth of fibro blasts and endothelial cells in culture. Am. J. Pathol. 81, 337-348.

337. Eisenstein, R., Kuettner, K.E., Soble, L.W., and Sorgente, N. (1976): Tissue inhibitors are cell growth regulators. In Protides of the Biological Fluids, 23rd Colloquium (Peeters, H., Ed.), Pergamon Press, Oxford, pp. 217-219.

338. Langer, R., Brem, H., Falterman, K., Klein, M., and Folkman, J. (1976): Isolation of a cartilage factor that inhibits tumor neovascularization. Science 193, 70-72.

339. Mansfield, P.B., Wechezak, A.R., and Sauvage, L.R. (1975): Preventing thrombus on artificial vascular surfaces: true endothelial cell linings. Trans. Am. Soc. Artif. Int. Organs 21, 264-272.

340. Brais, M., and Braunwald, N.S. (1976): Acceleration of tissue ingrowth on materials implanted in the heart. Ann. Thorac. Surg. 21, 221-229.

341. Minick, C.R., Stemerman, M.B., and Insull, W., Jr. (1977): Effect of regenerated endothelium on lipid accumulation in the arterial wall. Proc. Natl. Acad. Sci. USA 74, 1724-1728.

342. Bondjers, G., and Bjorkerud, S. (1973): Cholesterol accumulation and content in regions with defined endothelial integrity in the normal rabbit aorta. Atherosclerosis 17, 71-83.

343. Schwartz, S.M., Stemerman, M.B., and Benditt, E.P. (1975): The aortic intima. II. Repair of the aortic lining after mechanical denudation. Am. J. Pathol. 81, 15-42.

344. Spaet, T.H., Stemerman, M.B., Veith, F.J., and Lejnieks, I. (1975): Intimal injury and regrowth in the rabbit aorta; medial smooth muscle cells as a source of neointima. Circ. Res. 36, 58-70.

345. Stemerman, M.B., Spaet, T.H., Pitlick F., Cintron, J., Lejnieks, I., and Tiell, M.L. (1977): Intimal healing. The pattern of reendothelialization and intimal thickening. Am. J. Pathol. 87, 125-142.

346. Stemerman, M.B. (1977): Factors governing the healing response of injured arteries. Ann. N.Y. Acad. Sci. 283, 310-316.

347. Fishman, J.A., Ryan, G.B., and Karnovsky, M.J. (1975): Endothelial regeneration in the rat carotid artery and the significance of endothelial denudation in the pathogenesis of myointimal thickening. Lab. Invest. 32, 339-351.

348. Fry, D.L. (1968): Acute vascular endothelial changes associated with increased blood velocity gradients. Circ. Res. 22, 165-197.

349. Baumann, F.G., Imparato, A.M., and Geun-Eum, K. (1976): The evolution of early fibromuscular lesions hemodynamically induced in the dog renal artery. I. Light and transmission electron microscopy. Circ. Res. 39, 809-827.

350. Stehbens, W.E. (1974): Subendothelial edema. Haemodynamic production of lipid deposition, intimal tears, mural dissection and thrombosis in the blood vessel wall. Proc. Roy. Soc. Lond. Biol. 185, 357-373.

351. Stehbens, W.E. (1974): The ultrastructure of the anastomosed vein of experimental arteriovenous fistulae in sheep. Am. J. Pathol. 76, 377-400.

352. Cerra, F.B., Raza,S., Andres, G.A., and Siegel, J.H. (1977): The endothelial damage of pulsatile renal preservation and its relationship to perfusion pressure and colloid osmotic pressure. Surgery 81, 534-541.

353. Rabb, J.M., Renaud, M.L., Brandt, P.A., and Witt, C.W. (1974): Effect of freezing and thawing on the microcirculation and capillary endothelium of the hamster cheek pouch. Cryobiology 11, 508-518.

354. Bowers, W.D., Jr., Hubbard, R.W., Daum, R.C., Ashbaugh, P., and Nilson, E. (1973): Ultrastructural studies of muscle cells and vascular endothelium immediately after freeze-thaw injury. Cryobiology 10, 9-21.

355. Malczak, H.T., and Buck, R.C. (1977): Regeneration of endothelium in rat aorta after local freezing. A scanning electron microscopic study. Am. J. Pathol. 86, 133-148.

356. Kanan, M.W., and van Diest, P. (1976): Endonasal venular permeability in rats exposed to the cold. Acta Otolaryngol. 82, 118-122.

357. Gabbiani, G., and Badonnel, M-C. (1975): Early changes of endothelial clefts after thermal injury. Microvasc. Res. 10, 65-75.

358. Sholley, M.M., Cavallo, T., and Cotran, R.S. (1977): Endothelial proliferation in inflammation. I. Autoradiographic studies following thermal injury to the skin of normal rats. Am. J. Pathol. 89, 277-296.

359. Smith, J.B., MacIntosh, G.H., and Morris, B. (1970): The migration of cells through chronically inflamed tissues. J. Pathol. 100, 21-29.

360. Stewart, G.J., Ritchie, W.G.M., and Lynch, P.R. (1974): Venous endothelial damage produced by massive sticking and emigration of leukocytes. Am. J. Pathol. 74:507-532.

361. Gschnait, F.G., Wolff, K., and Konrad, K. (1975): Erythropoietic protoprophyria--submicroscopic events during the acute photo-sensitivity flare. Br. J. Dermatol. 92, 545-557.

362. Reinhold, H.S., and Buisman, G.H. (1973): Radiosensitivity of capillary endothelium. Br. J. Radiol. 46, 54-57.

363. Reinhold, J.S., and Buisman, G.H. (1975): Repair of radiation damage to capillary endothelium. Br. J. Radiol. 48, 727-731.

364. De Gowin, R.L., Lewis, L.J., Hoak, J.C., Mueller, A.L., and Gibson, D.P. (1974): Radiosensitivity of human endothelial cells in culture. J. Lab. Clin. Med. 84, 42-48.

365. DeGowin, R.L., Lewis, L.J., Mason, R.E., Borke, M.K., and Hoak, J.C. (1976): Radiation-induced inhibition of human endothelial cells replicating in culture. Radiat. Res. 68, 244-250.

366. Fallon, J.T., Stehbens, W.E., and Eggleton, R.C. (1973): An ultrastructural study of the effect of ultrasound on arterial tissue. J. Pathol. 111, 275-284.

367. Wiedeman, M.P. (1974): Vascular reactions to laser in vivo. Microvasc. Res. 8, 132-138.

368. Jaenke, R.S., and Alexander, A.F. (1973): Fine structural alterations of bovine peripheral pulmonary arteries in hypoxia-induced hypertension. Am. J. Pathol. 73, 377-398.

369. Kjeldsen, K., and Thomsen, H.K. (1975): The effect of hypoxia on the fine structure of the aortic intima in rabbits. Lab. Invest. 33, 533-543.

370. Smith, P., and Heath, D. (1977): Ultrastructure of hypoxic hypertensive pulmonary vascular disease. J. Pathol. 121, 93-100.

371. Morrison, A.D., Orci, L., Berwick, L., Perrelet, A., and Winegrad, A.I. (1977): The effects of anoxia on the morphology and composite metabolism of the intact aortic intima-media preparation. J. Clin. Invest. 59, 1027-1037.

372. Nelson, E., Gertz, S.D., Rennels, M.L., Forbes, M.S., and Kawamura, J. (1975): Scanning and transmission electron microscopic studies of arterial endothelium following experimental vascular occlusion. In The Cerebral Vessel Wall (Cervós-Navarro, J., Betz, E., Matakas, F. and Wüllenweber, R., Eds.), Raven Press, New York, pp. 33-39.

373. Nelson, E., Sunaga, R., Shimamoto, T., Kawamura, J., Rennels, M.L., and Hebel, R. (1975): Ischemic carotid endothelium. Scanning electron microscopical studies. Arch. Pathol. 99, 125-131.

374. Bhawan, J., Joris, I., DeGirolami, U., and Majno, G. (1977): Effect of occlusion on large vessels. I. A study of the rat carotid artery. Am. J. Pathol. 88, 355-380.

375. Cunha-Vaz, J.G., and Shakib, M. (1967): Ultrastructural mechanisms of breakdown of the blood-retina barrier. J. Pathol. Bact. 93, 645-652.

376. Majno, G., Ames, A., III, Chiang, J., and Wright, R.L. (1967): No reflow after cerebral ischemia. Lancet, 569-570.

377. Ames, A., III, Wright, R.L., Kowada, M., Thurston, J.M., and Majno, G. (1968): Cerebral ischemia. II. The no-reflow phenomenon. Am. J. Pathol. 52, 437-453.

378. Chiang, J., Kowada, M., Ames, A., III, Wright, R.L., and Majno, G. (1968): Cerebral ischemia. III. Vascular changes. Am. J. Pathol. 52, 455-476.

379. Strock, P.E., and Majno, G. (1969): Microvascular changes in acutely ischemic rat muscle. Surgery 129, 1213-1224.

380. Willms-Kretschmer, K., and Majno, G. (1969): Ischemia of the skin. Electron microscopic study of vascular injury. Am. J. Pathol. 54, 327-353.

381. Armiger, L.C., and Gavin, J.B. (1975): Changes in the microvasculature of ischemic and infarcted myocardium. Lab. Invest. 33, 51-56.

382. Camilleri, J.P., Joseph, D., Fabiani, J.N., Deloche, A., Schlumberger, M., Relland, J., and Carpentier, A. (1976): Microcirculatory changes following early reperfusion in experimental myocardial infarction. Virchows Arch. A Path. Anat. Histol. 369, 315-333.

383. Ashraf, M., Livingston, L., and Bloor, C.M. (1977): Ultrastructural alterations in myocardial vessels after coronary artery occlusion. In Scanning Electron Microscopy, Vol. II, ITT Research Institute, Chicago, pp. 500-506.

384. Johnston, W.H., and Latta, H. (1977): Glomerular mesangial and endothelial cell swelling following temporary renal ischemia and its role in the no-reflow phenomenon. Am. J. Pathol. 89, 153-166.

385. Powell, W.J., Jr., DiBona, D.R., Flores, J., Frega, N., and Leaf, A. (1976): Effects of hyperosmotic mannitol in reducing ischemic cell swelling and minimizing myocardial necrosis. Circulation 53 (Suppl. 1), 45-49.

386. Vardi, J., and Fields, G.A. (1975): Pathophysiology of micro-angiopathic hemolytic anemia in severe pre-eclampsia. Am. J. Obstet. Gynecol. 122, 905-906.

387. Stout, C., and Lemmon, W.B. (1969): Glomerular capillary endo-thelial swelling in a pregnant chimpanzee. Am. J. Obstet. Gynecol. 105, 212-215.

388. Harrison, M.W., Connell, R.S., Campbell, J.R., and Webb, M.C. (1975): Microcirculatory changes in the gastrointestinal tract of the hypoxic puppy: an electron microscopy study. J. Pediatr. Surg. 10, 599-608.

389. Barrios, R., Inoue, S., and Hogg, J.C. (1977): Intercellular junctions in "shock lung." A freeze-fracture study. Lab. Invest. 36, 628-635.

390. Tedder, E., and Shorey, C.D. (1965): Intimal changes in venous stasis. Lab. Invest. 14, 208-218.

391. Renkin, E.M., Joyner, W.L., Sloop, C.H., and Watson, P.D. (1977): Influence of venous pressure on plasma-lymph transport in the dog's paw: convective and dissipative mechanisms. Microvasc. Res. 14, 191-204.

392. Bowden, D.H., and Adamson, I.Y.R. (1974): Endothelial regen-eration as a marker of the differential vascular responses in oxygen-induced pulmonary edema. Lab. Invest. 30, 350-357.

393. Bonikos, D.S., Bensch, K.G., Ludwin, S.K., Northway, W.H., Jr. (1975): Oxygen toxicity in the newborn. The effect of pro-longed 100 percent O_2 exposure on the lungs of newborn mice. Lab. Invest. 32, 619-635.

394. Constantinides, P., and Robinson, M. (1969): Ultrastructural injury of arterial endothelium. I. Effects of pH, osmolarity, anoxia, and temperature. Arch. Pathol. 88, 99-117.

395. Gabbiani, G., Badonnel, M-C., Mathewson, S.M., and Ryan, G.B. (1974): Acute cadmium intoxication. Early selective lesions of endothelial clefts. Lab. Invest. 30, 686-695.

396. Hirano, A., and Kochen, J.A. (1975): Some effects of intra-cerebral lead implantation in the rat. Acta Neuropathol. 33, 307-315.

397. Margolis, F. (1970): Pathogenesis of contrast media injury: insights provided by neurotoxicity studies. Invest. Radiol. 5, 392-406.

398. Waldron, R.L. II, and Bryan, R.N. (1975): Effects of contrast agents on the blood-brain barrier. Radiology 116, 195-198.

399. Chan, W.C., O'Mahoney, M.G., Yu, D.Y.C., and Yu, R.Y.H. (1975): Renal failure during intermittent rifampicin therapy. Tubercle 56, 191-198.

400. Gottlob, R. (1972): Endothelschädigung durch intravasale Injektion vaon Arzneimitteln. Arzneim.-Forsch. 22, 1970-1975.

401. Adamson, I.Y.R. (1976): Pulmonary toxicity of bleomycin. Environ. Health Perspect. 16, 119-125.

402. Balis, J.U., Gerber, L.I., Rappaport, E.S., and Neville, W.E. (1974): Mechanisms of blood-vascular reactions of the primate lung to acute endotoxemia. Exp. Mol. Pathol. 21, 123-137.

403. McGrath, J.M., and Stewart, G.J. (1969): The effects of endotoxin on vascular endothelium. J. Exp. Med. 129, 833-848.

404. Gerrity, R.G., Caplan, B.A., Richardson, M., Cade, J.F., Hirsch, J., and Schwartz, C.J. (1975): Endotoxin-induced endothelial injury and repair. I. Endothelial cell turnover in the aorta of the rabbit. Exp. Mol. Pathol. 23, 379-385.

405. Evensen, S.A., Pickering, R.J., Batbouta, J., and Shepro, D. (1975): Endothelial injury by bacterial endotoxin: effect of complement depletion. Europ. J. Clin. Invest. 5, 463-469.

406. Pietra, G.G., Szidon, J.P., Carpenter, H.A., and Fishman, A.P. (1974): Bronchial venular leakage during endotoxin shock. Am. J. Pathol. 77, 387-406.

407. Freudenberg, N., and Riese, K.H. (1976): Characterization of cells of the normal aortic endothelium of adult rats and changes due to endotoxin shock. I. Communication: light microscopy, autoradiography, DNA cytophotometry, and enzyme histochemistry. Beitr. Pathol. 159, 125-142.

408. Factor, S.M. (1976): Intramyocardial small-vessel disease in chronic alcoholism. Am. Heart J. 92, 561-575.

409. Asmussen, I., and Kjeldsen, K. (1975): Intimal ultrastructure of human umbilical arteries. Observations on arteries from newborn children of smoking and nonsmoking mothers. Circ. Res. 36, 579-589.

410. Osaka, A., Suzuki, K., and Oashi, M. (1975): The spurting of erythrocytes through junctions of the vascular endothelium treated with snake venom. Microvasc. Res. 10, 208-213.

411. Hurley, J.V., and Jago, M.V. (1975): Pulmonary edema in rats
     given dehydromonocrotaline: a topographic and electron-micro-
     scope study. J. Pathol. 117, 23-32.

412. Weber, G., Fabbrini, P., and Resi, L. (1974): Scanning and
     transmission electron microscopy observations on the surface
     lining of aortic intimal plaques in rabbits on a hyperdoles-
     terolic diet. Virchows Arch. A Path. Anat. Histol. 364, 325-
     331.

413. Silkworth, J.B., McLean, B., and Stehbens, W.E. (1975): The
     effect of hypercholesterolemia on aortic endothelium studied en
     face. Atherosclerosis 22, 335-348.

414. McMillan, G.C., and Stary, H.C. (1968): Preliminary experience
     with mitotic activity of cellular elements in the atherosclerot-
     ic plaques of cholesterol-fed rabbits studied by labeling with
     tritiated thymidine. Ann. N.Y. Acad. Sci. 149, 699-709.

415. Stary, H.C. (1974): Proliferation of arterial cells in athe-
     rosclerosis. In Arterial Mesenchyme and Arteriosclerosis,
     Proc. Int. Workshop on Arterial Mesenchyme and Arteriosclero-
     sis, New Orleans, 1973. Adv. Exp. Med. Biol. Vol. 43, Plenum,
     New York, pp. 59-81.

416. Stary, H.C. (1974): Cell proliferation and ultrastructural
     changes in regressing atherosclerotic lesions after reduction
     of serum cholesterol. In Atherosclerosis III (Schettler, G.
     and Weizel, A., Eds.), Springer-Verlag, Berlin, pp. 187-190.

417. Henriksen, T., Evensen, S.A., and Carlander, B. (1977):
     Injury of endothelial cells in culture induced by low density
     lipoproteins. Thromb. Haemost. 38, 138.

418. Still, W.J.S. (1971): The effect of triton WR 1339 on the
     arterial intima of the rat. Lab. Invest. 24, 373-382.

419. Maca, R.D., and Hoak, J.C. (1974): Endothelial injury and
     platelet aggregation associated with acute lipid mobilization.
     Lab. Invest. 30, 589-595.

420. Ham, K.N., Hurley, J.V., Lopata, A., and Ryan, G.B. (1970):
     A combined isotopic and electron microscopic study of the
     response of the rat uterus to exogenous estradiol. J. Endocr.
     46, 71-81.

421. Almén, T., Härtel, M., Nylander, G., and Olivecrona, H. (1975):
     The effect of estrogen on the vascular endothelium and its pos-
     sible relation to thrombosis. Surg. Gynec. Obstet. 140, 938-
     940.

422. Lough, J., and Moore, S. (1975): Endothelial injury induced by thrombin or thrombi. Lab. Invest. 33, 130-135.

423. Harker, L.A., Ross, R., Slichter, S.J., and Scott, C.R. (1976): Homocystine-induced arteriosclerosis. The role of endothelial cell injury and platelet response in its genesis. J. Clin. Invest. 58, 731-741.

424. Bauer-Sič, P. (1966): Das Vorkommen von Vitamin-E-Mangel-pigment in Sinusendothelien, insbesondere der Milz, beim experimentallen Vitamin-E-Mangel der Ratte. Zbl. Vet. Med. Reihe A, 13, 541-546.

425. Yu, W.A., Yu, M.C., and Young, P.A. (1974): Ultrastructural changes in the cerebrovascular endothelium induced by a diet high in linoleic acid and deficient in vitamin E. Exp. Mol. Pathol. 21, 289-299.

426. El-Ghazzawi, E.F., and Malaty, H.A. (1975): Electron microscopic observations on extraneuronal lipofuscin in the monkey brain. Cell Tissue Res. 161, 555-565.

427. Hasan, M., Glees, P., and Spoerri, P.E. (1974): Dissolution and removal of neuronal lipofuscin following dimethylaminoethyl p-chlorophenoxyacetate administration to guinea pigs. Cell Tissue Res. 150, 369-375.

428. McKinney, R.V., Jr. (1976): The structure of scorbutic regenerating capillaries in skeletal muscle wounds. Microvasc. Res. 11, 361-379.

429. Hüttner, I., More, R.H., and Rona, G. (1970): Fine structural evidence of specific mechanism for increased endothelial permeability in experimental hypertension. Am. J. Pathol. 61, 395-405.

430. Suzuki, K., Ookawara, S., and Ooneda, G. (1971): Increased permeability of the arteries in hypertensive rats: an electron microscopic study. Exp. Mol. Pathol. 15, 198-208.

431. Wiener, J., and Giacomelli, F. (1973): The cellular pathology of experimental hypertension. VII. Structure and permeability of the mesenteric vasculature in angiotensin-induced hypertension. Am. J. Pathol. 72, 221-240.

432. Hüttner, I., Boutet, M., Rona, G., and More, R.H. (1973): Studies on protein passage through arterial endothelium. III. Effect of blood pressure levels on the passage of fine structural protein tracers through rat arterial endothelium. Lab. Invest. 29, 536-546.

433. Forthomme, D., and Cantin, M. (1976): The retinal capillaries of the rat in deoxycorticosterone hypertension. Am. J. Pathol. 85, 263-276.

434. Siperstein, M.D., Unger, R.H., and Madison, L.L. (1968): Studies on muscle capillary basement membranes in normal subjects, diabetic, and prediabetic patients. J. Clin. Invest. 47, 1973-1999.

435. Siperstein, M.D. (1972): Capillary basement membranes and diabetic microangiopathy. In Advances in Internal Medicine, Vol. 18 (Stollerman, G.H., Ed.), Yearbook Medical Publishers, Inc., pp. 325-344.

436. Raskin, P., Marks, J.F., Burns, H., Jr., Plumer, M.E., and Siperstein, M.C. (1975): Capillary basement membrane width in diabetic children. Am. J. Med. 58, 365-372.

437. Siperstein, M.D., Raskin, P., and Burns, H. (1973): Electron microscopic quantification of diabetic microangiopathy. Diabetes 22, 514-527.

438. Aronoff, S.L., Bennett, P.H., Siperstein, M.D., and Williamson, J.R. (1976): Muscle capillary basement membrane thickening in prediabetic and diabetic Pima Indians. Proc. 1st Internat. Symp. on Biol. and Chem. of Basement Membranes, Philadelphia, PA, Nov. 29 - Dec. 1 (Abstr.).

439. Vracko, R., and Benditt, E.P. (1970): Capillary basal lamina thickening. Its relationship to endothelial cell death and replacement. J. Cell Biol. 47, 281-285.

440. Vracko, R. (1974): Basal lamina layering in diabetes mellitus. Evidence for accelerated rate of cell death and cell regeneration. Diabetes 23, 94-104.

441. Sosula, L. (1975): Retinal capillary junctions: ultrastructural tight junction artifacts induced by sodium ions and membrane reduction in streptozotocin diabetes. Cell Tissue Res. 161, 393-411.

442. Prineas, J.W., Ouvrier, R.A., Wright, R.G., Walsh, J.C., and McLeod, J.G. (1976): Giant axonal neuropathy -- a generalized disorder of cytoplasmic microfilament formation. J. Neuropathol. Exp. Neurol. 35, 458-470.

443. Banker, B.Q. (1975): Dermatomyositis of childhood. Ultrastructural alterations of muscle and intramuscular blood vessels. J. Neuropathol. Exp. Neurol. 34, 46-75.

444. Suzuki, K., Ookawara, S., and Ooneda, G. (1971): Increased permeability of the arteries in hypertensive rats: an electron microscopic study. Exp. Mol. Pathol. 15, 198-208.

445. Goodman, J.H., Bingham, W.G., Jr., and Hunt, W.E. (1976): Ultrastructural blood-brain barrier alterations and edema formation in acute spinal cord trauma. J. Neurosurg. 44, 418-424.

446. Persson, L., and Hansson, H.A. (1976): Reversible blood-brain barrier dysfunction to peroxidase after a small stab wound in the rat cerebral cortex. Acta Neuropathol. 35, 333-342.

447. Spaet, T.H., and Gaynor, E. (1970): Vascular endothelial damage and thrombosis. Adv. Cardiol. 4, 47-66.

448. Baumgartner, H.R. (1974): The subendothelial surface and thrombosis. Thrombl Diath. Hemorrh. 59 (Suppl.), 91-105.

449. Baumgartner, H.R., and Muggli, R. (1976): Adhesion and aggregation: morphological demonstration and quantitation in vivo and in vitro. In Platelets in Biology and Pathology (Gordon, Ed.), Elsevier, North-Holland, Biomedical Press, pp. 23-60.

450. Read, S. (1974): Basement membrane diseases: a review. Guy's Hosp. Rep. 123, 53-66.

451. Gonzalez-Crussi, F., Hull, M.T., and Grosfeld, J.L. (1976): Idiopathic pulmonary hemosiderosis: evidence of capillary basement membrane abnormality. Am. Rev. Resp. Dis. 114, 689-698.

452. Sotto, M.N., Langer, B., Hoshino-Shimizu, S., and De Brito, T. (1976): Pathogenesis of cutaneous lesions in acute meningococcemia in humans: light, immunofluorescent, and electron microscopic studies of skin biopsy specimens. J. Infect. Dis. 133, 506-514.

453. Greenberger, N.J., DeLor, C.J., Fisher, J., Perkins, R.L., Murad, T., and Kapral, F. (1971): Whipple's disease. Characterization of anaerobic Corynebacteria and demonstration of bacilli in vascular endothelium. Am. J. Dig. Dis. 16, 1127-1136.

454. De Brito, T., Hoshino-Shimizu, S., Pereira, M.O., and Rigolon, N. (1973): The pathogenesis of the vascular lesions in experimental rickettsial disease of the guinea pig (Rocky Mountain Spotted Fever group). Virchows Arch. Abt. A Pathol. Anat. 358, 205-214.

455. Walker, D.H., Harrison, A., Henderson, F., and Murphy, F.A. (1977): Identification of Rickettsia rickettsii in a guinea pig model by immunofluorescent and electron microscopic techniques. Am. J. Pathol. 86, 343-358.

456. Haas, J.E., and Yunis, E.J. (1970): Viral crystalline arrays in human Coxsackie myocarditis. Lab. Invest. 23, 442-446.

457. Margolis, G., Jacobs, L.R., and Kilham, L. (1976): Oxygen tension and the selective tropism of K-virus for mouse pulmonary endothelium. Am. Rev. Resp. Dis. 114, 45-51.

458. Kilham, L., and Margolis, G. (1966): Spontaneous hepatitis and cerebellar "hypoplasia" in suckling rats due to congenital infections with rat virus. Am. J. Pathol. 49, 457-475.

459. Margolis, G., and Kilham, L. (1970): Parvovirus infections, vascular endothelium, and hemorrhagic encephalopathy. Lab. Invest. 22, 478-488.

460. Margolis, G., and Kilham, L. (1975): Problems of human concern arising from animal models of intrauterine and neonatal infections due to viruses: a review. II. Pathologic studies. Progr. Med. Virol. 20, 144-179.

461. Eady, R.A.J. (1975): Tubular aggregates: viral or not? Transact. St. John's Hosp. Dermatol. Soc. 61, 102-104.

462. Baringer, J.R., and Swoveland, P. (1972): Tubular aggregates in endoplasmic reticulum: evidence against their viral nature. J. Ultrastruc. Res. 41, 270-276.

463. Kimura, A., Tosaka, K., and Nakao, T. (1975): Measles rash. I. Light and electron microscopic study of skin eruptions. Arch. Virol. 47, 295-307.

464. Baringer, J.R. (1971): Tubular aggregates in endoplasmic reticulum in Herpes simplex encephalitis. N. Engl. J. Med. 285, 943-945.

465. Baringer, J.R., and Griffith, J.F. (1970): Experimental Herpes simplex encephalitis: early neuropathologic changes. J. Neuropathol. Exp. Neurol. 29, 89-104.

466. Kristensson, K. (1976): Experimental Herpes simplex virus infection in the immature mouse brain. Acta Neuropathol. 35, 343-351.

467. Norton, W.L. (1969): Endothelial inclusions in active lesions of systemic lupus erythematosus. J. Lab. Clin. Med. 74, 369-379.

468. Fraire, A.E., Smith, M.N., Greenberg, S.D., Weg, J.G., and Sharp, J.T. (1971): Tubular structures in pulmonary endothelial cells in systemic lupus erythematosus. Am. J. Clin. Pathol. 56, 244-248.

469. Haas, J.E., and Yunis, E.J. (1970): Tubular inclusions of systemic lupus erythematosus. Ultrastructural observations regarding their possible viral nature. Exp. Mol. Pathol. 12, 257-263.

470. Bloodworth, J.M.B., Jr., and Shelp, W.D. (1970): Endothelial cytoplasmic inclusions. Arch. Pathol. 90, 252-258.

471. Bariéty, J., Richer, D., Appay, M.D., Grossetete, J., and Callard, P. (1973): Frequency of intraendothelial 'virus-like' particles: an electron microscopy study of 376 human renal biopsies. J. Clin. Pathol. 26, 21-24.

472. Gambarelli, D., Pellissier, J.F., and Hassoun, J. (1974): Structures tubulo-réticulaires dans les cellules endothéliales et péricytaires, les lymphocytes et les cellules satellites du muscle dans un cas de sclérodermie. C.R. Soc. Biol. (Paris) 168, 308-310.

473. Norton, W.L., Velayos, E., and Robinson, L. (1970): Endothelial inclusions in dermatomyositis. Ann. Rheum. Dis. 29, 67-72.

474. Banker, B.Q. (1975): Dermatomyositis of childhood. Ultrastructural alterations of muscle and intramuscular blood vessels. J. Neuropathol. Exp. Neurol. 34, 46-75.

475. Macadam, R.F., Vetters, J.M., and Saikia, N.K. (1975): A search for microtubular inclusions in endothelial cells in a variety of skin diseases. Br. J. Dermatol. 92, 175-182.

476. Eady, R.A.J., and Odland, G.F. (1975): Intraendothelial tubular aggregates in experimental wounds. Br. J. Dermatol. 93, 165-173.

477. Schumacher, H.R., Jr. (1970): Tubular paramyxovirus-like structures in synovial vascular endothelium. Ann. Rheum. Dis. 29, 445-447.

478. Oliveira Soares, J., Chaves Serras, A., and Moura Nunes, J.F. (1975): Tubuloreticular structures in hepatic endothelial cells in a case of malignant melanoma liver metastasis. Experientia 31, 1345-1346.

479. Antal, M., and Németh, B. (1976): Tubuläre Strukturen in den Endothelien der Retina und in Retinoblastomen. Klin. Monatsbl. Augenheilkd. 169, 496-499.

480. Landolt, A.M., Ryffel, U., Hosbach, H.U., and Wyler, R. (1976): Ultrastructure of tubular inclusions in endothelial cells of pituitary tumors associated with acromegaly. Virchows Arch. A Path. Anat. Histol. 370, 129-140.

481. Kovacs, K., Horvath, E., Pritzker, K.P.H., and Schwartz, M.L. (1977): Pituitary growth hormone cell adenoma with cytoplasmic tubular aggregates in the capillary endothelium. Acta Neuro-Pathol. 37, 77-79.

482. Datsis, A.G. (1973): Endothelial inclusions in congenital infantile nephrosis. Virchows Arch. Abt. A Path. Anat. 359, 105-109.

483. Kojimahara, M. (1977): Filaments and rod-shaped tubulated bodies in the endothelia of anterior cerebral arteries in young rats. Cell Tissue Res. 182, 505-511.

484. Pothier, L., Uzman, B.G., Kasac, M.M., Saito, H., and Adams, R.A. (1973): Immunoglobulin synthesis and tubular arrays in the endoplasmic reticulum in transplanted human tumors of lymphoid origin. Lab. Invest. 29, 607-613.

485. Sengel, A., and Stoebner, P. (1972): Pseudocrystalline inclusions in muscular endothelial cells. Virchows Arch. Abt. B Zellpathol. 10, 354-358.

486. Spear, G.S., Slusser, R.J., Garvin, A.J., Horger, E.O. III, Bailey, R.P., and Schneider, J.A. (1975): A cytoplasmic body in human fetal endothelium. Am. J. Pathol. 78, 333-342.

487. Clearkin, K.P., and Enzinger, F.M. (1976): Intravascular papillary endothelial hyperplasia. Arch. Pathol. Lab. Med. 100, 441-444.

488. Winkelmann, R.K., Van Heerden, J.A., and Bernatz, P.E. (1971): Malignant vascular endothelial tumor with distal embolization. A new entity. Am. J. Med. 51, 692-697.

489. Spence, A.M., and Rubinstein, L.J. (1975): Cerebellar capillary hemangioblastoma: its histogenesis studied by organ culture and electron microscopy. Cancer 35, 326-341.

490. Gokel, J.M., Kürzl, R., and Hübner, G. (1976): Fine structure and origin of Kaposi's sarcoma. Pathol. Europ. 11, 45-47.

491. Gimbrone, M.A., Jr., and Fareed, G.C. (1976): Transformation of cultured human vascular endothelium of SV40 DNA. Cell 9, 685-693.

492. Hirano, A., and Matsui, T. (1975): Vascular structures in brain tumors. Hum. Pathol. 6, 611-621.

493. Suzuki, Y. (1969): Fenestration of alveolar capillary endothelium in experimental pulmonary fibrosis. Lab. Invest. 21, 304-308.

494. Campbell, G.R., and Uehara, Y. (1972): Formation of fenestrated capillaries in mammalian vas deferens and ureter transplants. Z. Zellforsch. 134, 167-173.

495. Snyder, D.H., Hirano, A., and Raine, C.S. (1975): Fenestrated CNS blood vessels in chronic experimental allergic encephalomyelitis. Brain Res. 100, 645-649.

496. Bhawan, J., Edelstein, L., and Jacobs, J.B. (1975): Endothelial fenestrations in cellular blue naevus and halo naevus. Lancet 1, 1350-1351.

497. Wolff, J.R. (1977): Ultrastructure of the terminal vascular bed as related to function. In Microcirculation, Vol. 1, (Kaley, G. and Altura, B.M., Eds.), University Park Press, Baltimore, pp. 95-130.

498. Boyd, W.H. (1970): Proliferation of glomerular capillary endothelial cells under the influence of hypophyseal intermediate lobe materials. Z. Anat. Entwicklungsgesch. 130, 306-315.

499. Williams, G.M., Krajewski, C.A., Dagher, F.J., ter Haar, A.M., Roth, J.A., and Santos, G.W. (1971): Host repopulation of endothelium. Transplant. Proc. 3, 869-872.

500. Szulman, A.E. (1972): A, B, H blood-group antigens in human placenta. N. Engl. J. Med. 286, 1028-1031.

501. Szulman, A.E., and Marcus, D.M. (1973): The histologic distribution of the blood group substance in man as disclosed by immunofluorescence. VI. The Le[a] and Le[b] antigens during fetal development. Lab. Invest. 28, 565-574.

502. Gibofsky, A., Jaffe, E.A., Fotino, M., and Becker, C.G. (1975):
     The identification of HL-A antigens on fresh and cultured human
     endothelial cells. J. Immunol. 115, 730-733.

503. Moraes, J.R., and Stastny, P. (1976): Eight groups of human
     endothelial cell alloantigens. Tissue Antigens 8, 273-276.

504. Moraes, J.R., and Stastny, P. (1977): Human endothelial cell
     antigens: molecular independence from HLA and expression in
     blood monocytes. Transplantation Proc. 9, 605-607.

505. Moraes, J.R., and Stastny, P. (1977): A new antigen system
     expressed in human endothelial cells. J. Clin. Invest. 60,
     449-454.

506. Cerilli, J., Jesseph, J.E., and Miller, A.C. (1972): The
     significance of antivascular endothelium antibody in renal
     transplantation. Surg. Gynecol. Obstet. 135, 246-252.

507. Cerilli, G.J., Holliday, J.E., and Lee, I.C. (1975): Antivas-
     cular endothelium antibody in renal transplantation. Surg.
     Forum 26, 341-342.

508. Cerilli, J., Holliday, J.E., Fesperman, D.P., and Folger, M.R.
     (1977): Antivascular endothelial cell antibody -- its role in
     transplantation. Surgery 81, 132-138.

509. Hirschberg, H., Evensen, S.A., Henriksen, T., and Thorsby, E.
     (1974): Stimulation of human lymphocytes by allogeneic endo-
     thelial cells in vitro. Tissue Antigens 4, 257-261.

510. Hirschberg, H., Evensen, S.A., Henriksen, T., and Thorsby, E.:
     The human mixed lymphocyte-endothelium culture interaction.
     Transplantation 19, 495-504.

511. de Bono, D. (1976): Endothelial-lymphocyte interactions in
     vitro. I. Adherence of nonallergised lymphocytes. Cell. Im-
     munol. 26, 78-88.

512. Williams, M., Harr, A., Parks, L., and Roth, J. (1976):
     Rejection and repair of endothelium in major vessel transplants.
     J. Cardiovasc. Surg. 17, 94-95.

513. de Bono, D.P. (1972): Host repopulation of endothelium in
     human kidney transplants. Transplantation 14, 438-441.

514. Williams, G.M., ter Haar, A., Krajewski, C., Parks, L.C., and
     Roth, J. (1975): Rejection and repair of endothelium in major
     vessel transplants. Surgery 78, 694-706.

515. de Bono, D. (1974): Effects of cytotoxic sera on endothelium in vitro. Nature 252, 83-84.

516. de Bono, D.P., MacIntyre, D.E., White, D.J.G., and Gordon, J.L. (1977): Endothelial adenine uptake as an assay for cell- or complement-mediated cytotoxicity. Immunology 32, 221-226.

517. Hirschberg, J., Thorsby, E., and Rolstad, B. (1975): Antibody-induced cell-mediated damage to human endothelial cells in vitro. Nature 255, 62-64.

518. Kingston, D., and Glynn, L.E. (1971): A cross-reaction between Str. pyogenes and human fibroblasts, endothelial cells and astrocytes. Immunology 21, 1003-1016.

519. Williamson, N., Asquith, P., Stokes, P.L., Jowett, A.W., and Cooke, W.T. (1976): Anticonnective tissue and other antitissue "antibodies" in the sera of patients with coeliac disease compared with the findings in a mixed hospital population. J. Clin. Pathol. 29, 484-494.

520. Wiener, J., Pearl, J.S., Lattes, R.G., and Spiro, D. (1969): Endothelial cell-leukocyte bridges in skin allografts. Transplantation 7, 439-443.

521. Gaynor, E., Bouvier, C.A., and Spaet, T.H. (1968): Circulating endothelial cells in endotoxin-treated rabbits. Clin. Res. 16, 535.

522. Bouvier, C.A. (1973): Endothelium and the GSR. Bibl. Anat. 12, 92-97.

523. Payling-Wright, H., and Giacometti, N.J. (1972): Circulating endothelial cells and arterial endothelial mitoses in anaphylactic shock. Brit. J. Exp. Pathol. 52, 1-4.

524. Brais, M.P., and Braunwald, N.S. (1974): Tissue acceptance of materials implanted within the circulatory system. Arch. Surg. 109, 351-358.

525. Akert, K.,Sandri, C., Weibel, E.R., Peper, K., and Moor, H. (1976): The fine structure of the perineural endothelium. Cell Tissue Res. 165, 281-295.

526. Weibel, E.R. (1974): On pericytes, particularly their existence on lung capillaries. Microvasc. Res. 8, 218-235.

527. Björkerud, S., and Bondjers, G. (1971): Arterial repair and atherosclerosis after mechanical injury. I. Permeability and light microscopic characteristics of endothelium in non-atherosclerotic and atherosclerotic lesions. Atherosclerosis 13, 355-363.

528. Baumgartner, H.R., Stemerman, M.B., and Spaet, T.H. (1971): Adhesion of blood platelets to subendothelial surface: distinct from adhesion to collagen. Experientia 27, 283-285.

529. Casley-Smith, J.R., and Chin, J.C. (1971): The passage of cytoplasmic vesicles across endothelial and mesothelial cells. J. Microscopy 93, 167-189.

530. Sinclair, R.A. (1972): Origin of endothelium in human renal allografts. Brit. Med. J. 4, 15-16.

531. Sinclair, R.A. (1972): The sex chromatin marker in the endothelium of paraffin-embedded renal and cardiac tissue. J. Anat. 112, 215-221.

532. Morrison, F.S., and Baldini, M.G. (1969): Antigenic relationship between blood platelets and vascular endothelium. Blood 33, 46-56.

533. Anderson, R.G.W., Brown, M.S., and Goldstein, J.L. (1977): Role of the coated endocytic vesicles in the uptake of receptor-bound low density lipoprotein in human fibroblasts. Cell 10, 351-364.

534. Maca, R.D., Fry, G.L., Hoak, J.C., and Loh, P.T. (1977): The effects of intact platelets on cultured human endothelial cells. Thromb. Res. 11, 715-727.

535. D'Amore, P.A., Hechtman, H.B., and Shepro, D. (1978): Ornithine decarboxylase activity in cultured endothelial cells stimulated by serum, thrombin and serotonin. Thromb. Haemostas. In press.

536. Joó, F. (1972): Effect of N^6O^2-dibutyryl cyclic 3'5'-adenosine monophosphate on the pinocytosis of brain capillaries of mice. Experientia 28, 1470-1471.

APPENDIX B

WORKSHOP PARTICIPANTS
AUTHOR INDEX
SUBJECT INDEX

Dr. Nathan Back
School of Pharmacy
State University of New York
  at Buffalo
H355 Hochstetter Hall
Buffalo, New York   14260

Dr. Peter G. Barton
Department of Biochemistry
University of Alberta
  School of Medicine
Edmonton, Alberta, T6G ON2
Canada

Dr. Carl G. Becker
Department of Pathology
The New York Hospital -
  Cornell Medical Center
525 East 68th Street, Room C-440
New York, New York   10021

Dr. Thomas P. Bersot
Laboratory of Experimental
  Atherosclerosis
National Heart, Lung, and
  Blood Institute
National Institutes of Health
Building 10, Room 5N204
Bethesda, Maryland   20014

Dr. E. J. Walter Bowie
Hematology Research
Mayo Clinic
200 First Street, S.W.
Rochester, Minnesota   55901

Dr. K. M. Brinkhous
Department of Pathology
School of Medicine
University of North Carolina
711 Preclinical Education
  Building, 228-H
Chapel Hill, North Carolina   27514

Dr. A. Bleakley Chandler
Department of Pathology
Medical College of Georgia
Augusta, Georgia   30902

Dr. Shu Chien
Department of Physiology
College of Physicians and Surgeons
Columbia University
17th Floor, Room 454
630 West 168th Street
New York, New York   10032

Dr. Robert W. Colman
Department of Medicine
Hospital of the University of
  Pennsylvania
3400 Spruce Street
Philadelphia, Pennsylvania   19104

Dr. Kathleen D. Curwen
Department of Pathology,
Room RB607
Peter Bent Brigham Hospital
721 Huntington Avenue
Boston, Massachusetts 02115

Dr. Rita Dougherty
Lipid Nutrition Laboratory
Agriculture Research Service
Department of Agriculture
BARC-East, Building 308,
Room 125
Beltsville, Maryland 20705

Dr. Theodore Dubin
Department of Pathology,
Room C-440
Cornell University Medical
  College
1300 York Avenue
New York, New York 10021

Dr. Hans Eibl
Immuno Ag - Aktiengesellschaft
  Furchemistrich Medizinische
  Produkte
Industriestrasse 72
A 1220 Vienna, Austria

Dr. Karl Eurenius
Division of Blood Diseases
  and Resources
National Heart, Lung, and
  Blood Institute
National Institutes of Health
Bethesda, Maryland 20014

Dr. Michael D. Ezekowitz
Department of Cardiology
The Johns Hopkins Hospital
The Johns Hopkins School of
  Medicine
Baltimore, Maryland 21205

Dr. David N. Fass
Department of Hematology
Mayo Clinic
200 First Street, S.W.
Rochester, Minnesota 55901

Dr. Richard J. Forstrom
Hospital Group/Applied Research
American Hospital Supply
  Corporation
1015 Grandview Avenue
Glendale, California 91201

Dr. Joseph C. Fratantoni
Division of Blood Diseases and
  Resources
National Heart, Lung, and
  Blood Institute
National Institutes of Health
Building 31, Room 4A05
Bethesda, Maryland 20014

Dr. Robert J. Friedman
Albert Einstein College of
  Medicine
51 Lawrence Road
Scarsdale, New York 10583

Dr. Donald L. Fry
Laboratory of Experimental
  Atherosclerosis
National Heart, Lung, and
  Blood Institute
National Institutes of Health
Building 10, Room 5N204
Bethesda, Maryland 20014

Dr. Helmuth Gastpar
Associate Dean and Professor
Univ.-Ent-Hospital
Pettenkoferstrasse 8
D-8000 Munich 2, West Germany

Dr. Edward Genton
Faculty of Health Sciences
McMaster University
1200 Main Street West
Hamilton, Ontario, L8S 4J9
Canada

Dr. Jonathan M. Gerrard
Department of Pediatrics
University of Minnesota
  Medical School, Box 446
Minneapolis, Minnesota 55455

Dr. Ross G. Gerrity
Cleveland Clinic Foundation
9500 Euclid Avenue
Cleveland, Ohio 44106

Dr. Michael A. Gimbrone, Jr.
Department of Pathology
Peter Bent Brigham Hospital
721 Huntington Avenue
Boston, Massachusetts 02115

Dr. Antonio M. Gotto, Jr.
Department of Medicine
Baylor College of Medicine
1200 Moursund Avenue
Houston, Texas 77030

Dr. Thomas R. Griggs
Division of Cardiology
Department of Medicine
University of North Carolina
    School of Medicine
805 Preclinical Educational
    Building, 228H
Chapel Hill, North Carolina
    27514

Dr. Donald J. Hanahan
Department of Biochemistry
University of Texas Health
    Science Center at San Antonio
7703 Floyd Curl Drive
San Antonio, Texas 78284

Dr. M. Daria Haust
Department of Pathology
Faculty of Medicine
University of Western Ontario
London, Ontario, Canada

Dr. Susan Haynes
Epidemiology Branch
National Heart, Lung, and
    Blood Institute
National Institutes of Health
Federal Building, Room 2C16
Bethesda, Maryland 20014

Dr. Peter M. Henson
Department of Pediatrics
National Jewish Hospital and
    Research Center
3800 East Colfax Avenue
Denver, Colorado 80206

Dr. Gerard Hornstra
Unilever Research
Vlaardingen/Duiven
Olivier Van Noortlaan 120
Vlaardingen, Postbus 114
Netherlands

Dr. James M. Iacono
Agriculture Research Service
U.S. Department of Agriculture
Room 338-A
Administrative Building
Washington, D.C. 20250

Dr. Eric A. Jaffe
Department of Medicine
Division of Hematology - Oncology
The New York Hospital -
    Cornell Medical Center
525 East 68th Street
New York, New York 10021

Dr. Russell Jaffe
Clinical Center
National Institutes of Health
Building 10, Room 4N309
Bethesda, Maryland 20014

Dr. Mary Jane Jesse
Division of Heart and Vascular
    Diseases
National Heart, Lung, and
    Blood Institute
National Institutes of Health
Bethesda, Maryland 20014

Dr. J. H. Joist
Division of Laboratory Medicine
Washington University School of
    Medicine
Barnes Hospital
St. Louis, Missouri 63110

Dr. Isabelle Joris
Department of Pathology
University of Massachussetts
  Medical School
Worcester, Massachusetts 01605

Dr. Joseph T. Judd
Lipid Nutrition Laboratory
Agriculture Research Service
Department of Agriculture
BARC-East, Building 308
Room 125
Beltsville, Maryland 20705

Dr. Morris J. Karnovsky
Department of Pathology
Harvard Medical School
25 Shattuck Street
Boston, Massachusetts 02115

Dr. Raelene L. Kinlough-Rathbone
Department of Pathology
Faculty of Health Sciences
McMaster University
1200 Main Street West
Hamilton, Ontario, L8S 4J9
Canada

Dr. Craig S. Kitchens
University of Florida
  College of Medicine
Gainesville, Florida 32610

Dr. Bruce A. Kottke
Cardiovascular Research Unit
Mayo Clinic and Foundation
200 First Street, S.W.
Rochester, Minnesota 55901

Dr. Hau C. Kwaan
Department of Medicine
Northwestern University Medical
  School
V. A. Lakeside Hospital
333 East Huron Street
Chicago, Illinois 60611

Dr. Herbert Lau
Sidney Farber Cancer Institute
35 Binney Street
Boston, Massachusetts 02115

Dr. K. T. Lee
Department of Pathology
Albany Medical College of Union
  University
47 New Scotland Avenue
Albany, New York 12208

Dr. Woong Man Lee
Department of Pathology
Albany Medical College
Albany, New York 12208

Dr. Robert S. Lees
Arteriosclerosis Center
Massachusetts Institute of
  Technology
40 Ames Street
Cambridge, Massachusetts 02142

Dr. Jon C. Lewis
Department of Pathology
Bowman Gray School of Medicine
Winston-Salem, North Carolina
  27103

Dr. Robert W. Mahley
Laboratory of Experimental
  Atherosclerosis
National Heart, Lung, and
  Blood Institute
National Institutes of Health
Building 10, Room 5N115
Bethesda, Maryland 20014

Dr. Guido Majno
Department of Pathology
University of Massachusetts
  Medical School
55 Lake Avenue North
Worcester, Massachusetts 01605

Dr. Manuel R. Malinow
Section of Cardiovascular
  Diseases
Oregon Regional Primate
  Research Center
505 N.W. 185th Avenue
Beaverton, Oregon 97005

Dr. Henry C. McGill, Jr.
Department of Pathology
University of Texas
Health Science Center at
  San Antonio
7703 Floyd Curl Drive
San Antonio, Texas 78284

Dr. Gardner C. McMillan
Division of Heart and
  Vascular Diseases
National Heart, Lung, and
  Blood Institute
National Institutes of Health
Federal Building, Room 516
Bethesda, Maryland 20014

Dr. D. C. B. Mills
Center for Thrombosis Research
Temple University School
  of Medicine
2400 North Broad Street
Philadelphia, Pennsylvania 19140

Dr. C. Richard Minick
Department of Pathology
The New York Hospital -
  Cornell Medical Center
525 East 68th Street
New York, New York 10021

Dr. J. R. A. Mitchell
Department of Medicine
General Hospital
University of Nottingham
Nottingham, NG1 6HA England

Dr. Sean Moore
Department of Pathology
Faculty of Health Sciences
McMaster University
1200 Main Street West
Hamilton, Ontario, L8S 4J9
Canada

Dr. Robert H. More
Department of Pathology
McGill University
3775 University Street
Montreal, Quebec H3A 2B4
Canada

Dr. J. F. Mustard
Faculty of Health Sciences
McMaster University
1200 Main Street West
Hamilton, Ontario, L8S 4J9
Canada

Dr. Ralph L. Nachman
Department of Medicine
Division of Hematology - Oncology
The New York Hospital -
  Cornell Medical Center
525 East 68th Street
New York, New York 10021

Dr. Curtis B. Nelson
Division of Scientific Affairs
American Heart Association
7320 Greenville Avenue
Dallas, Texas 75231

Dr. Robert M. Nerem
University Hall - Room 250
Ohio State University
230 North Oval Mall, Room 250
Columbus, Ohio 43210

Dr. Arne Nordoy
University of Tromso
Tromso, Norway

Dr. Hymie L. Nossel
Department of Medicine
College of Physicians and
   Surgeons of Columbia
   University
630 West 168th Street
New York, New York   10032

Dr. Thomas A. Pearson
The Johns Hopkins University
   School of Medicine
5817 Clearspring Road
Baltimore, Maryland   21212

Dr. Frances A. Pitlick
Department of Molecular Bio-
   physics and Biochemistry
Yale University Medical Center
Sterling Hall of Medicine
333 Cedar Street
New Haven, Connecticut   06510

Dr. Peter W. Ramwell
Department of Physiology
   and Biophysics
Georgetown University
   School of Medicine
Washington, D.C.   20007

Dr. Robert L. Reddick
National Cancer Institute
National Institutes of Health
Building 10, Room 2A29
Bethesda, Maryland   20014

Dr. Choo Y. Rhee
Montefiore Hospital
111 East 210th Street
Bronx, New York   10467

Dr. Abel L. Robertson, Jr.
Case Western Reserve University
   School of Medicine
2119 Abington Road
Cleveland, Ohio   44106

Dr. Robert D. Rosenberg
Sidney Farber Cancer Institute
Harvard Medical School
35 Binney Street
Boston, Massachusetts   02115

Mr. William E. Sanders
Information Specialist
National Heart, Lung, and
   Blood Institute
National Institutes of Health
Building 31, Room 5A03
Bethesda, Maryland   20014

Dr. Norberta Schoene
Lipid Nutrition Laboratory
Agriculture Research Service
Department of Agriculture
BARC-East, Building 308
Room 111
Beltsville, Maryland   20705

Dr. Colin J. Schwartz
Research Division
Cleveland Clinic
9500 Euclid Avenue
Cleveland, Ohio   44106

Dr. Hal Siegel
Department of Biochemical
   Pharmacology
State University of New York
   at Buffalo
313 Hochstetter Hall
Amherst, New York   14260

Dr. Kim Solez
The Johns Hopkins Hospital
601 North Broadway
Baltimore, Maryland   21205

Dr. J. Bryan Smith
Cardeza Foundation
Department of Pharmacology
Thomas Jefferson University
1015 Walnut Avenue
Philadelphia, Pennsylvania   19107

Dr. Louis C. Smith
Department of Biochemistry
Baylor College of Medicine
Brown Fondren Building #202
6516 Bertner Boulevard
Houston, Texas 77030

Dr. Helge Stormorken
Institute for Thrombosis
  Research
Rikshospital
Oslo 1, Norway

Dr. Jack P. Strong
Department of Pathology
Louisiana State University
  School of Medicine in
  New Orleans
1542 Tulane Avenue
New Orleans, Louisiana 70112

Dr. M. T. Ravi Subbiah
Cardiovascular Research Unit
Mayo Clinic
200 First Street, S.W.
Rochester, Minnesota 55901

Dr. Fletcher B. Taylor
Department of Pathology -
  MS 137
University of Oklahoma Health
  Science Center
Box 26901, 801 N.E., 13th
Oklahoma City, Oklahoma 73190

Dr. Wilbur A. Thomas
Department of Pathology
Albany Medical College of
  Union University
47 New Scotland Avenue
Albany, New York 12208

Dr. Mel Tiell
Research Associate
Department of Hematology
Montefiore Hospital and Medical
  Center
111 East 210th Street
Bronx, New York 10067

Dr. William D. Wagner
Department of Comparative
  Medicine
Bowman Gray School of Medicine
300 South Hawthorne Road
Winston-Salem, North Carolina
  27103

Dr. Bernard I. Weigensberg
Pathology Institute, Room 205
McGill University
3775 University Street
Montreal, Quebec H3A 2B4 Canada

Dr. Harvey Weiss
Division of Hematology
The Roosevelt Hospital
428 West 59th Street
New York, New York 10019

Dr. Babette B. Weksler
Department of Medicine
Division of Hematology - Oncology
The New York Hospital -
  Cornell Medical Center
525 East 68th Street
New York, New York 10021

Dr. Stanford Wessler
Department of Medicine
New York University
550 First Avenue
New York, New York 10016

Dr. Stanley Wiener
Department of Medicine
Long Island Jewish Hospital -
  Hillside Medical Center
New Hyde Park, New York 10019

Dr. Thomas N. Wight
University of New Hampshire
Kendall Hall
Durham, New Hampshire   03824

Dr. Hans J. Wilkens
State University of New York
   at Buffalo
School of Pharmacy
H355 Hochstetter Hall
Buffalo, New York   14260

Dr. Robert W. Wissler
Department of Pathology and
   Specialized Center of Research
   in Atherosclerosis
University of Chicago
Chicago, Illinois   60637

Dr. Harvey Wolinsky
Departments of Medicine and
   Pathology
Albert Einstein College of
   Medicine
1300 Morris Park Avenue
Bronx, New York   10461

Dr. Neville Woolf
Bland-Sutton Institute of
   Pathology
Middlesex Hospital
London, WIN 8AA, England

Dr. Donald B. Zilversmit
Division of Nutritional Sciences
Cornell University
Savage Hall
Ithaca, New York   14853

AUTHOR INDEX

Becker, Carl G., 371
Beeler, David, 449
Bowie, E. J. W., 385
Brinkhous, K. M., 385

Carvalho, Angelina, C. A., 301, 309
Chandler, A. Bleakley, 111
Colman, Robert W., 421

Dougherty, Rita M., 309

Eggen, Douglas, A., 11

Ferro-Luzzi, Anna, 309
Fry, Donald L., 353

Galli, Claudio, 309
Genton, Edward, 437
Gerrity, Ross G., 111
Gotto, Antonio M., Jr., 61

Hanahan, Donald J., 337
Haust, M. Daria, 33

Iacono, James M., 309

Joris, Isabelle, 169, 227

Keys, Ancel 309
Kinlough-Rathbone, R., 127
Kwaan, Hau C., 295

Lau, Herbert, 449
Lees, Robert, 301

Majno, Guido, 169, 227
McGill, Henry C., Jr., 273
McMillan, Gardner C., 3
Mitchell, J. R. A., 281
Mustard, J. F., 127

Nachman, R. L., 247
Naito, Herbert K., 111
Nelson, Gary J., 309
Nossel, Hymie L., 459

Packham, M. A., 127
Paoletti, Rudolfo, 309

Rosenberg, Judith S., 449
Rosenberg, Robert D., 449

Schwartz, Colin J., 111
Smith, J. Bryan, 343
Strong, Jack P., 11

Therriault, Donald G., 309
Thomas, W. A., 257
Tracy, Richard E., 11

Wessler, Stanford, 409
Wissler, Robert W., 77
Woolf, Neville, 145

SUBJECT INDEX